Designing
Clinical Research

AN EPIDEMIOLOGIC APPROACH

Designing Clinical Research

AN EPIDEMIOLOGIC APPROACH

BY

Stephen B. Hulley, MD, MPH

Professor of Epidemiology, Medicine, and Health Policy
University of California, San Francisco

Steven R. Cummings, MD

Assistant Professor of Medicine and Epidemiology
University of California, San Francisco

WITH MAJOR CONTRIBUTIONS BY

Warren S. Browner, MD, MPH

Assistant Professor of Epidemiology and Medicine
University of California, San Francisco

Thomas B. Newman, MD, MPH

Assistant Professor of Pediatrics and Epidemiology
University of California, San Francisco

Norman Hearst, MD, MPH

Clinical Assistant Professor of Epidemiology and Family Medicine
University of California, San Francisco

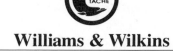

Williams & Wilkins

BALTIMORE • PHILADELPHIA • HONG KONG
LONDON • MUNICH • SYDNEY • TOKYO

A WAVERLY COMPANY

Editor: Nancy Collins
Associate Editor: Carol Eckhart
Copy Editor: Megan Shelton
Design: JoAnne Janowiak
Illustration Planning: Lorraine Wrzosek
Production: Theda Harris

Printed in the United States of America

Library of Congress Cataloging in Publication Data

Designing clinical research.
   Includes bibliographies and index.
    1. Clinical trials—Technique. 2. Medicine—Research—Methodology.
3. Biological chemistry—Research—Methodology. I. Hulley, Stephen B.
II. Cummings, Steven R. [DNLM: 1. Epidemiologic Methods. 2. Research
Design. WA 950 D457]
R853.C55D47 1988   610'.72   87-19015
ISBN 0-683-04249-1

95 96 97

10

11 12 13 14 15

Introduction

"On being asked to talk on the principles of research, my first thought was to arise after the chairman's introduction, to say, 'Be careful', and to sit down . . .

That principles of research do in fact exist, or that there are persons qualified to expound on them, are not self-evident . . . "

J. Cornfield (1)

This is a book about the science of doing applied clinical research. Despite the wry beginning of Cornfield's seminal essay on the same topic 30 years ago, we all know that there is such a science and that it works. The evidence is unmistakable: the effectiveness of modern medicine in preventing and treating many diseases. But what is this science and how does it work? Codifying the best way to do research on clinical and public health problems is not an easy task, and there is no single approach that everyone agrees is best. The approach set out in this book uses epidemiologic terms and principles, and emphasizes the value of being systematic. It is straightforward and practical, as close to a cookbook as we could make it.

The approach is somewhat idealized, the real world of research being more haphazard than that portrayed here. But these ideals are worth striving towards: despite improvements in the quality of clinical research over the past two decades, most published studies still contain avoidable errors. Our goal, therefore, is to foster further improvements by presenting a system of excellence; we leave the reader to discover for himself* where practical realities require some bending of ideals.

This book avoids statistical notation. An investigator must understand the principles of statistical analysis, but he need not be master all of its technical aspects. This is even true for biometric tasks like sample size estimation. Excessive technical detail can be harmful if it serves as a barrier to communication or distracts the investigator from more important tasks.

What are these more important tasks? One is **being creative**, recognizing important research questions and devising clever approaches to getting the correct answer. Another is **using good judgment** for the tradeoffs between the competing scientific and practical goals that challenge the architect of a study. Difficult choices are everywhere, and a good investigator distinguishes himself with his **common sense** in formulating the research question and in settling on a particular design, source of subjects, sample size, and set of measurements. Our main goal in writing this book has been to develop guidelines for making these judgments.

The book works well as a chapter-by-chapter companion to the process of creating a study. We base this view on our experience with earlier versions in five years of teaching clinical research methods at the graduate and post-graduate level. Each of our students has designed a real study, and many have gone on to carry it out. We recommend this degree of active involvement, even for those who are studying the topic chiefly to develop an understanding of research rather than the skills to do it. A small study can be done in a summer if the investigator finds the right mentor and existing program to attach himself to, and a real-life experience in the research world is far more instructive than an armchair venture.

---

*Or herself! We use the masculine pronoun for scientists of either gender in the first half of the book and the feminine pronoun in the second half, a sequence that was randomly assigned by coin toss, with three witnesses (all male) present.

Besides, many people find that they *like* doing research. For those with inquiring minds, the pursuit of truth can become a lifelong fascination. For perfectionists and craftsmen, there are endless challenges in the effort to create the most elegant study. And for those with the ambition to make a lasting contribution to society, there is the prospect that skill, tenacity and luck may lead to important advances.

Overview of the research process and where this book fits in:

This book begins with the philosophic cornerstone of research, the process of drawing inferences about truth in the universe from events observed in the study sample (Chapter 1). It ends with pragmatic guidelines for writing a proposal for research funding (Chapter 17). In between is the nitty gritty of designing and implementing a research project. This can be divided into six steps (Figure 1).

The first is the choice of the research question, the question about a health problem in the real world that the investigator wants to answer with the study. Settling on a good research question is often the biggest challenge facing a new investigator. Chapter 2 sets forth some ideas on how to go about the task, the most important of which is the choice of a wise mentor.

The second step, developing the study protocol, is the topic of most of this book. The objective is to design a feasible and inexpensive study that will produce a correct answer to the research question. The pursuit of this objective includes deciding how to recruit study subjects (Chapter 3), choosing the measurement approaches (Chapters 4 and 5) and study design (Chapters 7 to 11), estimating the sample size (Chapters 12 & 13), addressing ethical concerns (Chapter 14), planning the data management and analysis (Chapter 15).

The third and fourth steps, pretesting and carrying out the study, are addressed in Chapter 16. Because the implementation phase is costly in time and money, we give special attention (Chapter 6) to the secondary analysis shortcut in the Figure. By attaching himself to an existing research team or accessing an existing data file, a young investigator can often find ways to answer new questions with information that has already been collected.

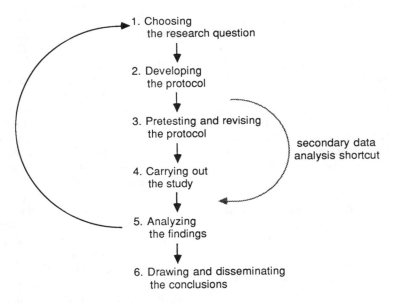

1. Choosing
   the research question

2. Developing
   the protocol

3. Pretesting and revising
   the protocol

secondary data
analysis shortcut

4. Carrying out
   the study

5. Analyzing
   the findings

6. Drawing and disseminating
   the conclusions

Figure 1:   The sequence and cycle of research

The fifth and sixth steps, analyzing the study and disseminating its conclusions, are discussed only briefly (in Chapter 15). The reader must consult other works for information on drawing the correct conclusions from research and deciding how they apply to clinical and public health decisions. We recommend a companion to this book entitled "Clinical Epidemiology", by Fletcher, Fletcher and Wagner (2), and several other excellent books (3-5).

Benediction

Figure 1 sets out in linear sequence the six steps that characterize a single research project. The Figure also shows a cycle, with the fifth step leading naturally to the next project. Most studies generate more questions than they answer, and many investigators find that their awareness of researchable questions grows as they gain experience.

There are other benefits that come with experience. Clinical research becomes easier and more rewarding as the investigator gains familiarity with the particulars of recruitment, measurement, and design that pertain to his area of specialization. A higher percentage of his applications for funding are successful. He acquires a staff and junior colleagues, and develops lasting friendships with scientists working on the same topic in distant places. And because most increments in knowledge are small and uncertain—major scientific breakthroughs are rare indeed—he begins to see substantial advances in the state of medicine as an aggregate result of his efforts.

These are reassuring thoughts when we set out to design a research project. There is no need to solve the whole puzzle all at once. It will suffice to join the many first-rate scientists at work, adding small but true pieces of knowledge, one at a time.

REFERENCES

1. Cornfield J. Principles of research. *Am J Ment Deficiency* 1959;64:240–252
2. Fletcher R., Fletcher S., Wagner. *Clinical Epidemiology, Ed 2.* Baltimore, Williams & Wilkins, 1987.
3. Friedman GD. *Primer of Epidemiology, Ed 3.* New York, McGraw Hill, 1987.
4. Gehlbach SH. *Interpreting the Medical Literature: A Clinician's Guide.* Lexington, MA, DC Heath & Co, 1982.
5. Sackett DL, Haynes RB, Tugwell P. *Clinical Epidemiology: A Basic Science for Clinical Medicine.* Boston, Little, Brown & Co, 1985.

Acknowledgement

We gratefully acknowledge our families for years of patience and support, Hal Holman, MD, and Philip Lee, MD, for getting it all started, our students for sharpening the relevance of our approach, microcomputers for making it fun through endless iterations, figures and text, and the Clinical Epidemiology Training Grant from the Andrew P. Mellon Foundation which brought us together and allowed us to spend time on these ideas.

Contributors

Dennis Black, PhD
Assistant Professor of Biostatistics
University of California, San Francisco

Warren Browner, MD, MPH
Assistant Professor of Epidemiology and
  Medicine
University of California, San Francisco

Steven Cummings, MD
Associate Professor of Medicine and
  Epidemiology
University of California, San Francisco

Virginia Ernster, PhD
Associate Professor of Epidemiology
University of California, San Francisco

David Feigal, MD, MPH
Assistant Professor of Medicine and
  Epidemiology
University of California, San Francisco

Cary Fox, MA
Senior Programmer, Clinical Epidemiology
  Program
University of California, San Francisco

Sandra Gove, MD, MPH
Assistant Professor of Epidemiology and
  International Health
University of California, San Francisco

Norman Hearst, MD, MPH
Assistant Professor of Family Medicine and
  Epidemiology
University of California, San Francisco

Stephen Hulley, MD, MPH
Professor of Epidemiology, Medicine, and
  Health Policy
Vice-Chairman, Department of
  Epidemiology and International Health
University of California, San Francisco

Christine Ireland, MA
Administrator, Clinical Epidemiology
  Program
University of California, San Francisco

Bernard Lo, MD
Associate Professor of Medicine and
  Medical Ethics
University of California, San Francisco

Michael Martin, MD, MPH, MBA
Clinical Assistant Professor of Epidemiology
  and Medicine
University of California, San Francisco

Michael Nevitt, PhD
Assistant Professor of Social Epidemiology
University of California, San Francisco

Thomas Newman, MD, MPH
Assistant Professor of Pediatrics and
  Epidemiology
University of California, San Francisco

William Strull, MD
Attending Physician
Kaiser Permanente Medical Center,
  San Francisco
University of California, San Francisco

A. Eugene Washington, MD, MPH
Associate Adjunct Professor of Preventive
  Medicine and Epidemiology
University of California, San Francisco

Contents

Introduction   v

Acknowledgment   viii

Contributors   ix

CHAPTER   1__Getting Started: The Anatomy and Physiology of Research   1
Stephen B. Hulley, Thomas B. Newman, and Steven R. Cummings

CHAPTER   2__Conceiving the Research Question   12
Steven R. Cummings, Warren S. Browner, and Stephen B. Hulley

CHAPTER   3__Choosing the Study Subjects: Specification and Sampling   18
Stephen B. Hulley, Sandra Gove, Warren S. Browner, and Steven R. Cummings

CHAPTER   4__Planning the Measurements: Precision and Accuracy   31
Stephen B. Hulley and Steven R. Cummings

CHAPTER   5__Planning the Measurements: Questionnaires   42
Steven R. Cummings, William Strull, Michael C. Nevitt, and Stephen B. Hulley

CHAPTER   6__Using Secondary Data   53
Norman Hearst and Stephen B. Hulley

CHAPTER   7__Designing a New Study: I. Cohort Studies   63
Steven R. Cummings, Virginia Ernster, and Stephen B. Hulley

CHAPTER   8__Designing a New Study: II. Cross-sectional and Case-control Studies   75
Thomas B. Newman, Warren S. Browner, Steven R. Cummings, and Stephen B. Hulley

CHAPTER   9__Designing a New Study: III. Diagnostic Tests   87
Warren S. Browner, Thomas B. Newman, and Steven R. Cummings

CHAPTER   10__Enhancing Causal Inference in Observational Studies   98
Thomas B. Newman, Warren S. Browner, and Stephen B. Hulley

CHAPTER 11___Designing a New Study: IV. Experiments   110
Stephen B. Hulley, David Feigal, Michael Martin, and Steven R.
Cummings

CHAPTER 12___Getting Ready to Estimate Sample Size: Hypotheses
and Underlying Principles   128
Warren S. Browner, Thomas B. Newman, Steven R. Cummings,
and Stephen B. Hulley

CHAPTER 13___Estimating Sample Size and Power   139
Warren S. Browner, Dennis Black, Thomas B. Newman, and
Stephen B. Hulley

CHAPTER 14___Addressing Ethical Issues   151
Bernard Lo, David Feigal, and Stephen B. Hulley

CHAPTER 15___Planning for Data Management and Analysis   159
David Feigal, Dennis Black, Norman Hearst, Deborah Grady,
Cary Fox, Thomas B. Newman, and Stephen B. Hulley

CHAPTER 16___Implementing the Study: Pretesting, Quality Control,
and Protocol Revisions   172
Stephen B. Hulley, David Siegel, and Steven R. Cummings

CHAPTER 17___Writing and Funding a Research Proposal   184
Steven R. Cummings, A. Eugene Washington, Christine Ireland,
and Stephen B. Hulley

Appendix   197

Index   239

CHAPTER 1

Getting Started: The Anatomy and Physiology of Research

Stephen B. Hulley, Thomas B. Newman, and Steven R. Cummings

INTRODUCTION 1

THE ANATOMY OF RESEARCH: WHAT IT'S
  MADE OF 1

  The research question
  The significance
  The design
  The subjects
  The variables
  Statistical issues

THE PHYSIOLOGY OF RESEARCH: HOW IT
  WORKS 5

  Designing the study
  Implementing the study
  Drawing causal inference
  The errors of research

DESIGNING THE STUDY 9

  Developing the study protocol
  Trade-offs

SUMMARY 11

ADDITIONAL READINGS 11

APPENDIX 1. Outline of an AIDS study
  protocol 197

— — — — — — — — — — — —

INTRODUCTION

This chapter introduces clinical research from two viewpoints, setting up themes that run together through the book. One theme is the **anatomy** of research—what it's made of. This includes the tangible elements of the **study plan**: the research question, design, subjects, measurements, sample size calculation, and so forth. An investigator's goal is to create these elements in a form that will make the project fast, inexpensive, and easy to do.

The other theme is the **physiology** of research—how it works. Studies are useful to the extent that they yield valid **inferences**, first about the events that happened in the study sample (*internal validity*), and then about generalizing these events to people outside the study (*external validity*). The goal is to minimize the errors, random and systematic, that threaten conclusions based on these inferences.

Separating these two themes is artificial in the same way that the anatomy of the human body doesn't make much sense without some understanding of its physiology. But the separation also has the same advantage: it simplifies our thinking about a complex topic.

THE ANATOMY OF RESEARCH: WHAT IT'S MADE OF

The structure of a research project is set out in its **protocol**, the written plan of the study. Protocols are well known as devices for seeking grant funds, but they also have a vital scientific function: helping the investigator to organize his research in a logical, focused, and efficient way. Table 1.1 outlines the components of a protocol. We will introduce the whole set here, expand on each of them in the ensuing chapters of the book, and return in Chapter 17 to put the completed pieces together.

The research question

The **research question** is the objective of the study, the uncertainty about a health issue

Table 1.1
Outline of the study protocol

Element	Purpose
Research questions (objectives)	What questions will the study address?
Significance (background)	Why are these questions important?
Design	How will the study be carried out?
Time frame	
Epidemiologic approach	
Subjects	Who are the subjects, and how will they be
Selection criteria	selected?
Sampling design	
Variables	What measurements will be made?
Predictor variables	
Outcome variables	
Statistical issues	How large is the study, and how will it be
Hypotheses	analyzed?
Sample size estimation	
Analytic approach	

that the investigator wants to resolve. Research questions often begin with a vague and general concern that must be narrowed down to a concrete, researchable issue. For example,

> *Initial research question*: Are intravenous (i.v.) drug abusers likely to spread the AIDS epidemic to the general population?

This is a good place to start, but the question must be focused before planning efforts can begin. Often this involves breaking the whole question into its constituent parts, and singling out one or two of these to build the protocol around.

> *More specific research questions:*
> 1. What proportion of i.v. drug abusers have been infected by the AIDS virus?
> 2. What risk factors increase the chance of transmitting the infection?

A good research question should pass the "so what" test—getting the answer should contribute usefully to our state of knowledge. The question must also be feasible to study. Deciding what is **feasible** is a complicated issue that we will come to in the second, physiologic half of this chapter.

The significance

The **significance** section of a protocol sets the proposed study in context and gives its rationale. What is known about the topic at hand, why is the research question important, and what kind of answers will the study provide? This section cites previous research that is relevant (including the investigator's own work), and indicates the problems with that research and what questions remain. It makes clear how the findings of the proposed study will help resolve these uncertainties and influence clinical and public health policy.

The design

The design of a study is a complex topic that involves a number of decisions (Fig. 1.1). The most fundamental is whether to stand apart from the events taking place in the study subjects (in an **observational study**), or to test the effects of an intervention on these events (in an **experiment**). If the investigator chooses an observational design, his next decision is whether to make the measurements on a single occasion (in a **cross-sectional** study) or over a period of time (in a **longitudinal** study). A third aspect of the design decision (not shown explicitly in the figure) is whether to deal exclusively with past and present events in a **retrospective** study, or to follow study subjects **prospectively** for events that have not yet occurred when the study begins.

No one approach is always better than the others; for each research question a judgment must be made as to which design is the most efficient way to get a satisfactory answer. The randomized trial is often held up as the ultimate standard, but there are many situations for which an observational study is a better choice. The relatively low cost of retrospective case-control studies, for example, makes them particularly attractive for questions they can answer satisfactorily. Figure 1.1 shows how four of the most basic study designs—the *case-control study*, the *randomized control trial*, the *cross-sectional study*, and the *cohort study*—could be used to study four different AIDS-related research questions. These designs, and others, are presented in Chapters 7-11.

A typical sequence for studying a topic begins with relatively easy and open-ended observational studies of a type that is often called **descriptive**; these studies explore the lay of the land, describing distributions of diseases and health-related characteristics in the population (What is the prevalence of antibodies to AIDS virus in i.v. drug abus-

ers?). Descriptive studies are usually followed or accompanied by analytic studies that analyze associations in order to discover cause-and-effect relationships (What risk factors increase the likelihood of AIDS virus infection in this population?). The final step is often an **experiment** to establish the effects of an intervention (Does a health education program alter the incidence of infection?). Experiments usually occur later in the sequence of research studies because they tend to be more difficult and expensive, and to answer more narrowly focused questions.

It is useful to characterize the design in a single sentence that begins with its name, as illustrated in Figure 1.1. Some studies do not easily fit into these molds, however, and classifying them can be a surprisingly difficult exercise. It is worth the effort—a precise description of the type of study helps to clarify the investigator's thoughts and is useful for

<u>Design</u>   <u>Example</u>

Observational Study

The investigator   A case-control study
observes the events   comparing the needle-sharing
without altering them   history of i.v. drug-abusers
                                      who have AIDS virus
                                    antibodies with the history
                                       of those who do not

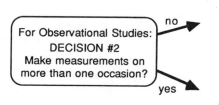
DECISION #1
Alter the events
under study?
no
yes

Experiment

He applies an   A randomized trial of the
intervention, and observes   impact of a health-
the effect on the outcome   education program on
                                    needle-sharing habits

Cross-sectional Study

Each subject is examined   A cross-sectional study of
on only one occasion   needle-sharing habits and
                                    AIDS virus antibodies
                                 measured at the same exam

For Observational Studies:
DECISION #2
Make measurements on
more than one occasion?
no
yes

Longitudinal Study

Each subject is followed   A cohort study that assesses
over a period of time   current needle-sharing habits
                                 of a group of i.v. drug-abusers,
                                   then observes who subsequently
                                   develops AIDS virus antibodies

Figure 1.1.   Some design decisions, illustrated by the four major epidemiologic prototypes: the case-control study, the randomized trial, the cross-sectional study, and the cohort study.

orienting colleagues and consultants. (This single sentence is the research analog to the opening sentence of a medical resident's report on a new hospital admission: "This 62 year old white policeman was well until 2 hours prior to admission, when he developed crushing chest pain radiating to the left shoulder.") If the study has two major phases, the design for each should be mentioned.

> *Research Design*: This is a cross-sectional study of the prevalence of antibodies to the AIDS virus among methadone clinic patients, followed by a prospective cohort study of the risk factors for seroconversion among those initially free of antibodies.

The subjects

There are two major decisions to be made in choosing the study subjects (Chapter 3). **Specifying the selection criteria** is the process of defining the study population: the kinds of patients best suited to the research question and where to recruit them. **Sampling** is the process of picking the subgroup of this population who will actually be the subjects of the study. An AIDS study might specify as selection criteria patients in the methadone program at San Francisco General Hospital, and sample consecutively the next 100 patients entering that program. These design choices represent trade-offs; drawing the same number of i.v. drug abusers from street sources might expand generalizability but be more difficult and costly.

The variables

Another major set of decisions in designing any study concerns the choice of which **variables**—characteristics of the study subjects—to measure (Chapter 4). In a descriptive study the investigator looks at individual variables, one at a time. A study of the prevalence of AIDS virus infection, for example, focuses on the distribution of a single variable: The presence or absence of AIDS virus antibodies in the study sample.

In an analytic study the investigator analyzes the relationships among two or more variables in order to predict outcomes and to draw inferences about cause and effect. In considering the association between two variables, the one that precedes the

other (or is presumed on biologic grounds to be antecedent) is called the **predictor variable**, and the other is called the **outcome variable**.[a] Most observational studies have many predictor variables (e.g., needle-sharing habits, socioeconomic status, age, race), and several outcome variables (AIDS virus antibodies, symptoms of AIDS).

Experiments have a special kind of predictor variable, termed the **intervention**, which the investigator manipulates (e.g., a health education program about needle-sharing). This design allows him to observe the effects on the outcome variable (seroconversion) while controlling for the influence of **confounding** variables—other predictors like socioeconomic status that can confuse the interpretation of the outcome (Chapter 10).

Statistical issues

The investigator must develop plans for managing and analyzing the study data. For analytic studies and experiments this always includes a hypothesis-testing component: specifying in advance at least one main **hypothesis**. A hypothesis is a version of the research question that has the purpose of providing the basis for testing the statistical significance of the findings.

> *Hypothesis*: I.v. drug abusers who cleaned their needles with bleach during the past year will be less likely to have antibodies to AIDS virus than those who did not.

Descriptive studies do not require a hypothesis because their purpose is to describe how variables are distributed (e.g., the prevalence of AIDS virus antibodies) rather than how they are associated with each other.

All studies should also have a **sample size estimation** (Chapters 12 and 13). For studies with prior hypotheses, this means estimating the number of subjects needed to consistently observe the expected difference in outcome between study groups. For descriptive studies, an analogous approach considers the number of subjects needed to

---

[a] Predictor variables are often termed "independent" and outcome variables "dependent", but we find this usage confusing, particularly since "independent" means something quite different in the context of multivariate analyses.

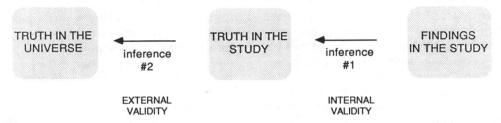

Figure 1.2. The two inferences involved in drawing conclusions from the findings of a study and applying them to the universe outside.

produce descriptive statistics (means, proportions, etc.) of adequate precision.

THE PHYSIOLOGY OF RESEARCH: HOW IT WORKS

One way to think about how research works is to consider the end result of a research project, the process of drawing and applying the study conclusions. Two major sets of inferences are involved (illustrated from right to left in Figure 1.2). One of these concerns the **internal validity** of the study, the degree to which the investigator's conclusions correctly describe what actually happened in the study. The other concerns the **external validity** (also called generalizability), the degree to which these conclusions are appropriate when applied to the universe outside the study.

When an investigator plans and carries out a study he needs to keep these two inferences in mind; the overall goal is to maximize their validity at the end of the study. The

logical order of the planning process is reversed, however, now going from left to right (bottom panel of Fig. 1.3). The first step is to settle on the health problem in the universe that is of interest (the research question). The investigator then designs a research plan that will provide inferences of satisfactory validity, and implements the study in a way that enhances these inferences.

In this section we will first address the design side of Figure 1.3, then turn to the implementation side, and finally consider the errors that threaten the validity of these inferences.

Designing the study

The **research question**, as noted earlier, is what the investigator really wants to answer (What proportion of i.v. drug abusers in San Francisco have been infected with the AIDS virus?). This question cannot be answered explicitly because it would be impossible to study all the i.v. drug abusers in San

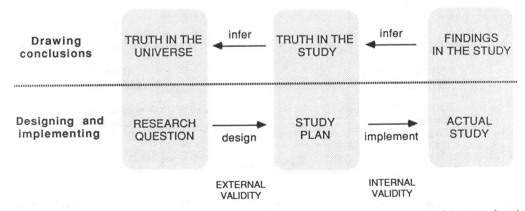

Figure 1.3. The process of designing and implementing a research project sets the stage for the process of drawing conclusions from it.

Francisco, and because our tests for infection are imperfect. So the investigator must settle for a related question that *can* be answered by the study (What proportion of the patients attending methadone clinics at San Francisco General Hospital have antibodies to the AIDS virus?). The transformation from research question to **study plan** is illustrated in Figure 1.4.

One major component of this transformation is the *choice of a sample of subjects that will represent the target population*. The group of subjects specified in the protocol can only be a subset of the population of interest because there are practical barriers to studying the entire population. In this example, the very large numbers of i.v. drug abusers (about 12,000 in San Francisco) would make it enormously expensive to study all of them, and their inaccessibility (most i.v. drug abusers are not known to medical authorities) would make it impossible. The decision to

study patients in the San Francisco General Hospital methadone clinic is a compromise: this is a sample that is feasible to study, but one that may produce a falsely low prevalence of AIDS virus infection if the i.v. drug abusers who come to the methadone clinic tend to have fewer high-risk habits than those who do not come there.

The other major component of the transformation is the *choice of variables that will represent the phenomena of interest*. The variables specified in the study plan are usually proxies for these phenomena. The decision to use antibodies as a proxie for AIDS virus infection provides a feasible way to measure this infection, but it may result in a falsely low prevalence because antibodies do not appear until several months after infection.

In short, each of the differences in Figure 1.4 between the research question and the study plan has the purpose of making the study more practical. The cost of this in-

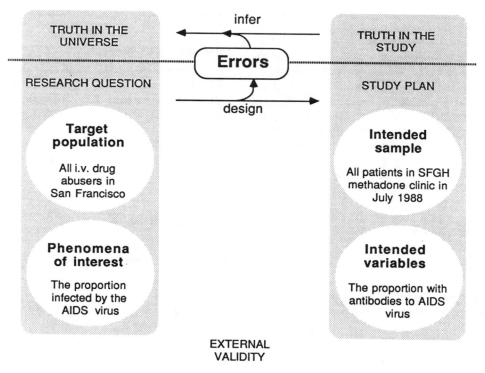

Figure 1.4. Design errors: if the intended sample and variables do not represent the target population and phenomena of interest, the errors that result will threaten the validity of drawing inferences about what is happening in the universe.

crease in practicality, however, is the risk that the study may produce a wrong answer to the research question—for example, a prevalence of AIDS virus antibodies in methadone clinic patients of 15%, when the prevalence of infected i.v. drug abusers in the population is really 30%. Figure 1.4 illustrates the important fact that errors in designing the study are a common reason for getting the wrong answer to the research question.

Implementing the study

Returning to Figure 1.3, the right hand side is concerned with implementation, and the degree to which the actual study matches the study plan. At issue here is the problem of a wrong answer to the research question because the way the sample was actually drawn and the measurements made differed in important ways from the way they were designed (Fig. 1.5).

The **actual sample** of study subjects is almost always different from the intended sample. The plans to study all methadone clinic patients, for example, would probably be disrupted by incomplete attendance (say only 150 of the 200 patients who are registered in the clinic show up during the month of the study), and by noncompliance (say only 100 of these agree to be studied). The 100 patients who volunteer to be tested may have a different prevalence of AIDS infection from those who do not show up or refuse to have the test. In addition to these problems with the subjects, the **actual measurements** often differ from the intended measurements. The ELISA assay is a reasonably sensitive and specific test for AIDS virus antibody in most populations, for example, but i.v. drug abusers often have biologically false-positive results—antibodies acquired nonspecifically, without any exposure to the AIDS virus. There can also be technical errors, such as a mix-up in the labeling of the specimens, or in carrying out the assay.

These differences between the study plan and the actual study could further distort the answer to the research question—for

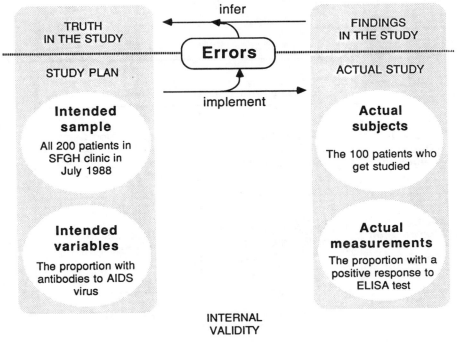

Figure 1.5. Implementation errors: if the actual subjects and measurements do not represent the intended sample and variables, the errors that result will threaten the validity of drawing inferences about what actually happened in the study.

example, the observed prevalence of positive ELISA tests might be 7.5% when the actual prevalence in all clinic patients is 15%. Figure 1.5 illustrates the important fact that errors caused by difficulties in implementing the study are the other common reasons (besides errors of design) for getting the wrong answer to the research question.

Drawing causal inference

A special kind of validity problem arises in studies that examine the **association** between a predictor and an outcome variable in order to draw **causal inference**. If the study finds an association between cleaning needles with bleach and the ELISA test result, does this represent a cause and effect relationship, or is there some other explanation? Reducing the likelihood of spurious associations and other rival explanations is one of the major challenges for the architect of an observational study (Chapter 10).

The errors of research

No study is free of errors, and the inferences that have been described are never perfectly valid. The goal is simply to maximize internal and external validity so that the inferences about what happened in the study sample can be usefully applied to the population. Erroneous inferences can be controlled either in the **analysis phase** of research or in the **design and implementation phases** (Fig. 1.6). This book deals mainly with design and implementation phase strategies: preventing errors from occurring in the first place, to the extent that it is practical and economic to do so.

The two main kinds of error that interfere with research inferences are **random error** and **systematic error**. The distinction is important because the strategies for minimizing them are quite different.

Random error is a wrong result due to chance—unknown sources of variation that are equally likely to distort the sample in either direction. If the true prevalence of antibodies to AIDS virus in the population is 30%, a well-designed sample of 100 patients from that population might contain exactly 30 patients with antibodies. More likely, however, the sample would contain some

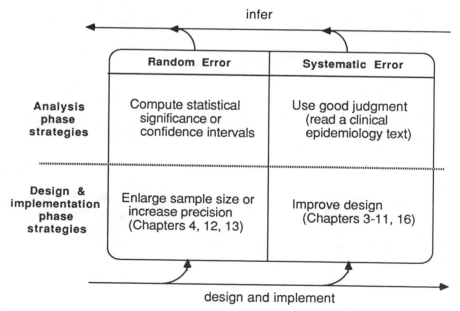

Figure 1.6. Research errors can have both random and systematic elements, as indicated in this blown up version of the error box in Figures 1.4 and 1.5; the box summarizes the strategies for minimizing the effects of these errors that are available in the design and analysis stages of research.

nearby number like 28, 29, 31, or 32. Occasionally chance would produce a substantially different number, like 19 or 42. Among several techniques for reducing the influence of random error (Chapter 12), the simplest and best known is to increase the sample size. The use of a larger sample diminishes the likelihood of a wrong result by increasing the **precision** of the estimate—the degree to which the observed prevalence approximates 30% each time a sample is drawn.

Systematic error is a wrong result due to **bias**—sources of variation that distort the study findings in one direction. An illustration is the decision in Figure 1.4 to use patients who come to the methadone clinic to represent all i.v. drug abusers. Increasing the sample size has no effect on systematic error. The only way to improve the **accuracy** of the estimate—the degree to which it approximates the true value—is to design the study in a way that either reduces the size of the various biases or gives some information about them. An example would be to draw a second sample of i.v. drug abusers by advertising for volunteers through street sources, and to compare the observed prevalence in the two samples.

The examples of random and systematic error in the preceding two paragraphs are components of **sampling error**, threatening the inference from the study subjects to the population. Both random and systematic errors can also be components of **measurement error**, threatening the inference from the study measurements to the phenomena of interest. An example of random measurement error is the variation in the titer of AIDS virus antibody observed when a single specimen is tested repeatedly. An example of systematic measurement error is the fact that testing for antibodies will consistently underestimate the prevalence of AIDS virus infection because patients who have been infected for less than 3 months will not yet have antibodies.

The concepts presented in the last several pages are summarized in Figure 1.7. Here is an important bottom line: Getting the right answer to the research question is a matter of designing and implementing the study in a fashion that keeps the extent of the inferential errors at an acceptable level.

DESIGNING THE STUDY

Developing the study protocol

The first step in designing a study is to establish the research question. This task is discussed at length in Chapter 2. Once the research question is in hand, the process of developing the study plan can begin.

There are **four versions** of the study plan

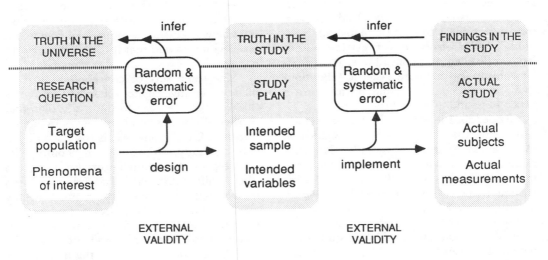

Figure 1.7. Summary of how research works.

that are produced in sequence, each larger and more detailed than the preceding one.

The first version is the **study question**, a one-sentence analogue of the research question that specifies what the study will actually answer if it is successful.

The second version is a **1–2 page outline** of the elements of the study. We recommend the sequence in Table 1.1. It does what the review of systems does in a clinical examination—serves as a **standardized checklist** that reminds the investigator to include all the components. Just as important, the sequence has an orderly logic that helps clarify the investigator's thinking on the topic.

The third version is the **study protocol**, a fleshed in version of the 1–2 page outline that can range from 5 to several hundred pages. The full protocol is the main document used to plan the study and to apply for grant support; we discuss parts of it throughout this book, and put them all together in Chapter 17.

The fourth version is the **operations manual**, a collection of specific procedural instructions, questionnaires, and other materials designed to assure a uniform and standardized approach to carrying out the study with good quality control (Chapters 4 and 16).

The study question and 1–2 page outline should be written out at an early stage. Putting thoughts down on paper leads the way from vague ideas to specific plans, and provides a concrete basis for getting advice from colleagues and consultants. It's a challenge to do it—ideas are easier to talk about than to write out—but the rewards are a faster start and a better project.

Appendix 1 illustrates the 1–2 page study plan using the AIDS example discussed in this chapter. As usual, this study plan deals more with the anatomy of research (Fig. 1.1) than with its physiology (Fig. 1.7), so the investigator must remind himself to worry about the internal and external validity that will result when it comes time to draw inferences about what happened in the study sample and formulate conclusions for the population. A study's virtues and problems can be revealed by explicitly considering how the question the study is likely to answer differs from the research question, given the plans for acquiring subjects and making measurements, and given the likely problems of implementation.

With the 1–2 page outline in hand and the internal and external validity inferences in mind, the investigator can proceed with fleshing out the details of his protocol. He will discover that this includes getting advice from colleagues, drafting specific recruitment and measurement methods, changing the study question and outline, pretesting specific recruitment and measurement methods, making more changes, getting more advice, and so forth. This iterative process is the nature of research design and the topic of the rest of this book.

Trade-offs

We have seen that errors are an inherent part of all studies, and that the main issue is whether the errors will be large enough to change the conclusions in important ways. The investigator, when designing a study, is in much the same position as a labor union official bargaining for a new contract. The union official begins with a wish list—shorter hours, more pay, parking spaces, and so forth. He must then make concessions, holding onto the things that are most important and relinquishing those that are not essential. At the end of the negotiations is a vital step: he must look at the best contract he was able to negotiate and decide if it has become so bad that it is no longer worth having.

The same sort of concessions must be made by an investigator when he transforms the research question to the study plan and considers the potential problems in implemention. On the one side is the issue of scientific validity, on the other, feasibility. The last step of the union negotiator is all too often omitted. Once the study plan has been formulated, the investigator must decide whether it adequately addresses the research question, and whether it can be implemented with acceptable levels of error. Often, the answer is "no," and the investigator must begin the process anew. But take heart!

Good scientists distinguish themselves not so much by their uniformly good research ideas as by their tenacity in turning over those that won't work at an early stage and trying again.

SUMMARY

1. The *anatomy of research* is the set of tangible elements that make up the study plan: the research question, design, study subjects, measurement approaches, and statistical plans. The challenge is to design a study plan with elements that are fast, inexpensive, and easy to implement.
2. The *physiology of research* is how the study works: the study findings are used to draw *inferences* about what actually happened in the study sample (*internal validity*), and about events in the world outside (*external validity*). The challenge here is to design and implement a study plan with adequate control over two major threats to these inferences: *random error (chance)* and *systematic error (bias)*.
3. A good way to develop the study plan is to write a *one-sentence* summary and to expand this into a *1-2 page outline* that sets out the study elements in a standardized sequence. Later on the study plan will be expanded into the *protocol* and the *operations manual*.
4. The next step is to consider the main inferences that will be drawn from the study subjects to the population, and from the study measurements to the phenomena of interest. At issue here are the relationships between the *research question* (what the investigator really wants to answer in the world outside), the *study plan* (what the study is designed to answer), and the *actual study* (what the study will actually answer, given the errors of implementation that can be anticipated).
5. Good judgment by the investigator and advice from colleagues are needed for the many *trade-offs* involved and for determining the overall viability of the project.

ADDITIONAL READINGS

Babbie E. *The Practice of Social Research*. Belmont, CA, Wadsworth, 1983. (*A well-organized and sensible social science research text.*)

Friedman LM, Furberg CD, DeMets DL. *Fundamentals of Clinical Trials*, ed 2. Littleton, MA, PSG Publishing Co, 1985. (*An excellent book on clinical trials, with good examples and a special emphasis on large-scale collaborative studies.*)

Kelsey JF, Thompson WD, Evans AS: *Methods in Observational Epidemiology*. New York, Oxford University Press, 1986. (*An excellent and thoughtful text on designing observational studies.*)

Kleinbaum DG, Kupper LL, Morgenstern H. *Epidemiologic Research: Principles and Quantitative Methods*. Belmont CA, Lifetime Learning Publications, 1982. (*A challenging text that emphasizes quantitative methodology.*)

Meinert, C. *Clinical Trials*. New York, Oxford University Press, 1986. (*An advanced but readable book that comprehensively sets out the practical details of designing a clinical trial.*)

Pocock SJ. *Clinical Trials: A Practical Approach*. Chichester, John Wiley & Sons, 1983. (*A sound book on experiments by one of Britain's leading statisticians.*)

Polit D, Hungler B. *Nursing Research: Principles and Methods*, ed 2. Philadelphia, JB Lippincott Co, 1983. (*A practical and comprehensive text, easy to read and well organized, combining social and medical sciences in a fashion that is relevant to all health researchers.*)

Rose G, Blackburn H, Prineas R. *Cardiovascular Survey Methods*. Geneva, WHO, 1982. (*A good, concise presentation of the special concerns of cardiovascular researchers.*)

Schlesselman JJ. *Case-Control Studies: Design, Conduct, Analysis*. New York, Oxford University Press, 1982. (*An excellent standard reference on case-control studies, with two good chapters on research strategies by Paul Stolley.*)

Silverman WA. *Human Experimentation: A Guided Step into the Unknown*. Oxford, England, Oxford University Press, 1985. (*This book glories in relevant historic events and the lessons for clinical research that we may learn from them.*)

Spilker B. *Guide to Clinical Studies and Developing Protocols*. New York, Raven Press, 1984. (*A step-by-step manual with some useful check lists and examples.*)

CHAPTER 2

Conceiving the Research Question

*Steven R. Cummings, Warren S. Browner, and
Stephen B. Hulley*

INTRODUCTION **12**

ORIGINS OF A RESEARCH QUESTION **12**
  Build on experience
  Be alert to new ideas
  Keep the imagination roaming

CHARACTERISTICS OF A GOOD RESEARCH
  QUESTION **14**
  Feasible
  Interesting
  Novel
  Ethical
  Relevant

DEVELOPING THE RESEARCH QUESTION AND
  STUDY PLAN **15**
  Problems and solutions
  Primary and secondary questions

SUMMARY **17**

REFERENCES **17**

ADDITIONAL READINGS **17**

APPENDIX 2. Developing the Research
  Question: A Hypothetical Example **198**

— — — — — — — — — — — —

INTRODUCTION

The **research question** is the uncertainty
about something in the population that the
investigator wants to resolve by making
measurements on his study subjects (Fig.
2.1). There is no shortage of questions in the
universe. Even as we succeed in producing
good answers to some questions, we remain
surrounded by others. Recent clinical trials,
for example, have established that β-block-
ers reduce mortality for at least the first 2
years after a myocardial infarction (1). But
now there are new questions: Are some β-
blockers more effective than others? Do all
patients benefit (2)? How long should treatment be continued after the infarction?

The challenge in searching for a research
question is not a shortage of uncertainties in
the universe; it is the difficulty of finding an
important one that can be transformed into
a *feasible and valid* **study plan.**

ORIGINS OF A RESEARCH QUESTION

Build on experience

For an established investigator, the best research questions usually emerge from the
findings and problems he has observed in his
own prior studies and in those of other
workers in the field. A new investigator has
not yet developed this base of experience.
Although a fresh perspective can sometimes
be useful, allowing a creative person to conceive new approaches to old problems, lack
of experience is largely an impediment.

A good way to start is to master the published literature in an area of study; *scholarship* is a necessary ingredient to good research. But no amount of reading can
substitute for first hand experience in guiding
the many judgments of clinical research.
Therefore an essential strategy for a young
investigator is to apprentice himself to an experienced senior scientist who has the time
and interest to work with him regularly. A
good relationship of this sort also provides
the tangible resources a young investigator
needs—office space, computer facilities, support for supplies and laboratory tests, etc.
The *choice of a mentor* is the single most important decision a new investigator makes.

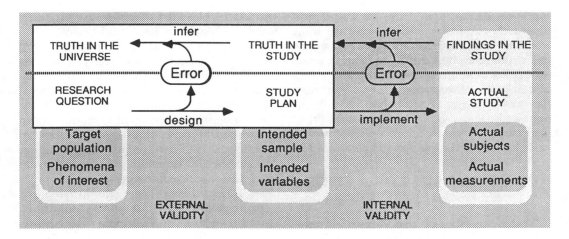

Figure 2.1. Choosing the research question and designing the study plan.

Be alert to new ideas

In addition to the **medical literature** and **journal clubs** as a source of ideas for research questions, all investigators find it very helpful to attend **national meetings** in which recent work is presented. The discussion of the work in the meeting can be supplemented by informal conversations with other scientists during the breaks. A new investigator who overcomes his shyness and engages a speaker over coffee will often find the experience richly rewarding.

A **skeptical attitude** about prevailing beliefs can stimulate good research questions. For example, surgery was formerly recommended for patients with asymptomatic gallstones because studies had claimed that up to 50% of such patients eventually developed symptoms or complications. However, one research group critically reviewed these studies and observed that some had included patients with symptomatic gallstones. Other studies had counted symptoms that were probably not due to gallstones. Using better criteria for gallstone-related symptoms in a well-defined cohort of patients with asymptomatic gallstones, the investigators found that only 15% of the patients suffered any biliary pain during 15 years of follow-up (3).

The application of **new technologies** often helps generate new research questions about familiar clinical problems. The development of assays that measure very small

concentrations of cotinine (a metabolite of nicotine) in urine, for instance, has stimulated new questions and studies about the effects of second-hand exposure to cigarette smoke (see Appendix 2). Similarly, taking a concept or technique from one field and applying it to a problem in a different field can lead to new insights and advances. One recent study applied the concept of "social support," developed primarily in social science research, to the study of survival after myocardial infarction. It found that patients with less social support had a higher mortality rate during the three years following their infarctions (4).

Careful **observation of patients** has historically been one of the major sources of descriptive studies and is still a fruitful source of research questions. **Teaching** is also an excellent source of inspiration; ideas for studies often occur while preparing presentations or during discussions with inquisitive students. Because there is usually not enough time to develop these ideas on the spot, it is useful to keep them in a notebook for future reference.

Keep the imagination roaming

There is a major role for **creativity** in the process of conceiving the research question, imagining new answers to old questions and having fun with ideas. There is also a need for **tenacity**, for returning to a troublesome problem repeatedly until there is a resolution that feels comfortable. Some creative ideas come to mind during informal conversations with colleagues over lunch, and others occur in brainstorming sessions. Many inpirations are solo affairs that strike while preparing a lecture, showering, or just sitting and thinking. The trick is to put an unresolved problem clearly in view and turn on the mental switch that lets the mind run freely toward it.

CHARACTERISTICS OF A GOOD RESEARCH QUESTION

The characteristics of a good research question, which have the mnemonic **FINER**, are summarized in Table 2.1.

Table 2.1.
Criteria for a good research question

Feasible

    Adequate number of subjects
    Adequate technical expertise
    Affordable in time and money
    Manageable in scope

Interesting to the investigator

Novel

    Confirms or refutes previous findings
    Extends previous findings
    Provides new findings

Ethical

Relevant

    To scientific knowledge
    To clinical and health policy
    To future research directions

Feasible

It is best to know the practical limits and problems of studying a question early on, before wasting much time and effort along unworkable lines.

The number of subjects: Many studies do not achieve their intended purposes because they are unable to enroll enough subjects. The first step is to make a preliminary estimate of the sample size requirements of the study (Chapter 13). The next step is to estimate the number of subjects likely to be available for the study, the number who would be excluded or refuse to participate, and the number who would be lost to follow-up. Even careful planning often produces estimates that are overly optimistic, and the investigator should be very certain that there are enough willing subjects. It is sometimes necessary to carry out a pilot survey to be sure. If the number of subjects appears insufficient, there are a number of strategies the investigator can consider. These include expanding the inclusion criteria, eliminating unnecessary exclusion criteria, lengthening the time-frame for enrolling subjects, acquiring additional sources of subjects, developing more precise measurement approaches (Chapter 4), and using a different study design.

Technical expertise: The investigators must have the skills, equipment and experience needed for recruiting the subjects, measuring the variables, and managing and analyzing the data. The easiest strategy is to use familiar and established approaches, because the process of developing new methods and skills is time consuming and uncertain. When it is necessary to develop an approach such as a new questionnaire for the study, expertise in how to accomplish the innovation should be available. Consultants can help to shore up technical aspects that are unfamiliar to the investigators, but for *major* areas of the study it is better to have an experienced colleague as a co-investigator. For example, it is often wise to include a statistician as a regular part-time member of the research team from the beginning of the planning process.

Cost in time and money: It is important to estimate the costs of each component of the project, bearing in mind that the time and money needed will generally exceed the amounts projected at the outset. If the costs are prohibitive, the only options are to consider a less expensive design or to develop additional sources of funding. If the study will be too expensive or time-consuming it is best to know this early, when the question can be modified or abandoned before a great deal of effort has been expended.

Scope: Problems often arise when an investigator attempts to accomplish too much, making many measurements on a large group of subjects in an effort to answer too many research questions. The solution is to narrow the scope of the study and focus only on the most important goals. Many scientists find it difficult to give up the opportunity to answer interesting side questions, but the reward will be a better answer to the main question at hand.

Interesting

An investigator may have many motivations for pursuing a particular research question: because it will provide financial support, because it is a logical or important next step in building a career, or because getting at the truth of the matter seems interesting. We like this last reason; it is one that grows as it is exercised, and that provides the intensity of effort needed for overcoming the many hurdles and frustrations of the research process.

Novel

Good clinical research is novel; it contributes new information. A study that merely reiterates what is already established is not worth the effort and cost. On the other hand, a question need not be totally original in order to be worth studying. It may ask whether a previous observation can be replicated, whether the findings in one population also apply to a different group of subjects, or whether improved measurement techniques can clarify the relationship between known risk factors and a disease. A confirmatory study is particularly useful if it avoids the weaknesses of previous studies.

Ethical

A good research question must be ethical. If the study poses unacceptable physical risks or invasion of privacy (Chapter 14), the investigator must seek other ways to answer the research question. If there is uncertainty about whether the study is ethical, it may help to discuss it with the institutional review board that will ultimately review the study plans.

Relevant

Among the characteristics of a good research question, none is more important than its relevance. A good way to decide about relevance is to imagine the various outcomes that are likely to occur and consider how each possibility might advance scientific knowledge, influence clinical management and health policy, or guide further research.

DEVELOPING THE RESEARCH QUESTION AND STUDY PLAN

It is important to write down the research question and a **1-2 page outline** of the study plan at an early stage. This requires some self-discipline, but it forces the investigator to clarify his own ideas about the plan and to discover specific problems that need attention. The 1-2 page outline also provides a basis for colleagues to react to with specific suggestions.

Problems and solutions

The potential problems in choosing the research question and developing the study plan are recapped, with their solutions, in Table 2.2. Two general kinds of solutions deserve special emphasis. The first is the importance of getting **good advice**. We recommend a research team that includes representatives of each of the major aspects of the study, and that includes at least one senior scientist. In addition, it is a good idea to consult with specialists who can guide the discovery of previous research on the topic and the choice and design of measurement techniques. Sometimes a local expert will do, but it is often useful to contact individuals in other institutions who have published pertinent work on the subject. A new investigator may be intimidated by the prospect of writing or calling someone he knows only as an author in the *New England Journal of Medicine*, but most scientists respond favorably to such requests for advice.

The second thing to emphasize is the way the study plan should gradually emerge from an **iterative process** of designing, reviewing, pretesting and revising (Chapter 16). Once the 1-2 page study plan is written, advice from colleagues will usually result in important changes. As the protocol gradually takes shape, a small pretest of

Table 2.2.
The research question and study plan:
Problems and solutions

Potential problem	Solutions

1. Vague or inappropriate	• Write the research question at an early stage
	• Get specific in the 1-2 page study plan about
	  - how the subjects will be sampled
	  - how the variables will be measured
	• Think about ways to make
	  - the subjects more representative of the population
	  - the measurements more representative of the phenomena of interest

2. Not feasible	
Too broad	• Specify a smaller set of variables • Narrow the question
Not enough subjects available	• Expand the inclusion criteria • Eliminate exclusion criteria • Add other sources of subjects • Lengthen the time frame for entry into study • Use more efficient variables or designs
Methods inadequate or beyond the skills of the investigator	• Consult experts and review the literature for alternative methods • Learn the skills • Collaborate with colleagues who have the skills
Too expensive	• Consider less costly study designs and measurement methods • Seek additional financial support
3. Not relevant or novel	• Modify the research question
4. Uncertain ethical suitability	• Consult with institutional review board • Modify the research question to avoid potentially unethical elements

the number and willingness of the potential subjects may lead to a new accessible population. The preferred blood test may turn out to be prohibitively costly, and a less expensive alternative must be sought. And so on. This iterative process, which requires tenacity and attention to detail, is illustrated in Appendix 2.

Primary and secondary questions

Many studies have more than one research question. Experiments often address the effect of the intervention on several outcomes (for example, the Multiple Risk Factor Intervention Trial [MRFIT] asked whether lowering risk factors would prevent heart attacks *and* whether it would lower total mortality (6)). It is also common to look separately at the results in various subgroups of study subjects (the MRFIT investigators decided in advance to look at the effects of treatment in the healthiest subgroup—those with normal electrocardiograms at the outset (6)). Many research projects also include ancillary studies (the MRFIT contained a study of the relationship between psychologic factors and heart disease (7)).

The advantage of designing a study with several research questions is the efficiency that can result, with several answers emerging from a single study. The disadvantages are the increased complexity of designing and implementing the study, and of drawing statistical inferences from a study with multiple hypotheses (see Chapter 12). A sensible strategy is to establish a single **primary** research question around which to focus the development of the study plan. This can be supplemented with **secondary** research questions that may also produce valuable conclusions.

SUMMARY

1. All studies should start with a *research question* that addresses what the investigator would like to know. The goal is to find an *important* one that can be transformed into a *feasible and valid study plan*.
2. Two important ingredients for developing a research question are *scholarship* and *experience*. The single most important decision for an investigator who is not yet experienced is his *choice of a senior scientist* to serve as his mentor.
3. Good research questions often *arise* from medical articles and conferences, from critical thinking about clinical practices and problems, from applying new concepts or methods to old issues, and from alert observations during patient care and teaching.
4. Before committing much time and effort to writing a proposal or carrying out a study, the investigator should consider whether the research question and study plan are "FINER": *feasible, interesting, novel, ethical* and *relevant*.
5. Early on, the research question should be developed into a written 1-2 page *study plan* that specifically describes how the subjects will be selected and the measurements made.
6. Developing the research question and study plan is an *iterative process* that includes consultations with advisors and friends, a growing familiarity with the literature, and pilot studies for testing the recruitment and measurement approaches. The qualities needed in the investigator are *judgment, tenacity* and *creativity*.
7. Most studies have more than one question, but it is useful to focus on a *single primary* question in designing and implementing the study.

REFERENCES

1. Yusuf S, Peto R, Lewis J, et al: Beta blockade during and after myocardial infarction: an overview of the randomized trials. *Prog Cardiovasc Dis* 27:335–371, 1985.
2. Furberg CD, Hawkins, CM, Lichstein E: Effect of propranolol in post-infarction patients with mechanical or electrical complications. *Circulation* 69; 761–765, 1984.
3. Gracie WA, Ransohoff DF: The natural history of gallstones: the innocent gallstone is not a myth. *N Engl J Med* 307:798–800, 1982.
4. Ruberman W, Weinblatt E, Boldberg JD, et al: Psychosocial influences on mortality after myocardial infarction. *N Engl J Med* 311:552–559, 1984.
5. The MRFIT Research Group: Coronary heart disease death, nonfatal acute myocardial infarction and other clinical outcomes in the MRFIT. *Am J Cardiol* 58:1–13, 1986.
6. Shekelle RB, Hulley SB, Neaton JD, et al: The MRFIT Behavior Pattern Study: II. Type A behavior and incidence of CHD. *Am J Epidemiol* 122:559–570, 1985.

ADDITIONAL READINGS

Friedman LM, Furberg CD, DeMets DL: *Fundamentals of Clinical Trials*, ed 2. Littleton, MA, PSG Publishing Co, Inc., 1985, pp 11–22. (*A good discussion of primary and secondary questions, and of how to choose the intervention and outcome variables in an experiment.*)

Kuhn TS: *The Structure of Scientific Revolutions*. Chicago, University of Chicago Press, 1962. (*A seminal work on the origin of revolutionary research ideas.*)

Polit D, Hungler B: *Nursing Research: Principles and Methods*, ed 2. Philadelphia, JB Lippincott Co, 1983, pp 59–138. (*A detailed discussion, relevant to all health sciences, of how to conceive, evaluate and modify research questions.*)

Silverman WA: *Human Experimentation: A Guided Step into the Unknown*. Oxford, England, Oxford University Press, 1985, pp 14–29. (*Interesting historical and philosophical background.*)

CHAPTER 3

Choosing the Study Subjects: Specification and Sampling

Stephen B. Hulley, Sandra Gove, Warren S. Browner, and Steven R. Cummings

INTRODUCTION 18

BASIC TERMS AND CONCEPTS 18
Target and accessible populations
Generalizing the study findings
Steps in designing the protocol for acquiring
    study subjects

SPECIFICATION 21
Establishing inclusion criteria
Establishing exclusion criteria
Choosing the accessible population

SAMPLING 24
Probability sampling
Nonprobability sampling
Summarizing the choice among sampling design
    options

RECRUITMENT 26
The goals of recruitment
Enhancing the response rate
General recruitment approaches

RECAPPING THE ERRORS IN CHOOSING THE
    STUDY SUBJECTS 27
Design errors
Implementation errors

SUMMARY 29

REFERENCES 30

ADDITIONAL READINGS 30

APPENDIX 3.   Drawing a random sample 200

— — — — — — — — — — — —

INTRODUCTION

A good choice of study subjects serves the vital purpose of assuring that the findings in the study accurately represent what is going on in the population (Fig. 3.1). The protocol must specify a sample of subjects that can be studied at an acceptable cost in time and money, yet one that is large enough to control random error in generalizing the study findings to the population and representative enough to control systematic error in these inferences.

These are conflicting goals that challenge the judgment of the investigator. We will come to the issue of choosing the appropriate *number* of study subjects in Chapter 13. In this chapter we address the process of specifying and sampling the *kinds* of subjects who will be representative and feasible.

BASIC TERMS AND CONCEPTS

Target and accessible populations

A **population** is a complete set of people with a specified set of characteristics, and a sample is a subset of the population. In the lay usage, the characteristics that define a population are geographic; we speak, for example, of the population of Canada. In research the characteristics are also clinical, demographic, and temporal, and they are used to define two kinds of populations:

1. The **clinical** and **demographic** characteristics define the **target population**, the large set of all patients throughout the world to which the results will be generalized: all teenagers with asthma, for example.
2. The **geographic** and **temporal** characteristics define the **accessible population**, the subset of the target population that is available for study: teenagers with asthma living in the investigator's town in 1989.

18

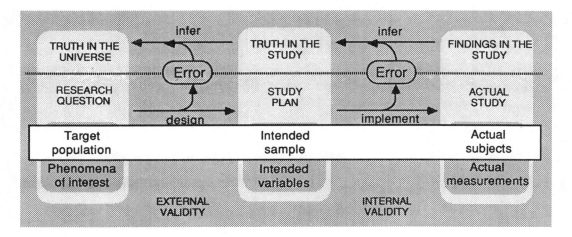

Figure 3.1. Choosing study subjects that represent the population.

Generalizing the study findings

The subclassification into two kinds of populations, target and accessible, expands the left-hand side of the basic clinical research model (Fig. 3.1) into two parts. This is illustrated in Figure 3.2 (next page) with a finding in the Framingham Study, the association between hypertension and coronary heart disease (CHD).

In deciding whether this finding in the sample of Framingham residents represents an association in the general population, the **internal validity inference** is from the actual subjects to the intended sample. Unfortunately, one-third of the Framingham residents selected for the study refused to participate, and in their place the Framingham investigators put other residents who happened to hear about the study and volunteered (1). Because nonrespondents are often less healthy than average, and volunteers more healthy, the actual sample is probably somewhat unrepresentative of the intended sample. Every sample has some errors, however, and the issue is whether they are large enough to cause a wrong answer to the research question. Most experts would agree that the Framingham Study sampling errors are too small to invalidate the conclusions.

The **first external validity inference** in Figure 3.2 is the generalization from the intended sample to the accessible population.

The Framingham sampling design called for listing all the residents of that town and then asking every second person to participate. This is a systematic sampling design, and it provides a scientific basis for saying that the intended sample represented the accessible population.

The **second external validity inference** in Figure 3.2 is the generalization from the accessible population to target populations that are geographically or temporally remote. This inference is more subjective. The town of Framingham was selected from the universe of towns in the world, not with a scientific sampling design, but because it seemed a fairly typical middle-class residential community and it was convenient to the investigators. The validity of generalizing the results to all suburban U.S. residents is based on the general knowledge that patterns of disease tend to be similar in demographically similar populations.

Whether generalizations apply to more remote target populations is always less certain, and it is an issue that depends a good deal on the nature of the research question. In general, analytic studies that examine biologic relationships can be more widely generalized than descriptive studies that describe distributions of health factors. (For example, the *strength* of hypertension as a risk factor for CHD tends to be more consis-

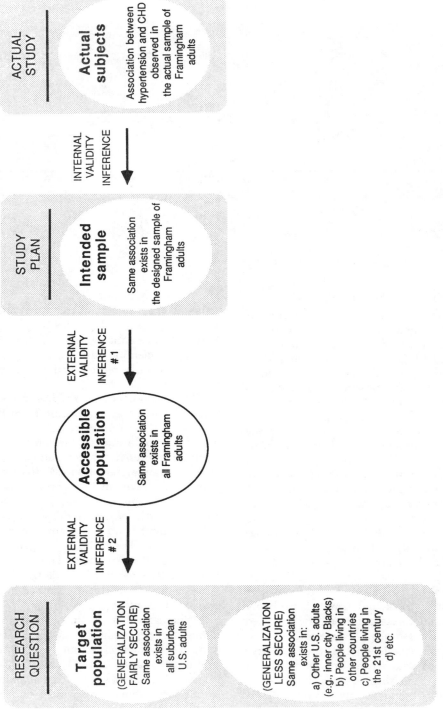

Figure 3.2 Inferences in generalizing from the study subjects to the accessible and target populations, using a finding from the Framingham study as an illustration.

tent among diverse populations than the *prevalence* of hypertension.) The uncertainty of drawing inferences to other target populations illustrates the fact that in clinical research, generalizability is rarely a simple yes-or-no matter; it is usually a qualitative judgment about the validity of these inferences.

Steps in designing the protocol for acquiring study subjects

The inferences in Figure 3.2 are presented from right to left, the sequence used for interpreting the findings of a completed study. An investigator who is planning a study reverses this sequence (Fig. 3.3). He begins by **specifying** the clinical and demographic characteristics of target populations that will serve the research question well. He then uses temporal and geographic criteria to specify the choice of an accessible population that is representative and practical. These two steps together are the topic of the

next section of this chapter; later on we will come to the third step, a scientific and efficient approach to **sampling** from the accessible population.

SPECIFICATION

Suppose an investigator wants to study the efficacy of calcium supplements for preventing osteoporosis. He begins by creating two sets of selection criteria—inclusion and exclusion—that define the populations to be studied.

Establishing inclusion criteria

The **inclusion criteria** define the main characteristics of the target and accessible populations (Table 3.1). The task of specifying the **clinical characteristics** involves difficult judgments about what factors are important to the research question and how to define them. How does the investigator put into practice the criterion that the subjects be in

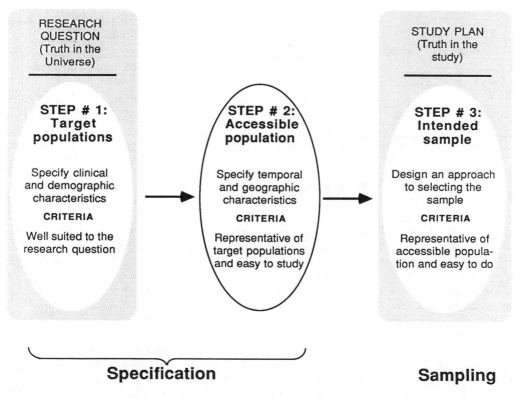

Specification   **Sampling**

Figure 3.3.   The three steps in designing the protocol for choosing the study subjects.

Table 3.1.
Designing Inclusion and Exclusion Criteria

	Considerations	Examples
Inclusion criteria (be specific)	Specifying the characteristics that define populations that are relevant to the research question and efficient for study:	A 5-year trial of calcium supplementation for preventing osteoporosis might specify that the subjects be:
Target population {	Demographic characteristics	White females age 45–50
	Clinical characteristics	In good general health: no known life-threatening disease not paraplegic or taking long-term corticosteroids[a]
Accessible population {	Geographic (administrative) characteristics	Patients attending the medical clinic at the investigator's hospital
	Temporal characteristics	Between January 1 and December 31, 1989
Exclusion criteria (be parsimonious)	Specifying subsets of the population that will *not* be studied because of:	The calcium supplementation trial might exclude subjects who are:
	A high likelihood of being lost to follow-up	Alcoholic or plan to move out of state
	An inability to provide good data	Disoriented or have a language barrier[b]
	Ethical barriers	Kidney stone formers (which would contraindicate oral calcium)
	The subject's refusal to participate	Unwilling to accept possibility of random allocation to placebo group

[a]An option that expands the target populations is to include those patients with special forms of osteoporosis and later to account for their different entry condition using special analytic approaches (see sections on stratification and adjustment in Chapter 10).
[b]Alternatives to exclusion (when these subgroups are important to the research question) would be collecting nonverbal data or using bilingual staff and questionnaires.

"good general health"? He may decide to include patients with diseases that are not strongly related to osteoporosis nor immediately life-threatening (e.g., hypertension), but not to include patients with diseases that may cause osteoporosis (e.g., paraplegia) or that may interfere with followup (e.g., lung cancer). The task of specifying the **demographic characteristics** (age, sex, and race) is even tougher, often involving trade-offs that balance generalizability against efficiency (2). Including men and black women in the study of osteoporosis, for example, would expand generalizability at the cost of an increase in the size or duration of the study (because osteoporosis develops more slowly in these populations).

On these kinds of issues there is no single course of action that is clearly right or wrong; the important thing is to make decisions that are sensible, that can be used consistently throughout the study, and that will provide a basis for applying the published conclusions to other populations. This is best accomplished by thinking about these issues during the design process (rather than having to deal with them after the study has begun) and resolving them with explicit criteria in the protocol.

The inclusion criteria that address the **geographic** (administrative) and **temporal characteristics** of the accessible population also involve trade-offs between scientific and practical goals. The investigator may find that patients at his own hospital are the most available and inexpensive source of subjects. The decision about whether peculiarities of the local population or environment might interfere with generalizing the results to all patients with the disease depends on the nature of the research question. Whereas a study of alcoholism would find rather different characteristics in patients attending a Veterans Administration Hospital than in those at a community hospital, a study of psoriasis might depend less on the location.

Establishing exclusion criteria

Exclusion criteria indicate subsets of individuals who meet the eligibility criteria, but are likely to interfere with the quality of the data or the interpretation of the findings (Table 3.1). Exclusion criteria may improve the feasibility of a study at the cost of generalizability, so the investigator should use them sparingly. Including alcoholics in the osteoporosis study would expand generalizability, for example, and allow the investigators to study excess alcohol consumption as a cause of demineralization. These advantages would come at the cost of greater problems with follow-up, however, and the investigator may decide to exclude alcoholics if he believes that preventing loss to follow-up is the more important consideration. (He will then face the difficult problem of developing specific criteria for classifying whether or not an individual is alcoholic.)

Some exclusions are mandated by ethical considerations, or by the patient's unwillingness to participate. Here the task for the investigator is to consider whether subjects excluded for these reasons will threaten external validity. If the number or kind of such exclusions becomes excessive (and what is

excessive depends a good deal on the research question), the generalizability of the study may be compromised.

Choosing the accessible population

The choice of accessible population presents two main options to the investigator. **Clinic-based samples** of patients are inexpensive and easy to recruit, but selection factors that determine who comes to the hospital or clinic may have an important effect. A common version of this problem is the specialty clinic at a tertiary care medical center, which tends to accumulate patients with serious or difficult varieties of a disease who give a distorted impression of the commonplace features and prognosis (3). Studies of the incidence of seizure disorders in children who have had febrile convulsions, for example, have yielded estimates that range from 1.5% in a general population to 58% in specialty clinic—a 40-fold difference (4)!

There are many research questions, however, for which clinic-based samples are an excellent choice. An example would be a study of the natural history of a discrete and uniformly severe disease like craniopharyngioma. Because nearly all patients with this diagnosis will be referred to a specialty clinic sooner or later, patients seen in this setting *are* representative of the target population of interest.

The other main option in choosing the accessible population is to select subjects in their homes, producing a sample that is representative of a specified region. Such "**population-based**" **samples** are particularly useful for guiding public health and clinical practice in the whole community. One of the largest and best examples is the Health and Nutrition Examination Survey (HANES), which used a probability sample of all U.S. residents (5). The chief disadvantages of choosing a population-based sample are the difficulty and expense involved, particularly for relatively uncommon diseases.

Accessible populations need not be geographically proximate if the data can be collected by mail or telephone (although these approaches may alter the validity of the responses (6)). The size and diversity of an accessible population can be increased by collaborating with colleagues in other hospitals and cities. Pre-existing data sets such as the HANES are electronically accessible populations that can be more representative and less time consuming than other possibilities (see Chapter 6).

SAMPLING

In clinical research it is sometimes possible to avoid sampling and its biases by studying the *entire* accessible population—all cases of Legionnaire's disease in the Philadelphia epidemic of 1976, for example. This is the best approach when it is feasible.

Usually, however, the accessible population is too large or too spread out over time, and there is a need to select a smaller group of individuals for study. The topic of sampling can be discussed at a highly technical level (7), but we favor a simpler approach. There are two main classes of sampling designs, probability and nonprobability. All an investigator needs for most research projects is an awareness of the main classes within these options, the judgment to choose one that will be practical and scientific, and the compulsiveness to carry it out well.

Probability sampling

A probability sample uses a random process to guarantee that each unit of the population has a specified chance of selection. It is a scientific approach, providing a rigorous basis for estimating the fidelity with which phenomena observed in the sample are representative of those in the population, and for computing statistical significance and confidence intervals (Chapter 15). There are several versions of the probability approach.

Simple random sampling is the process of enumerating every unit of the accessible population, and then selecting the sample at random. To take a simple random sample of the gallbladder surgery patients at his hospital, for example, the investigator could make a list of all such patients on the operating room schedules for the period of study, then use a table of random numbers to select a subset of these individuals for study. This last step is easy (Appendix 3) but the investi-

gator may have some difficulty obtaining an accurate listing of the population, and finding and enrolling those who are chosen.

Systematic sampling involves selecting by a periodic process, as in the Framingham approach of taking every second person from a list of town residents. Technically a form of probability sampling if the starting point is chosen at random, the systematic approach can be designed in a way that produces slightly more precise estimates than simple random sampling (7). However, systematic sampling is susceptible to errors caused by natural periodicities in the population, and it allows the investigator to predict and perhaps manipulate those who will be in the sample. It offers no logistic advantages over simple random sampling, and in clinical research it is rarely a better choice.

Stratified random sampling involves dividing the population into subgroups according to characteristics such as sex or race, and taking a random sample from each of these "strata." The subsamples in a stratified sample can be weighted to draw disproportionately from subgroups that are less common in the population but of special interest to the investigator. In studying the incidence of toxemia in pregnancy, for example, it would be possible to stratify the population according to racial group, and to sample equal numbers from each race. This would yield incidence estimates for blacks and whites that have comparable precision.

Cluster sampling is the process of taking a random sample of natural groupings (clusters) of individuals in the population. Cluster sampling is very useful when the population is widely dispersed and it is impractical or costly to list and sample from all of its elements. Consider, for example, the problem of reviewing the hospital records of patients with lung cancer selected randomly from a statewide list of discharge diagnoses; a larger number of patients could be studied at lower cost by choosing a random sample of the hospitals and taking all the cases from each. Community surveys often use a **two-stage cluster sample**: a random sample is drawn from city blocks enumerated on a map and a field team visits the blocks in the sample, lists all the addresses in each, and selects a subsample for study by a second random process.

The advantages of cluster sampling are well illustrated by the national HANES noted earlier (5), but they come at the cost of adding to the complexity of the data analysis (8). Another disadvantage is the fact that naturally occurring groups are often relatively homogeneous for the variables of interest; each city block, for example, tends to have people of uniform socioeconomic status. The goals in this form of sampling, therefore, are to seek clusters that are *heterogeneous* with respect to the variables of interest, and to sample a relatively large number of clusters in order to reduce the influence of any one of them.

Nonprobability sampling

Nonprobability sampling designs are more practical than probability designs for many clinical research projects. Because statistical significance tests are based on the assumption that a probability sample has been used, the objective in nonprobability sampling is to produce a facsimile, for the research question at hand, of a probability sample. (This is the same objective to keep in mind when choosing an accessible population that will be representative, i.e. a facsimile of a probability sample of the target populations.) There are three main nonprobability sampling designs.

Consecutive sampling involves taking every patient who meets the selection criteria over a specified time interval or number of patients. Consecutive sampling is the best of the nonprobability techniques, and one that is very often practical. It amounts to taking the complete accessible population over the duration of the study. The only problem arises when the duration is too short to adequately represent seasonal factors or other changes over time ("secular trends") that are important to the research question. A study of upper respiratory illness in patients seen during a 2-month period beginning in August , for example, would not be representative of viral syndromes occurring over the full year.

Convenience sampling is the process of taking those members of the accessible population who are easily available. Convenience sampling is widely used in clinical research because of its obvious advantages in cost and logistics. It is an acceptable choice for some research questions: a physiologic study of the effect of beta blockade on heart rate, for example, would probably produce the same results in almost any sample of healthy adults. For other research questions, however, the advantages of convenience sampling in cost and logistics are outweighed by the danger that volunteers may not adequately represent the population. The Multiple Risk Factor Intervention Trial (MRFIT), for example, sampled high-risk men by advertising free screening clinics; the resulting volunteer sample turned out to be healthier than the general population, and at the end of the study there were not enough deaths for an adequate statistical test of whether the intervention reduced mortality rates (9).

Judgmental sampling involves hand-picking from the accessible population those individuals judged most appropriate for the study. Judgmental sampling resembles convenience sampling, and has similar flaws. In a study of the effectiveness of a brochure about fat-controlled diets, for example, the investigator might choose from among his own patients those he considers likely to comply. Although the findings in this sample of well-motivated patients may suggest that the intervention is effective, it will be risky to apply this conclusion to other populations of patients.

Summarizing the choice among sampling design options

When it is feasible to recruit all available subjects over an intake period that is long enough to avoid unwanted periodicities and secular trends, a consecutive sample is usually the best choice (Fig. 3.4). If the only problem with using a consecutive sample is its excessive size, then a good strategy is to draw a random subsample from the consecutive series. If one or more subgroups of the population are of special interest the investigator can consider a stratified sample that draws disproportionately from these strata. If the size and extent of the population make

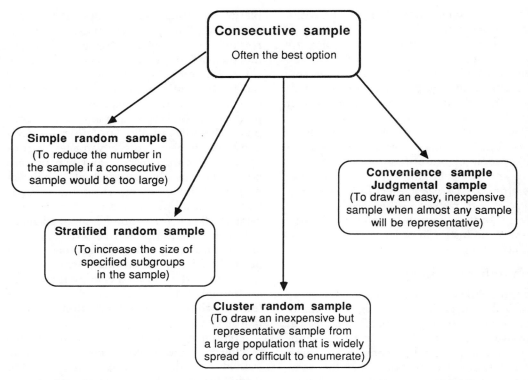

Figure 3.4. Choosing the sampling design for selecting study subjects from the accessible population.

it difficult to reach all its elements, he can consider cluster sampling.

Convenience or judgmental sampling designs are often cheaper and more practical. The decision on whether these are satisfactory requires a judgment on whether the proposed sample would serve as a facsimile for a random sample of the accessible population. For the research question at hand, would similar conclusions result?

RECRUITMENT

The goals of recruitment

An important factor to consider in choosing the accessible population and sampling approach is the feasibility of recruiting the subjects into the study (10,11). There are two main goals: (1) to recruit enough subjects to meet the sample size requirements of the study, and, (2) to recruit a sample that is unbiased.

The problem of falling short in the **num-** ber of subjects or rate of recruitment is one of the commonest in clinical research. It is safe to assume in planning a study that the number of subjects who meet the entry criteria and agree to enter the study will be fewer, often by several fold, than the number projected at the outset. The solutions to this problem are to estimate the magnitude of the recruitment problem empirically with a pretest, to plan the study with an accessible population that is larger than believed necessary, and to make contingency plans should the need arise for an even larger source of subjects. While the study is in progress it is important to tabulate the achievements in meeting the recruitment goals; examining the proportions of potential subjects lost to the study at various stages can lead to strategies for reducing some of these losses.

The solution to the problem of a **biased sample** is to choose populations and sampling methods wisely (using strategies discussed earlier in this chapter) and to minimize bias due to technical error or nonresponse. The proportion of subjects who agree to enter the study among those who are selected—the **response rate**—influences the validity of inferring that the sample represents the population. People who are difficult to reach and those who refuse to participate once they are contacted tend to be different from people who do respond.

Enhancing the response rate

The level of nonresponse that will seriously compromise the generalizability of the study depends on the research question, and on the reasons for not responding. A nonresponse rate of 25%, although a good achievement in many settings, can seriously distort the observed prevalence of a disease when the disease itself is a cause of nonresponse. The degree to which this bias will influence the conclusions of the study is often a difficult judgment, although it may be possible to estimate it during the study with an intensive effort to acquire additional information on a sample of nonrespondents. The best way to deal with nonresponse bias, however, is to minimize it at the outset.

The problem of failure to make contact with individuals who have been chosen for the sample can be reduced by designing a systematic series of repeated contact attempts, and by using alternative methods (mail, telephone, home visit). Among those who *are* contacted, refusal to participate can be minimized by improving the efficiency and attractiveness of the initial encounter, by using brochures and individual discussion to allay anxiety and discomfort, and by providing incentives such as reimbursing the costs of transportation and providing the results of tests. If language barriers are prevalent they can be circumvented by using bilingual staff and translated questionnaires.

General recruitment approaches

Sometimes recruitment involves selecting patients who are already known to the members of the research team, for example in a study of a new treatment in patients who are attending the investigator's clinic. Here the chief concern is to present the opportunity for participation in the study fairly, making clear the advantages and disadvantages. (In discussing the desirability of participation, the investigator must recognize the special ethical dilemmas that can arise when his advice as the patient's physician might conflict with his preferences as an investigator—see Chapter 14.)

Often recruitment involves contacting populations that are not known to the members of the research team. There are many approaches for contacting the prospective subjects. These include screening in work settings or public places such as shopping malls; using mailings and telephone calls; getting permission to examine potential subjects in extramural clinic and hospital settings; soliciting referrals from other clinicians; and carrying out retrospective record reviews.

It may be necessary to prepare for recruitment in advance by getting the support of important organizations, for example meeting with hospital administrators to discuss a clinic-based sample, and with the leadership of the medical society and county health department to plan a community screening operation. Endorsements should be obtained in writing and included as an appendix in any application for funding. For large studies it may be useful to create a favorable climate in the community by giving public lectures or by advertising through radio, TV, newspaper, fliers, or mass mailings.

RECAPPING THE ERRORS IN CHOOSING THE STUDY SUBJECTS

The advantage of sampling is efficiency: it allows the investigator to draw inferences about a large population at relatively small cost in time and effort. The disadvantage is the source of error it introduces: it can lead to conclusions about the population that are wrong. Errors that compromise the validity of applying the study's conclusions to the target populations can occur in either the design or implementation stages.

Design errors

Consider a study of the factors that cause people to start smoking. The investigator decides to sample eleventh-grade volunteers from the high school in the investigator's suburb. Design errors may occur at any of the levels we have discussed.

1. The **target population** (all eleventh graders, or more broadly, all high school students) may not be appropriate to the research question. If the antecedents of smoking take place at an earlier age, it might be better to study junior high students.
2. The **accessible population** (the students at this one high school) may not represent the target population; the causes of smoking differ in various cultural settings, and a better accessible population might be several high schools randomly selected from the whole region.
3. The **sampling design** (calling for volunteers) is likely to attract students who are not representative of the accessible population in their smoking behavior.

The strategies for preventing errors occurring at the first two levels are subjective (Table 3.2). The investigator must consider the kinds of subjects who would be most suitable for this research question, using advice from colleagues and data from pretests or the literature to reach a judgment about which of the available options is best. The strategy for preventing sampling error (the third level) can be more objective; it involves choosing the most scientific sampling design that is appropriate and feasible.

Implementation errors

Suppose that the investigator decided to avoid the bias associated with choosing volunteers by designing a 25% random sample of the entire eleventh grade, and that the actual sample turns out to be 70% female. If it is known that roughly equal numbers of boys and girls are enrolled in the school, then the disproportion in the sex distribution (and, therefore, in any sex-related antecedents of smoking) must represent an error in drawing the sample. There are two main types of implementation error, random and systematic (Table 3.3).

An unrepresentative sample may result from **random error** (chance). If the sample numbered only 10, a 7:3 disproportion would occur fairly often as a result of chance; in fact, the probability of finding at least seven heads in 10 tosses of a coin is

Table 3.2.
Design Errors in Choosing the Study Subjects and How to Prevent These Errors

Error	Preventive Strategies
1. The target population is not well suited to the research question.	• Design inclusion criteria that specify the age, sex, and clinical characteristics of appropriate subjects.
	• Design a parsimonious set of exclusion criteria that eliminate unwanted individuals.
	• Discuss alternatives with colleagues.
2. The accessible population does not sufficiently represent the target population.	• Design inclusion criteria that specify the time frame and the geographic characteristics of a suitable accessible population.
	• Discuss alternatives with colleagues.
3. The intended sample does not sufficiently represent the accessible population because of biased sampling design.	• Use a consecutive or probability sample whenever practical.
	• Otherwise, use good judgment in designing a convenience sample.
	• Draw a pretest sample to confirm the characteristics and availability of the subjects.

Table 3.3.
Implementation Errors in Choosing the Study Subjects and How to Prevent These Errors

Error	Preventive Strategies
The actual sample does not sufficiently represent the intended sample:	
1. Due to random sampling error (chance)	• Increase the number of subjects or use other strategies noted in Chapter 13.
	• Consider stratified sampling to enlarge specified subgroups.
2. Due to systematic sampling error (bias)	
Nonresponse bias	
a. Failure to make contact	• Use repeated attempts and/or alternative approaches.
b. Subject refuses to participate	• Provide written orientation in advance, and discuss potential source of anxiety.
	• Consider incentives such as transportation, reimbursement, and test results.
	• Consider special steps to inquire about the nonrespondents.
Mistakes	• Before the study, pretest the sampling methods.
	• During the study, control the quality of the recruitment process (see Chapter 16)

17%. But if the sample size were 100, the probability of finding at least 70 heads is less than 0.01%. This illustrates the facts that the investigator can estimate the magnitude of the random component of sampling error once the sample has been acquired, and that he can reduce it to any desired level by enlarging the sample size.

An unrepresentative sample may also result from **systematic error** (bias). There are two main sources of bias in the implementation phase. The large proportion of females could have been due to differential **nonresponse**—different rates of participation among boys and girls. The strategies for preventing nonresponse bias include the spectrum of techniques for enhancing recruitment that are summarized in Table 3.3. The large proportion of females could also represent a **technical mistake** in enumerating or selecting the names to be sampled. The strategies for preventing mistakes include the appropriate use of pretesting and quality control procedures that will be discussed in Chapter 16.

SUMMARY

1. One of the major objectives in clinical research is to prevent errors; another is to complete the study at a reasonable cost in time and money. The art of designing the protocol for acquiring study subjects is to find the best compromise between these goals.

2. The first step is to *conceptualize the target populations*, the large groups of people to which the results of the study will be generalized. This means formulating a specific set of *inclusion criteria* that establish the demographic and clinical characteristics of subjects well suited to the research question.

3. The second step is to *identify an accessible population* that will represent the target populations. This means formulating *more inclusion criteria* to establish where the subjects will be sought over what time period, and a parsimonious set of *exclusion criteria* that eliminate subjects who are unethical to study, unwilling to

participate, or seem likely to provide bad data.

4. The third step is to *design an approach to sampling* the accessible population if, as is nearly always the case, it cannot be studied in its entirety. A consecutive sample is often the best choice, using simple random sampling to reduce its size if necessary. Other *probability samples* (stratified and cluster) are useful in certain situations, and the easier *nonprobability samples* (convenience or judgmental) are satisfactory for some research questions.

5. Finally, the investigator must design approaches to *recruiting* the study subjects. The goals are to develop contact mechanisms for acquiring a sample of subjects that is large enough to meet the study needs, and that has acceptable levels of technical error and nonresponse bias.

REFERENCES

1. Dawber TR: *The Framingham Study.* Cambridge MA, Harvard University Press, 1980, pp 14–29.
2. Armitage P: Exclusions, losses to follow-up, and withdrawals in clinical trials. Shapiro SH, Louis TA (eds): In *Clinical Trials: Issues and Approaches.* New York, Marcel Dekker, Inc, 1983, pp 99–113.
3. Melton LJ: Selection bias in the referral of patients and the natural history of surgical conditions. *Mayo Clin Proc* 60:880–889, 1985.
4. Ellenberg JH, Nelson KB: Sample selection and the natural history of disease. Studies of febrile seizures. *JAMA* 243:1337, 1980.
5. National Center for Health Statistics: Plan and operation of the Health and Nutrition Examination Survey (HANES). *Vital and Health Statistics,* Series 1, Nos. 10a and 10b. DHEW Publication No. (HSM) 73–130. Washington, DC, US Government Printing Office, 1973.
6. Siemiatycki J, Campbell S, Richardson L, Aubert D: Quality of response in different population groups in mail and telephone surveys. *Am J Epidemiol* 120:302–314, 1984.
7. Kahn HA: *An Introduction to Epidemiologic Methods.* New York, Oxford University Press, 1983, pp 11–24.
8. Freeman JL, Freeman DH, Ostfeld AM: Analysis of data from successive complex sample surveys, with an example of hypertension prevalence from the US Health Examination Survey. *Int J Epidemiol* 12:230–237, 1983.
9. MRFIT Research Group: Multiple Risk Factor Intervention Trial (MRFIT): Risk factor changes and mortality results. *JAMA* 248:1465-1477, 1982.
10. Lipid Research Clinics Program: Recruitment for clinical trials. *Circulation* 66 (Suppl IV):1–78, 1982.
11. Baines CJ: Impediments to recruitment in the Canadian National Breast Screening Study: response and resolution. *Contr Clin Trials* 5:129–140, 1984.

ADDITIONAL READINGS

Babbie E: *The Practice of Social Research.* Belmont, CA, Wadsworth, 1983, pp 140–182. (*A sensible and readable description of the approach to selecting study subjects used by social scientists.*)
Friedman LM, Furberg CD, DeMets DL: *Fundamentals of Clinical Trials.* Boston, John Wright, 1985, pp 18–27. (*A good section on selection criteria that is relevant to all clinical research.*)
Hunninghake DB, Chairman: Workshop on Recruitment Experience in NHLBI-Supported Clinical Trials: Procedings. National Heart Lung and Blood Institute, NIH, 1987. (*An excellent compilation of experience in recruiting for clinical trials.*)
Levy PS, Lemeshow S: *Sampling for Health Professionals.* Belmont, CA, Lifetime Learning Publications, 1980. (*An advanced and technical description of probability sampling and its statistical implications.*)
Marks RG: *Designing a Research Project.* Belmont, CA, Lifetime Learning Publications, 1982, pp 99–114. (*An easy and practical description of sampling biases and how to avoid them.*)
Meinert CL: *Clinical Trials: Design, Conduct and Analysis.* New York, Oxford University Press, 1986, pp 149–152. (*A good summary of recruitment approaches for large scale clinical trials.*)
Pocock SJ: *Clinical Trials: A Practical Approach.* Chichester, NY, John Wiley & Sons, 1983, pp 35–38. (*An excellent discussion of the trade-offs involved in formulating selection criteria.*)
Polit DF, Hungler, BP: *Nursing Research: Principles and Methods,* ed 2. Philadelphia, JB Lippincott Co, 1983, pp 409–432. (*A readable text with a good overview of the whole topic of selecting and sampling.*)

CHAPTER 4

Planning the Measurements: Precision and Accuracy

Stephen B. Hulley and Steven R. Cummings

INTRODUCTION 31

MEASUREMENT SCALES 31
  Continuous variables
  Categorical variables
  Choosing a measurement scale

PRECISION 34
  Assessing precision
  Strategies for enhancing precision

ACCURACY 36
  Assessing accuracy
  Strategies for enhancing accuracy
  Blinding to eliminate differential bias
  Validity of abstract variables

OTHER DESIRABLE FEATURES OF
MEASUREMENT APPROACHES 39
  Individual measurements
  Measurements in the aggregate

SUMMARY 41

REFERENCES 41

ADDITIONAL READINGS 41

APPENDIX 4.   Operations manual: An
  example 201

— — — — — — — — — — — —

INTRODUCTION

Measurements are observations that describe phenomena in terms that can be analyzed statistically (Fig. 4.1). The **external validity** of a study depends in part on **how well the variables designed for the study represent the phenomena of interest.** How well does a fasting blood sugar level represent control of diabetes, for example, or a question about insomnia represent depression? The **internal validity** depends on **how well the actual**

measurements represent these variables. How well does the observed blood sugar level represent the true level, or the response about insomnia reflect actual sleeping habits?

The overall degree to which measurements in a sample represent the phenomena of interest in the population is a function of two sources of error; these are sampling error and measurement error, each of which has both random and systematic components. We have discussed in the preceding chapter the strategies for minimizing the sampling error in choosing the study subjects. We turn now to the strategies for minimizing measurement error: how to design measurements that will enhance the validity of drawing inferences from a study by being relatively **precise** (free of random error) and **accurate** (free of systematic error). Before coming to this we will begin by reviewing the scales for making measurements.

MEASUREMENT SCALES

Table 4.1 presents a simplified classification of measurement scales and the information that results. The classification is based on the *type* of variable that the measurement produces, and it is important because some types of variables are suitable for more informative and powerful statistics than others.

Continuous variables

Continuous variables have quantified intervals on an infinite arithmetic scale of values. The number of possible values of body

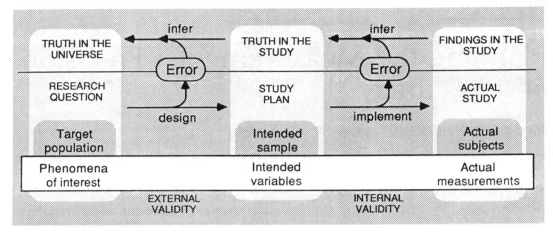

Figure 4.1. Designing measurements that represent the phenomena of interest.

weight, for example, is limited only by the sensitivity of the machine that is used to measure it. Continuous variables are rich in information and can be analyzed with powerful statistical tests.

A scale that has a finite number of quantified intervals (such as the number of cigarettes/day) is termed discrete. **Discrete variables** that have a considerable number of possible values resemble continuous variables in statistical analyses, and are equivalent for the purpose of designing research measurements.

Categorical variables

Phenomena that are not suitable for quantification can often be measured by classifying them in **categories**. It is useful to characterize categorical variables according to whether they have only two possible values (male or female sex, for example) or more than two (types of cancer); those with only two values are termed **dichotomous**.

It is also useful to characterize categorical variables according to the type of information they contain. **Nominal variables** are classifications that do not imply an ordering of the categories; type 0 blood, for example, is neither more nor less than type B. Nominal variables tend to have a qualitative and absolute character that makes them relatively straightforward to measure, but the options for statistical analysis are limited.

Ordinal variables are classifications that do have ordered positions, such as severe, moderate, and mild pain. They differ from discrete variables in having categories that are not numerical quantities specifying the amount of difference between one rank and the next. Ordinal variables tend to contain more information than nominal variables, but they are also more apt to require human judgment and to be susceptible to bias.

Choosing a measurement scale

A good general rule is to prefer measurements that produce continuous numerical values, because the additional information they contain improves efficiency. In a study comparing the antihypertensive effects of several treatments, for example, the strategy of measuring blood pressure in mm Hg allows the investigator to observe the magnitude of the change in every subject, whereas measuring it as a dichotomous variable would only allow him to assess whether or not each subject changed from the hypertensive category to the non-hypertensive one. The continuous variable obviously contains much more information, and the result, as we shall see in Chapter 13, is a study with more power and/or a smaller sample size.

The rule has some exceptions. The study of passive smoking and low birth weight discussed in Appendix 2 might be more concerned with babies whose weight is so low

Table 4.1.
Measurement scales

Type of measurement	Characteristics of variable	Example	Appropriate statistics	Information content and power
Categorical[a] Nominal	Unordered categories	Sex; blood type; vital status	Counts, rates, proportions, relative risk, chi-square, Mantel-Haentzel, regression	Low
Ordinal	Ordered categories with intervals that are not quantifiable	Degree of pain	In addition to the above: median, rank correlation	Intermediate
Continuous or Ordered discrete[b]	Ranked spectrum with quantifiable intervals	Weight; number of cigarettes/ day	In addition to the above: mean, standard deviation, t-test, analysis of variance, more powerful regression	High

[a]Categorical measurements that contain only two classes (e.g., sex) are termed dichotomous.
[b]Continuous variables have an infinite number of values (e.g., weight), whereas discrete variables have a finite scale (e.g., number of cigarettes/day). Discrete variables that are ordered (i.e., arranged in sequence from few to many) and that have a large number of possible values resemble continuous variables for practical purposes of measurement and analysis.

that their health is compromised than with differences observed over the full spectrum of birth weights. In this case the investigator is better off with a large enough sample to be able to analyze the results with a dichotomous outcome like the proportion of babies whose weight is below 2500 G. Even when the categorical data are more meaningful, however, it is still best to *collect* the data as a continuous variable. This leaves the analytic options open: to change the cutoff point that defines low birth weight (he may later decide that 2350 G is a better value for discriminating babies at increased risk of developmental abnormalities), or to fall back on the more powerful analysis of the predictors of the full spectrum of weight.

Similarly, when there is the option of designing the number of response categories in an ordinal scale, as in a question about food preferences, it is often useful to provide a half-dozen categories that range from "strongly dislike" through "neutral" to " extremely fond of." The results can later be collapsed into a dichotomy if appropriate (i.e. dislike and like), but the investigator has the option of using more powerful statistics on the full spectrum of responses if he wishes. Data can always be collapsed into fewer categories during the analysis phase, but they cannot be expanded.

Many characteristics are difficult to describe with categories or numbers, and the attempt to do so distorts reality. Pain, for example, can only be graded on an arbitrary and approximate scale, and many life-style characteristics are difficult to categorize. Even for these phenomena, however, the attempt to make measurements is an essential part of the scientific approach to description and analysis. An example is the structured interview that has been developed to classify the behavior pattern of people as Type A (hard driving) or Type B (easy going). The result is clearly an oversimplification—most people have a mixture of these characteristics—but the approach has the advantage of providing a systematic means for examining whether behavior pattern is associated with risk of developing a heart attack (1).

The processes of classification and measurement, if done well, can increase the objectivity of our knowledge, reduce bias, and provide a means of communication.

PRECISION

A very precise measurement is one that has nearly the same value each time it is measured. A beam scale can measure body weight with great precision, whereas an interview designed to measure quality of life is more likely to produce values that vary from one occasion to the next. Precision has a very important influence on the power of a study. The more precise a measurement, the greater the statistical power at a given sample size to estimate mean values and to test hypotheses (Chapter 13).

Precision, and the related concepts of reliability and consistency, are affected by **random error**: the greater the error, the less precise the measurement. There are three main sources of error in making measurements (Table 4.2). **Observer variability** refers to variability in measurement that is due to the observer, and includes such things as choice of words in an interview, or hand-eye coordination in using a mechanical instrument. **Subject variability** refers to intrinsic biologic variability in the study subjects due to such things as fluctuations in mood, circadian rhythms, and time since last medication. **Instrument variability** refers to variability in the measurement due to fluctuating environmental factors such as temperature and background noise.

Assessing precision

The precision of a variable is often described statistically using the **standard deviation** of repeated measurements. A useful statistic for comparing the precision of several variables is the **coefficient of variation**, the standard deviation divided by the mean. Imprecise measurement methods have large coefficients of variation.

Table 4.2.
Strategies for reducing random error in order to increase precision, with illustrations from a study of antihypertensive treatment (2)

Strategy to reduce random error	Source of random error	Example of random error	Example of strategy to prevent the error
1. Standardizing the measurement methods in an operations manual	Observer	Variation in blood pressure (BP) measurement due to variable rate of cuff deflation (sometimes faster than 2 mm Hg/second and sometimes slower)	Specify that the cuff be deflated at 2 mm Hg/sec
	Subject	Variation in BP due to variable length of quiet sitting	Specify that subject sit in a quiet room for 5 minutes before BP measurement
2. Training and certifying the observer	Observer	Variation in BP due to variable observer technique	Train observer in standard techniques
3. Refining the instrument	Instrument or observer	Variation in BP due to digit preference (e.g., the tendency to round numbers to a multiple of 5)	Use zero muddler to conceal BP reading until after it has been recorded
4. Automating the instrument	Observer	Variation in BP due to variable observer technique	Use automatic BP measuring device
	Subject	Variation in BP due to variable reaction to observer by subject	Use automatic BP measuring device
5. Repeating the measurement	Observer, subject, and instrument	All measurements and all sources of variation	Use mean of two or more BP measurements

Precision can also be assessed by the consistency of the results of paired measurements. The degree of concordance can be expressed as a simple **correlation coefficient**. (More complex but related approaches include the use of the kappa statistic, which expresses the degree of concordance beyond that due to chance (3), and Cronbach's alpha, which expresses internal consistency among three or more variables (4)). The paired measurements for these tests of precision are obtained in three ways:

Test-retest consistency: This is the concordance among repeated measurements on a sample of subjects. The time interval must be carefully selected; if it is too long, lack of agreement among results may be due to meaningful (nonrandom) changes in the characteristics being measured, and if it is too short there may be insufficient time for random fluctuations to occur.

Internal consistency: This is the concordance between two variables that measure the same general characteristic. If, for example, a questionnaire that measures functional status includes several questions about a subject's ability to walk (on flat ground, down a slope) the responses should be highly correlated with one another.

Inter- and intraobserver consistency: The interobserver consistency is the correlation among the values obtained by two or more observers on the same sample of subjects, and the intraobserver consistency is the correlation among repeated values obtained by a single observer.

Strategies for enhancing precision

There are five approaches to minimizing variance and increasing the precision of measurements (Table 4.2):

1. *Standardizing the measurement methods:* All study protocols should include **operational definitions**—specific instructions for making the measurements. There is a need to write out the directions for how, precisely, to prepare the environment and the subject, how to carry out and record the interview, how to calibrate the instrument, and so forth. This set of materials, termed the **operations manual**, is essen-

tial for large and complex studies and highly recommended for smaller ones (Appendix 4). Even when there is only a single observer, specific written guidelines for making each measurement will help his performance to be uniform over the duration of the study and serve as the basis for describing the methods when the results are reported.

2. *Training and certifying the observers:* Training will improve the consistency of measurement techniques, especially when several observers are involved. It is often important to test the mastery of the techniques specified in the operations manual and to certify that observers have achieved the prescribed level of performance (see Chapter 16).

3. *Refining the instruments:* Mechanical and electronic instruments can be engineered to reduce variability. Similarly, questionnaires and interviews can be written to increase clarity and to avoid potential ambiguities (see Chapter 5).

4. *Automating the instruments:* Variation in the way human observers make measurements can be eliminated with automatic mechanical devices and self-response questionnaires. This strategy will improve precision only if the automatic device is itself relatively precise, so that its measurements have less variability than those made by human observers.

5. *Repetition:* The impact of random error of any source is reduced by repeating the measurement and using the mean of the two or more readings. Precision can be substantially increased by this strategy, the primary limitation being the added cost and practical difficulties of repeating the measurements.

The decisions on how vigorously to pursue each strategy for each of the proposed measurements in the study should be based on the feasibility and cost of the strategy, the importance of the variable, and the magnitude of the potential problem with precision. In general, the first two strategies should always be used, and the fifth is an option that is guaranteed to improve precision when it is feasible and affordable.

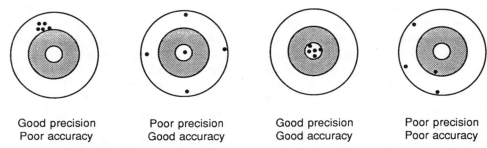

| Good precision | Poor precision | Good precision | Poor precision |
| Poor accuracy | Good accuracy | Good accuracy | Poor accuracy |

Figure 4.2. Illustration of the difference between precision and accuracy.

ACCURACY

The accuracy of a variable is the degree to which it actually represents what it is intended to represent (Fig. 4.2). This has a very important influence on the internal and external validity of the study—the degree to which the observed findings lead to the correct inferences about phenomena taking place in the study sample and in the universe.

Accuracy is different from precision in the ways shown in Table 4.3, and the two are not necessarily linked. If serum cholesterol were measured repeatedly using standards that had inadvertently been diluted twofold, for example, the result would be inaccurate but it could still be precise—consistently off by a factor of 2. This concept is further illustrated in Fig 4.2. Accuracy and precision do often go hand in hand, however, and many of the strategies for increasing precision will also improve accuracy.

Accuracy is a **function of systematic error**, or **bias**; the greater the error, the less accurate the variable. The three main classes of measurement error noted in the earlier section on precision each have counterparts here.

Observer bias is a consistent distortion, conscious or unconscious, in the perception or reporting of the measurement by the observer. It may represent systematic differences in the way an instrument is operated, such as a tendency to underestimate blood pressure in patients known to be receiving treatment. Or it may result from more intensive measurements in certain subjects—a more persistent search of medical records for a history of smoking cigarettes in a patient known to have lung cancer.

Subject bias is a consistent distortion of the measurement by the study subject. This may involve a true alteration in the phenomena under study, as in the "Hawthorne effect", a bias caused by the process of being studied. (This bias is named for the Hawthorne Western Electric Plant, where environmental manipulations to increase productivity caused a transient improvement

Table 4.3.
The precision and accuracy of measurement

	Precision	Accuracy
Definition	The degree to which a variable has nearly the same value when measured several times	The degree to which a variable actually represents what it is supposed to represent
Best way to assess	Comparison among repeated measures	Comparision with a reference standard
Value to study	Increase power to detect effects	Increase validity of conclusions
Threatened by	Random error (variance) contributed by: the observer the subject the instrument	Systematic error (bias) contributed by: the observer the subject the instrument

that disappeared when the novelty of being in an experiment wore off). Subject bias may also occur when only the perception of the phenomena has changed, as in the selective recall or reporting of an event (respondent bias). Breast cancer patients who believe that birth control pills are a cause of cancer, for example, may be more likely than those without cancer to remember using these medications or to imagine that they have used them.

Instrument bias can result from faulty function of a mechanical instrument—a white blood cell counter that has not been calibrated recently may drift downwards, for example, and begin to produce consistently lower readings. Instrument bias can also result from the use of techniques that are inappropriate to the objective of the measurement, such as leading questions on a questionnaire.

Assessing accuracy

The accuracy of objective measurements of concrete phenomena can usually be tested by comparison with reference techniques that are known be accurate (**gold standards**). The accuracy of a measurement of body weight, for example, can be checked by calibrating the scale with standard weights, and then expressed statistically as the mean difference between the standard value and the observed value, divided by the standard value.

Strategies for enhancing accuracy

The major approaches to increasing accuracy include the first four of the strategies listed earlier for precision, and three additional ones (Table 4.4):

5. *Making unobtrusive measures:* It is sometimes possible to design measurements that the subjects are not aware of, thereby eliminating the possibility that they will consciously bias the variable (5). A study of advice on healthy eating patterns for school children, for example, could measure the frequency of candy bar wrappers discovered in the trash after school.

6. *Blinding:* This classic strategy does not prevent an overall bias in the measure-

ments, but it can eliminate **differential bias** that affects one study group more than another (see below). In a classic double-blind experiment, neither the observer nor the subject knows whether active medicine or identical-looking placebo has been assigned. This assures that any bias that is present will affect measurements equally in the active and placebo groups.

7. *Calibrating the instrument:* The accuracy of many instruments, especially those that are mechanical or electrical, can be increased by periodic calibration using a gold standard.

The decision on how vigorously to pursue each of these seven strategies for each measurement rests, as noted earlier for precision, on the judgment of the investigator. The considerations are the feasibility and cost of the strategy, the importance of the variable, and the magnitude of the potential impact that the anticipated degree of inaccuracy will have on the conclusions of the study. The first two strategies should always be used, however, and the last is needed for any instrument that has the potential to change over time.

Blinding to eliminate differential bias

The strategy of blinding deserves further comment because of its value for controlling *differential* bias in explanatory studies. A technically successful double-blind study completely eliminates measurement error that affects one study group more than the other. A single-blind study in which the observer but not the subject knows the treatment assignment is better than no blinding at all, but it leaves open the possibility for observer bias that affects one group more than the other. Experiments that test intervention like exercise may be single blind in the other sense—only the observer does not know the treatment assignment. This does control differential bias, but unintended interventions can affect one group more than the other (see Chapter 11).

There are many designs that cannot be blinded at all. In a case-control study of whether birth control pills cause breast can-

Table 4.4.
Strategies for reducing systematic error in order to increase accuracy, with illustrations from a study of antihypertensive treatment (2)

Strategy to reduce systematic error	Source of systematic error	Example of systematic error	Example of strategy to prevent the error
1. Standardizing the measurement methods in an operations manual	Observer	Consistently high diastolic blood pressure (BP) readings due to using the point at which sounds become muffled	Specify the operational definition of diastolic BP as the point at which sounds cease to be heard
	Subject	Consistently high readings due to measuring BP right after walking upstairs to clinic	Specify that subject sit in quiet room for 5 minutes before measurement
2. Training and certifying the observer	Observer	Consistently high BP readings due to failure to follow procedures specified in operations manual	Trainer checks accuracy of observer's reading with a double-headed stethoscope
3. Refining the instrument	Instrument	Consistently high BP readings with standard cuff in subjects with very large arms	Use wide BP cuff in obese patients
4. Automating the instrument	Observer	Conscious or unconscious tendency for observer to read BP lower in treatment group	Use automatic BP measuring device
	Subject	BP increase due to proximity of attractive technician	Use automatic BP measuring device
5. Making unobstrusive measurements	Subject	Tendency of subject to overestimate compliance with study drug	Measure study drug level in urine without subject's knowledge
6. Blinding	Observer	Conscious or unconscious tendency for observer to read BP lower in treatment	Use double-blind placebo to conceal study group assignment
	Subject	Tendency of subject to overreport side effects if he knew he was on active drug	Use double-blind placebo to conceal study group assignment
7. Calibrating the instrument	Instrument	Consistently high BP readings due to scale being out of adjustment	Calibrate balance beam scale with 50-lb weight each week

cer, for example, it would be difficult to conceal from the observer (and impossible to conceal from the subject) whether the woman being interviewed was a cancer patient or a control subject. When the values of the variables cannot be blinded, it may be useful (if ethical) to try to keep the observers and respondents unaware of the objectives of the study. Another strategy is to include measurements of decoy variables that distract attention and can be used to estimate **attribution bias.** In the breast cancer study, for example, reported exposure to a diverse set of medications, dietary factors, and household cleansers would give an indication of the tendency to attribute the cancer to preferentially recalled or fabricated events.

Validity of abstract variables

Whether a variable represents what is intended is more difficult to assess when measurements are attempted for subjective and abstract phenomena like pain or quality of life (7). The issue here is external validity—how well the measurement represents the phenomenon of interest. Validity is an elusive and difficult topic that has 3 main aspects:

Predictive validity is the degree to which a measurement successfully predicts an outcome of interest. The validity of classifying men into Type A or Type B behavior pattern depends on how well this predicts subsequent coronary heart disease (1).

Criterion-related validity (convergence validity) is the degree to which the measurement agrees with other approaches for measuring the same characteristic. Is the subject's response to a question about stress concordant with the responses when relatives are questioned, with psychiatric diagnoses, and with urinary catecholamine levels?

Face validity (content validity) is a subjective judgment of whether a measurement makes sense intuitively, whether it seems to be a reasonable approach. Quality of life is an important outcome in many experiments, yet the the choice among approaches to assessing it (which deal variously with perceived life satisfaction and with measures of social, physical, emotional, and intellectual functioning (6)) is based largely on what seems best to the investigator and his consultants.

The general approach to validating an abstract measure is to begin by searching the literature and consulting with experts in an effort to find a suitable instrument that has already been validated. If one can be found, using it may bypass the need to further study the validity of the measurement approach. This strategy also has the advantage of making the results of the new study comparable to earlier work in the area. It has the disadvantage, however, that an instrument that is taken off the shelf may turn out to be outmoded or not appropriate for the research question at hand.

If existing instruments are not suitable for the needs of the study, then the investigator will need to develop a new measurement approach and validate it himself. This can be an interesting creative challenge that leads to new and valuable kinds of information, but it is fair to say that the process is often less scientific and conclusive than the word "validation" connotes. Predictive validity, the most substantive and convincing strategy, is often not feasible. Criterion-related validity is probably the next best approach, but in the absence of a good gold standard the investigator must often fall back on face validity. Although this is certainly subjective, with good judgment it can be reasonably satisfactory.

OTHER DESIRABLE FEATURES OF MEASUREMENT APPROACHES

There are number of other factors to consider when designing the approaches to making individual measurements, and to combining these in a measurement instrument.

Individual measurements

Measurements should be **sensitive** enough to detect differences in a characteristic that are important to the investigator. Just how much sensitivity is needed depends on the research question. For example, a study of whether or not Nicorette gum causes subjects to *quit* smoking can use an outcome measure that is relatively insensitive to the precise number of cigarettes smoked each day. On the other hand, if the question under study is the effect of reducing the nicotine content of cigarettes on the number of cigarettes smoked, the method would need to be sensitive to differences in daily habits of just a few cigarettes.

An ideal measurement is **specific**, representing only the characteristic of interest. The carbon monoxide level in expired air is a measure of smoking habits that is fairly specific, but that can also be affected by exposure to automobile exhaust. The overall specificity of assessing smoking habits can be increased by supplementing the carbon monoxide data with other measurements (such as self-report and serum thiocyanate) that are not effected by automobile exhaust (8).

Measurements should be **appropriate** to the objectives of the study. If the research question is vague or ambiguous, especially when the topic of the research is abstract, it may be unclear just what characteristics should be measured and how. This makes it difficult to choose a valid method of measurement, or to assess validity. A study of stress as an antecedent to thyrotoxicosis, for example, would need to consider which kind of stress (psychologic or physical, acute or chronic) was of interest before carefully setting out the operational definitions for measuring it.

Measurements should provide an adequate **distribution of responses** in the study population. A measure of functional status is most useful if it produces values that range from high in some subjects to low in others. One of the main functions of pretesting is to assure that the actual responses do not all cluster around one end of the possible range of response (Chapter 16).

Finally, there is the issue of **objectivity**. This is achieved by reducing the involvement of the observer and by increasing the structure of the instrument and the degree to which it addresses specific detail rather than vague generalization (Table 4.5). The danger in these strategies, however, is the consequent tunnel vision that limits the scope of the observations and the ability to discover unanticipated phenomena. The best design often compromises, including both an opportunity for acquiring subjective and qualitative data and a main set of more objective and quantitative measurements. In the SHEP

study of treating hypertension, for example, the subjects were asked whether they had had any trouble taking their medicine. This subjective and open-ended question was followed by specific queries about missed doses, and by counting the pills returned and testing the urine for the presence of the diuretic (2).

Measurements in the aggregate

Each individual measurement should be considered in the context of all the other study measurements. One useful tactic in designing measurement approaches is **supplementation**: measuring several different variables to represent the characteristic of interest. An index that combines several measurements can enhance the precision with which the characteristic is assessed. Congestive heart failure, for example, was diagnosed in the MRFIT if two of four major criteria (nocturnal dyspnea, rales, third heart sound, elevated jugular venous pressure) and two of four minor criteria (exertional dyspnea, ankle edema, hepetomegaly, and heart rate ≥ 120/minute) were present (9). Particularly in the case of abstract phenomena, the strategy of assessing a characteristic in a variety of ways (in effect surrounding it) will tend to improve validity.

There is also, however, the issue of **efficiency**. The full set of measurements should collect useful data at an affordable cost in time and money. Efficiency can be improved by increasing the quality of each item, and by reducing the number of items measured. Collecting more data than are needed is a very common error that can tire the subjects, overwhelm the research team, and clutter up data

Table 4.5.
Illustrations of the objective/subjective and qualitative/quantitative dimensions of measurement approaches

Involvement of observer	Structure of instrument	Advantages (sometimes)	Examples
Extensive	Minimal	More open to new things, qualitative phenomena	Unstructured interview Assessment of mood by inspection
Minimal	Extensive	More accurate, precise, and complete	Self-response questionnaires Automatic manometer
Extensive	Extensive	A mixture	Structured interview Standard neurologic exam

management and analysis. The result can be a study that is more expensive to carry out and produces less valid conclusions. A good rule for designing measurements is this: When in doubt, cut it out.

SUMMARY

1. Variables are either *continuous* (quantified on an infinite arithmetic scale), *discrete* (quantified on a finite numeric scale), or *categorical* (classified in categories). Categorical variables are further classified as *nominal* (unordered) or *ordinal* (ordered), and according to whether or not they are *dichotomous* (only two categories).

2. In designing a measurement scale, the investigator should usually *prefer continuous variables* (because they produce more information and power), followed by discrete and ordered categorical variables, and finally by dichotomous variables.

3. The *precision* of a measurement—the consistency of replicate measures—is another major determinant of power and sample size. Precision is reduced by random error (chance) from three sources of variability: the observer, the subject, and the instrument.

4. Two specific *strategies for increasing precision* that should be part of every study are to operationally define and standardize the methods in an operations manual, and to train and certify the observers. Other strategies that are often useful are refining the instruments, automating the instruments, and using the mean of repeated measurements.

5. The *accuracy* of a measurement—the degree to which it actually measures the characteristic it is supposed to measure—is a major determinant of the validity of the conclusions. Accuracy is *reduced by systematic error* (bias) from the same three sources: the observer, the subject, and the instrument.

6. The *strategies for increasing accuracy* include all those listed for precision, with the exception of repetition. In addition, accuracy is enhanced by calibration, by

unobtrusive measures, and (in comparisons between groups) by blinding.

7. Individual measurements should be *sensitive, specific, appropriate,* and *objective,* and they should detect differences over a *range of values.* In the aggregate, they should be deep but parsimonious, serving the research question well at moderate cost in time and money.

REFERENCES

1. Shekelle RB, Hulley SB, Neaton JD, et al: The MRFIT Behavior Pattern Study: II. Type A behavior and incidence of CHD. *Am J Epidemiol* 122:559–570, 1985.
2. Hulley SB, Furberg C, Gurland B, et al. The Systolic Hypertension in the Elderly Project (SHEP). *Am J Cardiol* 56:913–920, 1985.
3. Cohen J: A coefficient of agreement for nominal scales. *Educ Psychol Measurement* 20:37–46, 1960.
4. Cronbach LJ: Coefficient alpha and the internal structure of tests. *Psychometrika* 16:297–334, 1951.
5. Webb EJ et al: *Unobtrusive Measures.* Chicago, Rand Mcally, 1966.
6. Friedman LM, Furberg CD, DeMets DL: *Fundamentals of Clinical Trials.* Littleton, MA, PSG Publishing Co, Inc, 1985, pp 161–172.
7. Wenger NK, Mattson ME, Furberg CD, Elinson J: Assessment of quality of life in clinical trials of cardiovascular therapies. *Am J Cardiol* 54:908–914, 1984.
8. Vogt TM, Selvin S, Hulley SB. Comparison of biochemical and questionnaire measures of tobacco exposure. *Prev Med* 8:23–33, 1979.
9. The MRFIT Group. CHD death, nonfatal acute myocardial infarction and other clinical outcomes in the MRFIT. *Am J Cardiol* 58:1, 1986.

ADDITIONAL READINGS

Marks RG: *Designing a Research Project,* London, Lifetime Learning Publications, 1982, pp 31–48. (*A brief treatment of the main measurement issues.*)
Meinert, C: *Clinical Trials.* New York, Oxford University Press, 1986. (*Comprehensive and practical illustrations of research approaches to making measurements.*)
Nachmias D, Nachmias C: *Research Methods in the Social Sciences,* ed 2. New York, St. Martin's Press, 1981, pp 131–180. (*Good discussion of validity and other social science constructs.*)
Polit D, Hungler B: *Nursing Research: Principles and Methods,* ed 2. Philadelphia, JB Lippincott, Co, 1983, pp 253–408. (*A clear, comprehensive and readable description of measurements, with emphasis on both social and health science approaches.*)
Wenger NK, Mattson MD, Furberg CD, Elinson J: *Assessment of Quality of Life in Clinical Trails of Cardiovascular Therapies.* Le Jacq Publishing Co, 1984. (*Proceedings of a workshop reviewing the pros and cons of the available quality of life assessment tools.*)

CHAPTER 5

Planning the Measurements: Questionnaires

Steven R. Cummings, William Strull, Michael C. Nevitt, and Stephen B. Hulley

INTRODUCTION 42
  Interviews versus questionnaires
  Methods of administration

DESIGNING QUESTIONS AND
  INSTRUMENTS 43
  General
  Open-ended and closed-ended questions
  Instrument format
  Wording
  Codes, scores, and scales

STEPS IN WRITING QUESTIONNAIRES AND
  INTERVIEWS 48
  Decide which to use
  Make a list of variables
  Borrow from other instruments
  Write a draft
  Revise
  Pretest
  Shorten and revise again
  Precode

ADMINISTERING THE INSTRUMENT 50
  Getting complete and accurate data
  Enhancing the reliability of interviews

SUMMARY 51

REFERENCES 51

ADDITIONAL READINGS 52

APPENDIX 5. Smoking questionnaire 202

— — — — — — — — — — — —

INTRODUCTION

Much of the data in clinical research is gathered using questionnaires or interviews. For many studies, the validity of the results depends on the quality of these instruments. In this chapter we will examine the components of questionnaires and interviews and outline procedures for developing them.

Interviews versus questionnaires

There are two basic approaches to collecting data about people's attitudes, behaviors, knowledge, and personal history: **questionnaires** that the respondents administer to themselves and **interviews** that are administered verbally by a researcher. These two approaches have different advantages and disadvantages (Table 5.1). Questionnaires are generally more efficient and uniform, but interviews permit the interviewer to clarify questions and solicit complete and logical responses. Interviews have the disadvantage of being more costly and time consuming, and of being influenced by the relationship between the interviewer and the respondent (1). Both types of instruments can be standardized, but interviews are inevitably administered at least a little differently each time. Both methods of collecting information are susceptible to errors caused by imperfect memory, limited powers of observation, and respondents' desires to give socially acceptable answers.

For example, Type A personality (a style characterized by aggression and time urgency) can be measured by either the structured interview developed for the Western Collaborative Group Study or the Jenkins Activity Survey questionnaire (2). The interview appears to be better at identifying individuals who are at high risk of developing coronary heart disease (CHD), but the questionnaire can be applied less expensively and more uniformly.

Table 5.1.
Comparison of Questionnaire and Interviews

Advantages of Questionnaires	Advantages of Interviews
•**Economy:** Self-administration reduces staff time.	•**Clarity:** Interviewer can clarify questions, and avoid the problem of illiteracy.
•**Standardization:** Written instructions reduce biases from differences in administration or from interactions with interviewer.	•**Richness:** Interviewer can collect more complex answers and observations about the respondent's appearance and behavior.
•**Anonymity:** Privacy encourages candid and honest responses to sensitive questions.	•**Completeness:** Interviewer can minimize missing and inappropriate responses.
	•**Control:** Interviewer can control the order of questions.

Methods of administration

There are several different methods of administering questionnaires and interviews, each with advantages and disadvantages (3). Questionnaires can be mailed or given to subjects in person. Distributing questionnaires in person allows the researcher to clarify questions and review the responses to make sure that they are complete before the subject leaves. Mailed questionnaires, on the other hand, are usually less expensive; they do not require as much time from a research staff. A researcher can generally reach a wider population with a mailed questionnaire. Mailed questionnaires give respondents more time to think about their answers and to consult pertinent records.

Interviews can be conducted in person or over the telephone. Some studies show that telephone interviewing can reduce the costs associated with interviews while retaining most of the advantages listed in Table 5.1. In-person interviews, however, may be necessary if the study requires direct observation of participants, examinations, or visual cues such as response cards or rating scales (see below). Some elderly, ill, or low-income groups are best reached through in-person interviews in their residence or institutions.

DESIGNING QUESTIONS AND INSTRUMENTS

General

If the study has not already been explained, the instrument should begin by briefly describing the purpose of the study and why the person has been included. To assure accurate and standardized responses, all instruments must have instructions specifying how they should be filled out. This is true not only in self-administered questionnaires, but also for the forms on which responses are recorded by interviewers.

To improve the flow of the instrument, questions concerning major subject areas should be grouped together and introduced by headings or short descriptive statements. Simple questions about age, sex, birthdate, and so on are best put at the beginning of the instrument to "warm up" the respondent to the process of answering questions. For each question, particularly if its format differs from that of other questions on the instrument, instructions must indicate clearly how to respond. It may be helpful to start with an example to demonstrate how to answer that type of question.

Open-ended and closed-ended questions

Interviews and questionnaires frequently ask both open-ended and closed-ended questions to take advantage of the unique strengths of each approach. **Open-ended questions** seek an answer in the respondent's own words:

1. What habits do you believe increase a person's chance of having a heart attack?

_____

_____

Open-ended questions leave the respondent free to answer with fewer limits imposed by the researcher. The chief disadvantage to open-ended questions is that it is often difficult to code and analyze the responses.

Closed-ended questions ask respondents to choose one or more preselected answers:

2. Which *one* of the following do you think increases a person's chance of having a heart attack *the most*? (Check one.)
   [ ] smoking
   [ ] being overweight
   [ ] stress

Since closed-ended questions provide a list of possible alternatives from which the respondent may choose, they are quicker and easier to answer and the answers are easier to tabulate and analyze. In addition, the list of possible answers often helps clarify the meaning of the question.

Closed-ended questions have several disadvantages. They lead the respondent in certain directions and do not allow him to express his own, potentially unique, answers. Moreover, the potential responses listed by the researcher may not include an answer that is most appropriate for a particular respondent. This last problem can be minimized by conducting a pretest using an open-ended version of the questions to collect potential responses and using these responses to expand the list of potential answers to the question. Whenever there is a chance that the list of answers is not **exhaustive** (does not include all possible answers), it is important to include an option such as: "Other (please specify:)" or "None of the above." If the question requires the respondent to choose one "best" answer, then the list of possible responses should also be **mutually exclusive,** that is, the categories should not overlap (see example question 4, below).

When the question allows more than one answer, instructing the respondent to mark "all that apply" is not ideal. This does not force the respondent to consider each possible response, and a missing item may either represent an answer that does not apply, or an overlooked item. It is better, there-

fore, to ask respondents to mark each possible response as either "yes" or "no:"

3. Which of the following increases the chance of having a heart attack?

	yes	no	don't know
smoking	[ ]	[ ]	[ ]
being overweight	[ ]	[ ]	[ ]
stress	[ ]	[ ]	[ ]

Instrument format

The visual design of the instruments should make it as easy as possible for the respondent to complete all questions in the correct sequence. If the format is too complex, respondents or interviewers may skip questions, provide the wrong data, and even refuse to complete the instruments.

A neat format with plenty of space is more attractive and easier to use than one that is crowded or cluttered. People with visual problems, including many elderly subjects, will appreciate large type. Possible answers to closed-ended questions should be lined up vertically and preceded by boxes or brackets to check, or by numbers to circle, rather than open blanks:

4. How many different medicines do you take every day? (Check one)
   [ ] None
   [ ] 1–2
   [ ] 3–4
   [ ] 5–6
   [ ] 7 or more

5. Circle the number beside the *one* disease that you fear the most:
   1. stroke
   2. heart attack
   3. cancer
   4. pneumonia
   5. other (please specify): _____

Sometimes the investigator may wish to follow up certain answers with more detailed questions. This is best accomplished by a **branching question**. The respondent's answer to the initial question, often referred to as a "screener," determines whether he is directed to answer additional questions or skip ahead to later questions. For example:

6. Have you ever been told that you have high blood pressure?

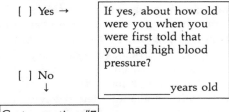

[ ] Yes → If yes, about how old were you when you were first told that you had high blood pressure?

[ ] No
↓
_____ years old

Go to question #7

Branching questions save time and allow respondents to avoid irrelevant or redundant questions. Directing the respondent to the next appropriate question is done by setting the follow-up questions on a different vertical margin, using arrows to point from response to follow-up questions, and including directions such as "Go to question #7".

Wording

Every word in a question can influence the validity and reliability of the responses. The objective should be to construct questions that are simple, free of ambiguity, and encourage accurate and honest responses without embarrassing or offending the respondent.

Clarity: The object of writing questions is to be as clear and specific as possible. In general, abstract words are more ambiguous than concrete words. For example, to measure the amount of exercise respondents get, asking "How much exercise do you usually get?" is more ambiguous than "How many flights of stairs do you climb during a typical day?"

Simplicity: Questions should use the simplest, most common words that convey the idea and avoid technical terms and jargon. For most people, for example, it is clearer to ask about "drugs you can buy without a prescription" than to ask about "over-the-counter medications." Sentences should also be simple; use the fewest words and simplest grammatical structure that convey the meaning.

Neutrality: Avoid "loaded" words and stereotypes that suggest that there is a most desirable answer. Asking "During the last month, how often did you drink an excessive amount of alcohol?" will discourage re-

spondents from admitting that they drink a lot of alcohol. "During the last month, how often did you drink more than 5 drinks in one day?" is a more factual, less judgmental (and less ambiguous) question.

Sometimes it is useful to set a tone that permits the respondent to admit behaviors and attitudes that may be considered undesireable. For example, when asking about a patient's compliance with prescribed medications, an interviewer or a questionnaire may use an introduction: "People sometimes forget to take medications their doctor prescribes. Do you occasionally forget to take your medication?" Wording of these introductions can be tricky: it is important to give the respondent permission to admit certain behaviors without encouraging him to exaggerate.

Collecting information about potentially sensitive areas like sexual behavior or income is especially difficult. Some people feel more comfortable answering these types of questions in self-administered questionnaires than in interviews, but a very skillful interviewer can sometimes encourage open and honest answers. In general, questions about sensitive subjects should be put toward the end of an instrument when a respondent is likely to be more comfortable with the interviewer or the questionnaire. It may also be useful to put potentially embarrassing responses on a card so that the respondent can answer by simply pointing to a response.

Double-barreled questions: Questions that use the words "or" or "and" sometimes lead to unsatisfactory responses. Consider this question that was designed to assess caffeine intake: "How many cups of coffee or tea do you drink during a day?" Coffee contains much more caffeine than tea, so a response that combines the two beverages is not as precise as it could be. When a question attempts to assess two things at one time, it is better to break it into two separate questions. "1) How many cups of coffee do you drink during a day?" and "2) How many cups of tea do you drink during a day?"

Setting the time frame: Many questions are designed to measure the amount or frequency of certain habitual or recurrent behaviors, like drinking alcohol or taking medications. In order to measure the behavior, it is essential to have the respondent describe it in terms of some unit of time, such as the number of cans of beer drunk during a day. If the behavior is usually the same day after day, such as taking one tablet of a diuretic every morning, the question can be very simple: "How many tablets do you take a day?"

Unfortunately, many behaviors change from day to day, season to season, or year to year. To measure these behaviors, the investigator must first decide just what aspect of the behavior is most important to the study: the average or the extremes. For example, a study of the effect of chronic alcohol intake on the risk of stroke may need a measurement of average consumption during a period of time. On the other hand, a study of the role of alcohol in the occurrence of falls may need to know how frequently the respondent drank enough alcohol to become intoxicated.

Questions about average behavior can be asked in two ways: counting actual behaviors during a period of time or asking about "usual" or "typical" behavior. For example, to determine average beer intake, an interviewer might try to quantify actual consumption:

> 7a. During the last 7 days, on how many days did you drink beer?
> 7b. For each day that you drank beer, how many 12 oz. cans did you have?

The interviewer could use a calendar to ask the respondent about each day during the particular period. This approach allows the investigator to calculate an average daily intake of beer. It may be a more accurate approach than asking about "usual" behaviors. It assumes, however, that the last seven days were a typical week. This approach can also be quite time consuming.

Alternatively, an investigator may determine average intake of beer by asking the respondent to estimate his usual intake:

> 8. About how many 12 oz. cans of beer do you have during a typical day?
> _____drinks per day

This format is simple and brief. It assumes, however, that the respondent can accurately average his behavior into a single estimate. Since drinking patterns often change markedly over even brief intervals, the respondent may have a difficult time deciding what is a "typical" day. Faced with questions that ask about usual or typical behavior, people often report modes of their behavior and ignore the extremes (4). They tend, for example, to underestimate their average intake of alcohol by forgetting days when they drank unusually large amounts.

In general, for behaviors that may change from time to time, it is better to ask about a specific period of time than to leave the time period unspecified. For example, it may be better to ask question #8 about usual beer intake as follows:

> 9. During the past month, how many 12 oz. cans of beer did you have on a typical day?
> _____drinks per day

Choosing the time period involves trade-offs. Focusing on a recent and brief period of time, such as the past week, may improve the respondent's recall and ability to average. On the other hand, the period of time defined in the question may not be typical of the rest of the year. If the period included holidays or special occasions, for example, this may overestimate the respondent's usual use of alcohol. When asking about actual behavior, the longer the time period, the more difficult it is for respondents to remember and the more they tend to bias their answer toward recent modes of behavior (4, 5).

Codes, scores, and scales

Numeric and alphabetic codes transform answers into variables that can be tabulated and analysed statistically. For nominal variables (categorical variables that have no ranking), code numbers are simply an abbreviated label for the answer; they have no inherent meaning. Race, for example, can be coded as "1" for black, "2" for white "3" for Hispanic, "4" for Asian and "5" for "other. For ordinal variables the numeric values have an inherent meaning that reflects the underlying rank order. Cigarette smoking, for example, could be coded as "1" for non-smoker, "2" for less than 1 pack per day, "3" for 1-2 packs per day, and "4" for more than 2 packs per day; each code number referring to a different rank of exposure to cigarette smoke.

Sometimes, the answers to a question are given a score as a way of measuring an abstract characteristic:

> 10. From 1 (very important) to 4 (not important), how important are these items for maintaining the health of women over age 65? (Circle one number for each item)

	importance			
	high			low
a. breast self-examination	1	2	3	4
b. annual flu vaccinations	1	2	3	4
c. high-calcium diet	1	2	3	4

In this case, the score (from 1 to 4) is a way of measuring an attitude.

Some characteristics, such as functional status, are best measured by asking several questions. For statistical analysis, answers to these multiple questions can be combined into a single overall score by using a consistent **scale** for the answers to all of the questions as in example 10, above. In order to be summarized in a single score, the scale must have only one *dimension*; that is, all of the questions must assess a single characteristic such as attitude about health behaviors. The two types of scales that are most widely used are Likert and Guttman scales.

Summative (Likert) scales Likert scales are commonly used to quantify attitudes and behaviors. Respondents are given a list of statements or questions and asked to select a response that best represents the rank or degree of their answer. Each response is assigned a number of points:

An investigator can compute an overall score for a respondent's answers by simply adding the points for each item. Simply adding up points, however, assumes that all of the items have a relatively high degree of "internal consistency," that is, that each item is measuring the same characteristic. This assumption can be tested statistically using measures such as Cronbach's alpha (6), which assess the correlations among items in a scale.

Relying on a single score to measure a characteristic is a convenient strategy but it can sometimes be misleading: the same total score can be obtained in many different ways and identical scores may have different meanings. The pattern of response may convey more information than the total score, but analyses of patterns can be a challenging and difficult task.

Cumulative ("Guttman") scales: Cumulative scales contain a series of statements that express increasing intensity of a characteristic. The respondent is asked to agree or disagree with each statement:

> 12. Circle the letter of every statement that you agree with:
> a. Smoking can cause illness.
> b. Smoking is an important cause of illness.
> c. Smoking is a very important cause of illness and death.
> d. Smoking is the most important cause of illness and death in the United States.

The respondent's score on a cumulative scale is the total number of items with which he agrees (or disagrees). Ideally, a respondent will give internally consistent answers: that is, he will endorse an item of a certain intensity and all items of lesser intensity. For example, if a person agrees with statement b) he would be expected to also agree with a). If he disagreed with statement c) he would be ex-

> 11. For each item, mark an "X" on the line that best represents your opinion:

	Strongly Agree (1)	Agree (2)	Neutral (3)	Disagree (4)	Strongly Disagree (5)
a. Smoking in public places should be illegal.	—	—	—	—	—
b. Advertisements for cigarettes should be banned.	—	—	—	—	—
c. Public funds should be spent for antismoking campaigns.	—	—	—	—	—

pected to also disagree with statement d). If responses have this sort of consistency, then the pattern of answers to individual questions can be inferred from the total score. The internal consistency of answers to Guttman scales can be analyzed statistically (7).

STEPS IN WRITING QUESTIONNAIRES AND INTERVIEWS

Decide which to use

If a variable is best collected by asking the respondent a question, then the investigator must first decide whether to use a self-administered questionnaire, an interview, or some combination of the two. The choice is often dictated by practical considerations; interviews may be prohibitively expensive or logistically impossible. When both methods are feasible, the choice generally involves tradeoffs between the greater cost-effectiveness, privacy, and standardization of questionnaires and the greater control over completeness, order of questions and qualitative information afforded by interviews.

Make a list of variables

Before designing an interview or questionnaire instrument, the researcher should construct a detailed outline of the information that will be needed. It is useful to think ahead to analyzing and reporting the results of the study and to include all of the items that will be necessary for answering the research questions.

Borrow from other instruments

In general, an investigator should use questions and instruments that have proven their clarity, reliability, and accuracy in other studies. Borrowing instruments also allows an investigator to compare his results with those of other studies that have used the same questions.

On the other hand, "standard" questionnaires are often unsatisfactory. An investigator may be able to improve the design or clarity of questions on existing instruments, tailoring them to the specific purposes of the study and to the special characteristics of the

respondents in that study. New questions may also produce novel and interesting data. For these reasons, many instruments include both standard and new questions. In general, the new questions are added at the end so as not to interfere with the sequence of the standard instrument.

For long instruments, such as scales to measure functional status, composing good new instruments can be a very time-consuming process. If it is necessary to test the reliability and accuracy of a new instrument, this can take months of additional study. In general, the creation of such instruments should be undertaken only when existing ones are not adequate for measuring the variables of interest, or when they are not appropriate for the people who will be included in the study.

Writing a single new question is a less time consuming process. However, all new questions should be pretested well to be sure that they are clear and produce appropriate answers. In some cases it may also be important to formally test their reliability and accuracy.

If an investigator decides to develop new questions, it is useful to start by collecting other questions about the same topic. They can be found by searching out and reviewing published studies about similar topics and by calling or writing to investigators who are working in the area of interest. It is useful to file each question or instrument by topic. As the researcher writes his questions, he can use these items as models or as a source of ideas for new questions.

Write a draft

The first draft of the instrument should include more questions about each topic than will eventually be included in the instrument. Because the instrument is likely to undergo several revisions, it is wise to write the first draft on a word processor. The first draft should include instructions for answering the questions and be set out in as clear and uncluttered a format as possible. Questions should be organized by topics, such as habits or medications, and topics should be organized in a way that maintains the flow of ideas and minimizes any adverse effects of sensitive topics on the subjects.

Revise

The investigator should read the first draft carefully as if he were a respondent and try to imagine all possible ways to misinterpret questions. He should look for words or phrases that might confuse or be misunderstood by even a few respondents and for abstract words or jargon that could be translated into simpler, more concrete terms. He should also look for questions that contain "and" or "or" and should be split into two or more questions.

It is useful to have colleagues and experts in questionnaire design review the instrument. In addition to considering the content of the items, they should also address the issue of clarity.

Pretest

The first draft should be tested for clarity of the questions and instructions. In general, the first pretest should be very small, perhaps including only 2 to 5 respondents. If the study is likely to include people with diverse cultural backgrounds, then respondents representing each different cultural group should be included in the pretests. A series of small pretests with revisions after each round is usually a more efficient strategy than one or two large pretests. It is useful to record the amount of time each instrument takes as a guide to deciding how much it will need to be shortened for the study.

After the wording of individual questions has been settled an investigator should, if possible, plan at least one larger pretest to to be certain that each question produces an adequate range of responses. At this stage it may also be useful to compare answers to similar questions to look for redundant information. If the pretests are large enough, statistical techniques (such as factor analysis) can be used to identify questions that are redundant. By retesting a group of respondents at different times or with different interviewers, these pretests can also describe the reproducibility of instrument. Large and well-funded studies sometimes employ experts in the field of survey research to con-

sult on the development of instruments and to conduct large scale pretests.

Shorten and revise again

Questionnaires and interviews are often too long. It is hard to resist the temptation to include additional questions "just in case" they might produce interesting data. In most studies, many such items are collected but never used.

Adding questions that that are not essential to answering the main research question can have a detrimental effect on the quality of the study. Long interviews or questionnaires may tire respondents and thereby decrease the accuracy and reliability of their answers. Extra questions also increase the cost and complexity of data analysis. To decide whether an item should be included, it is often helpful to think how the data will be used in analysing and writing the results of the study. If there is any doubt about whether an item will be used in later analyses, it is often best to leave it out.

At this stage, it can also be useful to rank or rate questions in terms of their importance to the primary aims of the study. Lower priority items can be removed until the instrument is pruned down to the desired length.

Another review of the instrument by colleagues who have experience in writing questionnaires may help polish the instrument for final use. If time allows, it is often useful to pretest the "final" version again with respondents who are typical of subjects in the study. It is better to take time to find unexpected bugs before the study begins than to have to revise the instruments after the study is underway.

Precode

All potential closed-ended responses should be *precoded*. For example, the following item from an interview about coffee has a series of precoded responses in the right-hand margin that will allow for rapid recording of data and rapid data entry:

> 13. How many cups of coffee does your wife drink during a typical day? (Circle one)
> None 1

Occasional cup, not every day	2
1-2	3
3-4	4
5 or more	5
Don't know	8

When appropriate, precoded responses should contain a code (with the same numeric value throughout the instrument) for "don't know" answers. A seperate code, usually "9" or "99," should be reserved to code missing data. To avoid errors, common responses, such as "yes" or "no" should always have the same order and same codes throughout the instrument.

Answers to open-ended items are often coded after the interview is completed. A coding manual which states explicitly how each item is to be categorized and coded is essential to assure consistent and reliable coding.

ADMINISTERING THE INSTRUMENT

Getting complete and accurate data

Once the study begins, the object is to collect 100% of the data from the subjects in the study and to record it in a computer without errors. The greater the amount of missing data, the greater the possibility that the results may not truly represent the intended subjects of the study. Furthermore, missing data make analysis of results more difficult and, by reducing the number of answers, reduce the statistical power of the study. Errors in the recording of data will increase the variability of responses, adding random error and decreasing the statistical power of the study. Errors in recording data can also be systematic, biasing the results of the study.

The strategies for **minimizing missing data and errors** are reviewed briefly here and discussed more fully in Chapters 16. The first is to *design* the instruments well, using the guidelines presented above. The instructions must be straightforward, and the questions clear, logically designed and attractively presented.

The second strategy is to develop a system for *administering* the instruments well.

All answers should be checked by the interviewer or researcher before the respondent leaves the site where the instrument was completed. Incomplete or ambiguous answers should corrected as soon as possible. If the respondent has left, she should be contacted by telephone to complete the items or, if necessary, asked to return to finish the instrument in person. Telephone interviews should be reviewed immediately after the call is completed. If the questionnaires are sent by mail, the response rate can be improved by enclosing stamped, addressed return envelopes, enclosing a small advance payment for cooperation, sending follow-up reminders, and making follow-up phone calls to nonrespondents. If mailed-in questionnaires are incomplete, the respondent should be contacted by telephone and/or a copy of the questionnaire should be returned with the incomplete items highlighted.

The third strategy is to *review the findings* periodically. The investigator can check a randomly selected set of completed forms for errors, and he can tabulate the results to look for missing or aberrant data. This requires that he enter the data into a computer soon after it is collected, an excellent practice that is discussed in Chapter 15.

Enhancing the reliability of interviews

The skill of the interviewer can have a substantial impact on the quality of the responses. Standardizing the interview procedure from one interview to the next is the key to maximizing reliability. The interview must be conducted with uniform wording of questions and uniform non-verbal signals during the interview. Interviewers must be careful to avoid introducing their own biases into the responses by changing the words or the tone of their voice. This requires practice and training.

The interview should be written in language that resembles common speech so that the interviewer can comfortably read or recite the questions *verbatim*. Questions that sound unnatural or stilted when they are said out loud will encourage interviewers to improvise their own more natural but less standardized way of asking the question.

Sometimes it is necessary to follow-up

on a respondent's answers to encourage him to give an appropriate answer or to clarify the meaning of a response. This "probing" can also be standardized by writing standard phrases in the margins or beneath the text of each question. For example, a question about how many cups of coffee a respondent drinks on a typical day may cause some respondents to say "I'm not sure; it's different from day to day." The instrument may include a standard follow-up "probe," such as: "Do the best you can: tell me *approximately* how many you drink on a typical day."

SUMMARY

1. For many clinical studies, the quality of the results depends on the quality of data collected by questionnaires and interviews. Investigators should take the time and care to be certain that the instruments are as clear, accurate, and reliable as possible before the study begins.
2. *Self-administered questionnaires* are more economical than interviews, and they are more readily standardized. *Interviews*, on the other hand, can improve clarity and produce more complete responses.
3. *Open-ended questions* are useful for developing new questions about new topics and describing the range of potential responses to a question. *Closed-ended questions*, however, are usually clearer and easier to answer and analyse. The potential answers to a closed-ended question should be exhaustive and mutually exclusive.
4. The instrument should be simple and easy to read. Interview questions should be comfortable to read out loud. Questions should be preceded by clear instructions and examples. The format should be spacious and uncluttered, with indentations and arrows that direct the respondent or interviewer.
5. All answers to closed-ended questions should be *coded in advance* and the codes or scores should be organized on the form in a way that will make data entry simple and efficient.
6. To measure abstract variables, such as attitudes or health status, questions can be combined into *summative (Likert)* or *cumulative (Guttman)* scales which can be summed to produce a total score. Such scores, however, assume that the questions measure a single characteristic and that the responses have a relatively high degree of internal consistency.
7. An investigator should try to use *existing instruments* that are known to produce accurate and reliable results. When it is necessary to devise a *new instrument*, the investigator should start by collecting existing instruments to be used as potential models and sources of ideas.
8. All instruments should be *pretested* before being used in the study. Initial pretests to improve the clarity of questions and instructions should include a small number of respondents who represent the range of potential respondents in the study. Later, larger pretests are useful to refine the range, reliability, efficiency, and statistical characteristics of the instrument.
9. Once the study begins, the investigator should aim for 100% *complete and error-free collection and entry of data*. This entails a check of all completed forms before the respondent leaves, follow-up of all missing or inappropriate answers, and a system of regular review of the data.

REFERENCES

1. Cannell C, Oksenberg L, Converse J: *Experiments in Interviewing Technique: Field Experiments in Health Reporting, 1971–1977*. Ann Arbor, Survey Research Center, Institute for Social Research, University of Michigan, 1979.
2. Jenkins CO, Zyzanski SJ. Prediction of clinical CHD by a test for the coronary-prone behavior pattern. NEJM 290: 1271–5, 1974.
3. Kelsey JL, Thompson WD, Evans AS: Measurement I: Questionnaires. in *Methods in Observational Epidemiology*. New York: Oxford University Press, 1986, pp 309–336.
4. Alanko T: An overview of techniques and problems in the measurement of alcohol consumption. In Smart S, et al. (eds), *Research Advances in Alcohol and Drug Problems*. New York , Plenum, 1984, pp 209–226.
5. Fienberg SE, Loftus EF, Tanur JM: Cognitive aspects of health survey methodology: an overview. *Milbank Mem Fund Q* 63:547–564, 1985.
6. Cronbach LJ: Coefficient alpha and the internal structure of tests. *Psychometrika* 16:297–334, 1951.

7. Seltiz C, Wrightsman L, Cook S: *Research Methods in Social Relations*, ed 3. New York, Holt, Rhinehart and Winston, 1976.

ADDITIONAL READINGS

Herrmann N: Retrospective information from questionnaires: II Interrater reliability and comparison of questionnaire types. *Am J Epidemiol* 121 (6): 948–953, 1985. (*A study comparing the reliability of self-administered questionnaires and interviews which asked about medical history and diet.*)

Hyman H: *Interviewing in Social Research.* Chicago, University of Chicago Press, 1975 (*A text on the importance of interviewing technique in survey research.*)

Oppenheim AN: *Questionnaire Design and Attitude Measurement.* New York, Basic Books, 1966. (*A classic, enjoyable and very readable treatise on the art of question writing.*)

O'Toole BI, Battistutta D, Long A, et al. A comparison of costs and data quality of three health survey methods: Mail, telephone and personal home interview. *Am J Epidemiol* 124 (2): 317–328, 1986. (*This study found mail questionnaires to have the lowest cost, but also the poorest data quality, in a comparison with phone and in-person interviews.*)

Schuman H and Pressler S. *Questions and answers in attitude surveys.* New York: Academic Press, 1981. (*A series of in-depth empirical investigations of the effect of question wording, form and context on answers to questions with a subjective component.*)

Seltiz C, Wrightsman L, Cook S: *Research Methods in Social Relations.* Third edition. New York: Holt, Rhinehart and Winston, 1976. (*This useful source book, which has stood the test of time, covers a broad range of survey research topics and includes a handbook on questionnaire design.*)

Siemiatycki J, Campbell S, Richardson L, et al: Quality of response in different population groups in mail and telephone surveys. *Am J Epidemiol* 120: 302–314, 1984. (*This study found the validity of health history questions to be greater in a mail than in a telephone survey format.*)

CHAPTER 6

Using Secondary Data

Norman Hearst and Stephen B. Hulley

INTRODUCTION 53
  Advantages and disadvantages

TYPES OF SECONDARY DATA SETS 53
  Aggregate data sets
  Individual data sets

GETTING STARTED 57
  Finding research questions to fit the data
  Finding data sets to fit a research question
  Types of study design

TERTIARY DATA ANALYSIS 60

SUMMARY 61

REFERENCES 61

ADDITIONAL READINGS 62

INTRODUCTION

Secondary data analysis is the use of an existing data base to investigate research questions other than those for which the data were originally gathered. A knowledge of when and how to use secondary data can be useful to anyone who does clinical research. With the rapidly increasing number of data bases available, researchers will use secondary data even more in the future. Nevertheless, surprisingly little has been written on how to go about this.

Advantages and disadvantages

The main **advantages** of secondary data are speed and economy. A research question that might otherwise require much time and money to investigate can sometimes be answered rapidly and inexpensively by analyzing existing data. For new investigators with limited support, this may be the best way to get started in research. For experienced re-searchers, the clever use of a data set collected for another purpose can sometimes produce important findings at little or no added cost.

In the MRFIT, for example, information about the smoking habits of the wives of the study subjects was recorded in order to examine whether social support influenced the men's ability to quit smoking. After the study was over, one of the investigators realized that the data provided an opportunity to investigate the health effects of passive smoking (a much more important research question!). A twofold excess in the incidence of heart disease was found in nonsmoking men married to smoking wives when compared with similar nonsmoking men married to nonsmoking wives (1).

Secondary data sets also have some serious **limitations**. The selection of which data to collect, the quality of the data gathered, and the method of entry and filing are all predetermined. The investigator may have to settle for a variable that is not what he would prefer to have measured (e.g., history of hypertension, a derived dichotomous variable, in place of the actual continuous blood pressure measurement). The quality of the data may be poor, with frequent missing or incorrect values. All of these factors contribute to the main disadvantage of secondary data: the investigator has no control over the data base.

TYPES OF SECONDARY DATA SETS

Secondary data sets are of two types: individual and aggregate. The term **individual data** means that there is separate information for each member of a list of individuals. Individual data may come from previous research studies, medical records, personnel files, death certificates, and many other sources. In such a data set, associations between characteristics can be measured among individual members of the study population, much as an investigator would do if gathering his own data.

When individual data are not available, aggregate data sets can sometimes be useful. The term **aggregate data** means that no information is available for specific individuals, only for groups (for example, death rates from cervical cancer in each of the 50 states.) With aggregate data, associations can only be measured among these groups, by comparing the prevalence of a risk factor with the rate of an outcome. Studies using aggregate data are called **ecological studies**.

Aggregate data sets

More has been written about ecological studies than about other types of secondary data analysis, and much of this has been critical (2). The major drawback of aggregate data is that associations are especially susceptible to confounding: groups of individuals, especially when separated by time or space, tend to differ from each other in many ways, not all of which are causally related. Furthermore, associations observed in the aggregate do not necessarily hold for the individual. For example, sales of cigarettes may be greater in states with high cervical cancer rates, but the women who get the cervical cancer may not be the same ones doing the smoking. This situation is referred to as the **ecological fallacy**. Nevertheless, ecological studies have produced many important results in the past, including some of the early evidence linking dietary fat intake with coronary heart disease (3). Aggregate data are most appropriately used to test the plausibility of a new hypothesis or to generate new hypotheses; interesting results can then be pursued in another study that uses individual data.

Aggregate data on various health, economic, and social factors are available for worldwide populations in the United Nations *Demographic Yearbook* (4) and *Statistical Yearbook* (5); for the U.S. population, they are found in the *Statistical Abstract of the United States* (6). Combined with data on the prevalence of risk factors, (e.g., per capita cigarette consumption), such statistics can form the basis for ecological studies. For example, one report used this type of data to analyze how social and economic factors affect infant mortality rates in 63 countries (7). Newspaper circulation per 1000 population (a proxy for educational status) was the factor most closely related to infant mortality, followed by level of economic development and number of physicians per 10,000 population. Data of this sort are useful for planning health and social policy, as well as for exploring etiology.

In the United States, the federal government publishes *Vital Statistics of the United States* (8), which includes various health statistics by state and by Standard Metropolitan Statistical Area (a geographic unit the size of a whole urban region, e.g., the San Francisco-Oakland Bay Area). For information by smaller geographic subunits, it is necessary to look to state and county health departments. Here, the information varies from state to state and from county to county. Generally, little is available for geographic subunits smaller than counties, although in some areas cause-specific mortality, incidence of reportable diseases, and perinatal statistics are available by zip code or census tract.

Data from **hospital discharge records** are available on computer tapes for all hospitalizations in some states (9) and for a representative sample of U.S. hospitals in the annual National Hospital Discharge Survey (see ref. 10, p. 38). These can be useful in health services research (e.g., determining local hospital utilization rates) and in some epidemiologic studies (e.g., examining mortality rates in hospitalizations for pneumonia by age, sex, and race). Publicly available tapes have been stripped of individual identifiers for reasons of confidentiality, and therefore cannot be used to study hospitalizations of specified individuals.

Individual data sets

Individual data bases that are likely to be useful to the health researcher generally fall into two categories. The first category includes **data collected in a previous research study** at the investigator's institution. Many studies collect more data than the investigators can analyze, and contain interesting findings that have gone unnoticed. Access to such data is controlled by the study's principal investigator, and the new researcher can explore this possibility with senior investigators at his institution with whom he would like to work.

The second category includes **large re-gional and national data sets** that are publicly available and do not have a principal investigator. Computerized data bases of this sort are a rapidly growing phenomenon, and as varied as the reasons people have for collecting information. Table 6.1 lists and describes some of the publicly available data sets most useful for epidemiologic research. For a more complete listing, readers may refer to several publications entirely devoted to the subject (10,19,20).

Table 6.1.
Examples of Secondary Data Sets

Type of Data	Where available
Aggregate data	
Vital statistics (international, national, state, and local)	In most university libraries
The United Nations *Demographics Yearbook* (4) Vital Statistics of the United States (8)	
Various economic, employment, demographic, and other factors	In most university libraries
The United Nations *Statistical Yearbook* (5) Statistical Abstract of Latin America (11) Statistical Abstract of the United States (6)	
Records of reportable disease incidence by geographic area	From the Centers for Disease Control, Atlanta, Georgia (see ref. 12)
The census	Summary data in most libraries (e.g., ref. 13); computer tapes from the U.S. Department of Commerce
Individual data	
Government statistics	
Death certificate data	
The National Death Index (national mortality follow-up for any cohort of individuals) (14) State death certificates registries (available in some states)	Example: California Automated Mortality Linkage System, Dept. of Epidemiology, 1699 HSW, University of California, San Francisco, CA 94143
Hospital discharge data	
The National Hospital Discharge Survey	See ref. 10, p 38
Computerized registries of hospital discharge data (available in some states)	Example: see ref. 9
The National Ambulatory Medical Care Survey	See ref. 10, pp 36–37

Table 6.1. continued

Type of Data	Where available
The HANES (Health and Nutrition Examination Survey, a periodic examination of a representative sample of the U.S. population)	See ref. 10, pp 17–25; see also ref. 15
The National Health Interview Survey (annual health surveys of a sample of the U.S. population)	See ref. 10, pp 26–30
Tumor registries (cancer incidence, treatment, and outcome)	From local tumor registries or nationally from the SEER program (see ref. 16)
Social Security records (vital status, work history, economic data)	From the Social Security Administration
Previous research studies	
Large cohort studies (e.g., Framingham, MRFIT)	Through the study's investigators
Smaller studies in your area of interest, which may have collected more data than they analyzed and reported	Through each study's principal investigator
Other medical data bases	
Computerized medical records from hospitals and ambulatory care practices	See refs. 17 and 18
Roswell Park Hospital (extensive data on cancer patients over several decades)	Contact Roswell Park Hospital, Buffalo, New York
Mayo Clinic data for Olmsted County (population-based morbidity and mortality data)	Contact Mayo Clinic, Rochester, Minnesota
Data from third-party payers: Medicare, Medicaid, private insurance companies, Workmen's Compensation, Health Maintenance Organizations	Through each program
Miscellaneous	
Trade union and company records (e.g., disability, injuries, absenteeism)	Through individual unions and companies
Military data (physical examinations and medical follow-up, mostly on young men)	From various military agencies. Example: Defense Manpower Data Center, 550 El Estero, #200, Monterey, CA 93940
Insurance company data (accidents, disability, mortality)	Through individual companies

We will discuss examples of the use of data sets included in Table 6.1 throughout this chapter, but several deserve special mention here. **Tumor registries** are government-supported agencies that collect complete statistics on cancer incidence, treatment, and outcome in defined geographic areas. The areas covered by these registries currently include about 10% of the U.S. population. One of the purposes of these registries is to provide access to outside investigators who wish to use the registry's data base. Combined data for all of the registries are also available in hard copy or on computer tapes from the Surveillance, Epidemiology, and End Results (SEER) Program (16).

Death certificate registries can be used to follow the mortality of any cohort of individuals defined in the past or in the present. In addition to a number of state registries, such as the CAMLIS system for California, there has been since 1978 a **National Death Index** (14), for all deaths occurring in the United States. This can be used to ascertain the vital status of individuals who have been the subject of an earlier study or are part of another data set that includes important predictor variables. One example of the usefulness of death certificate registries is the follow-up of men having heart attacks who were treated with high-dose nicotinic acid (or placebo) to lower serum cholesterol in the Coronary Drug Project: although there was no difference in death rates at the end of the 5-year intervention period (21), a mortality follow-up 7 years later using the National Death Index revealed a highly significant difference (22). This was the first clear-cut demonstration of an effect of cholesterol intervention on total mortality. Because the vital status of any U.S. resident is public information, this follow-up was complete even for men who had dropped out of the study.

The National Death Index can be used when any two of three basic individual identifiers (name, birthdate, social security number) are known. Ascertainment of the fact of death is 98.6% complete with this system (23), and additional information from the death certificates (notably cause of death) can then be obtained from state records. On the local level, some jurisdictions have moved toward automated vital statistics systems (24,25), in which individual data (such as information from birth or death certificates) are entered into computerized data bases as they are received, making up-to-the-minute analysis of individual data theoretically possible.

GETTING STARTED

Secondary data analysis can begin in two ways. An investigator may start with a research question of interest to him, and try to find a data set that can answer the question. This is the usual approach to clinical research, and the choice of an area of interest and of specific research questions has been discussed in Chapter 2. The other approach, unique to secondary data analysis, is to begin with a data set and try to find questions that it can answer. The challenge here is to discover useful findings in the piles of information that surround us.

With either approach, the help of a senior colleague experienced in clinical research is invaluable; choosing such a mentor is the most important decision that a new investigator makes. In secondary data analysis, this person can help not only in choosing a research question and designing a protocol, but also in identifying and gaining access to the appropriate data base.

Finding research questions to fit the data

This approach, which can be particularly useful to the new investigator looking for a research project, is summarized in Table 6.2. The investigator first chooses a data set and then thoroughly familiarizes himself with the information that has been gathered. It is useful to make a written list or flowchart of all the data collected, including the timing of variables that were measured more than once. The next step is to look for pairs or groups of variables whose relationship might be of interest. A brainstorming session involving others familiar with the data may help in this process.

Especially in large randomized controlled trials, the relationship between many variables may never be assessed as part of the original study, simply because the investigators do not find time to analyze all combinations. For example, in a study of treatment for hypertension, was blood pressure taken both sitting and standing? If so, was there any relationship between a postural change in blood pressure at baseline and prognosis or response to treatment? Was there any difference between blacks and whites in the natural progression of disease in the control group? What was the relationship between age, height, weight, and blood pressure among all those initially screened for the study?

Large national data sets provide a similar opportunity. The **Health and Nutrition Examination Survey** (HANES) includes medical histories, nutritional questionnaires, and physical examinations performed on a probability sample of the U.S. population (See ref. 10, pp. 17–25; see also ref. 15). Some investigators have built careers by analyzing these periodic surveys. The National Center for Health Statistics (NCHS), which collects the HANES data, limits its own analyses

Table 6.2.
Steps in Finding Research Questions to Fit an Existing Data Base

1. Choose a data base.
2. Become thoroughly familiar with the data base. Make a flow sheet of all variables and how they were measured.
3. Identify pairs or groups of variables whose association may be of interest.
4. Review the literature and consult experts to determine if these research questions would be novel and important.
5. Formulate specific hypotheses and settle on the statistical methods.
6. Analyze the data.

mainly to determining the prevalence of health conditions in the U.S. population, and encourages outside investigators to perform further analyses, such as examining potential risk factors for diseases. Any scientist with access to a mainframe computer and the competence to deal with the analytic implications of cluster sampling can arrange to purchase, at nominal cost, an analysis tape that includes any specified set of variables.

Research questions can also be built around aggregate data sets. Regional or national statistics can be analyzed to look for correlations among diseases, or between a disease and demographic, social, dietary, or economic indices. For example, an analysis of the mortality rates from different cancers among states of the United States provided the first indication that lung cancer and cervical cancer might have risk factors in common (26). This study began not with a specific hypothesis, but with the receipt in the mail of a book of cancer statistics and an informal discussion among the investigators about how these data might be profitably analyzed. Since then, several studies have confirmed cigarette smoking as a risk factor for cervical cancer (27).

Finding data sets to fit a research question

Familiarizing oneself with an existing data base in the hopes of finding new questions to answer may sound unexciting to some investigators, especially those who have already decided on a specific research question of interest to them. Such researchers may prefer the alternative approach: searching for a data set that can answer a particular ques-

tion they have in mind. This approach is less constrained, leaving the investigator free to choose among the full spectrum of research questions and data sets. It is suitable for any investigator with a research question, whether or not he has decided in advance to use secondary data.

Table 6.3 summarizes this approach to secondary data analysis. After choosing a research question and becoming familiar with the literature in that area (preferably with the help of a computerized literature search), the next step is to investigate whether the question can be addressed with an existing data base. This is important; it is better to spend days or weeks on the telephone and hundreds of dollars in long distance bills than to spend months or years and tens of thousands of dollars in unnecessary data collection. With the many computerized data bases now in existence, there may be one somewhere that can answer the research question. The challenge is to find it.

A useful way to begin is to draw up a list of pairs of predictor and outcome variables whose relationship might help to partially answer the research question. If there is no data set known to include the exact variable of interest, another closely associated variable might serve as a proxy. For example, census tract of residence can be used as a proxy for level of income because census data include median income by neighborhood. Data about taxes on cigarette sales can serve as a proxy for the prevalence of cigarette smoking in an ecological study. Religious preference can be used as a proxy for caffeine consumption if Mormons (for whom coffee is prohibited) are compared with members of other churches.

Table 6.3.
Steps in Finding Data Bases to Fit a Specified Research Question

1. Choose a research question and review the literature thoroughly.
2. List combinations of predictor and outcome variables whose relationship might help answer the research question.
3. Identify data bases that might include the variables of interest.
4. Become familiar with each of these data bases, and consult with individuals who know them well.
5. Choose the best data base(s) and gain access to the data.
6. Formulate specific hypotheses and settle on the statistical methods.
7. Analyze the data.

The next step is to locate data bases that include these predictor and outcome variables. A great ally in this effort is the telephone. The shoe-leather epidemiology made famous by John Snow and others has been supplemented today with telephone-wire epidemiology. A call to the authors of previous studies or government officials might result in access to files containing useful data. It is essential to conquer the anxiety that we all feel when contacting people we do not know to ask for help. In fact, most people will be surprisingly cooperative, either by providing data themselves or by suggesting other places to try.

It is often possible to link two data bases, one supplying information on the predictor variable and one on the outcome variable. This is relatively straightforward for ecological studies, so long as both data sets use the same boundaries for the groups being compared (e.g., counties, states). Sources of individual data are more difficult to link unless both data sets include the same unique individual identifiers, such as social security number or name and birthdate. Even when present in the original data sets, these personal identifiers may not be accessible to an investigator for reasons of confidentiality. In such circumstances, the holders of the data sets may be willing to carry out the analysis, or to prepare a merged file that includes the information needed with the personal identifiers deleted.

Once the data for answering the research question have been located, the next challenge is to obtain permission to use them. If the data set is publicly available, this task will be relatively straightforward, but if the data set is controlled by another

investigator it may require careful diplomacy. It is a good practice to use official letterhead on correspondence, and to adopt any institutional titles that are appropriate (e.g., instead of "I'm an epidemiology student at . . .," say, "I'm calling from the Department of Epidemiology at . . ."). If someone suggested the contact, it may be helpful to mention that person's name.

The investigation should be very specific about what information is sought, and the detailed request should be confirmed in writing. It is a good idea to keep the size of the request to a minimum. Offering to pay the cost of preparing data shows a seriousness of intent, and removes one potential reason for denying the request. The cost of preparing a data tape is usually only a few hundred dollars.

If the data set is controlled by another group of researchers, the most effective strategy may be to suggest a collaborative relationship. In addition to providing an incentive for others to share their data, having a coinvestigator who is familiar with the data base is helpful. It is important to clearly define such a relationship from the beginning, including who will be first author of the planned publications. Such arrangements are best made in a face-to-face meeting.

The two approaches to secondary analysis outlined above—beginning with a data base or beginning with a research question—represent extremes. What happens in practice is often a mixture of the two. An experienced researcher usually has defined areas of interest, in which he stays current on the literature and is aware of the important questions that need research. Whenever he becomes familiar with a new data base, he looks for questions that it might answer. Similarly, whenever he thinks of a new hypothesis, he looks for a data base with which to test it. In this way, a good researcher can contribute more to scientific knowledge than would be possible by only reporting results of the originally planned analyses of his own data.

Types of study design

Any type of study design can potentially be carried out with secondary data if an appropriate data set can be located. Secondary data have been most widely used for cross-sectional and case-control studies, but cohort studies are also an option when a single data set or combination of data sets permits an extended period of follow-up. Studies using life insurance company data to evaluate the long-term effects of obesity on mortality are a good example of a cohort study with a single data set (28). State and national mortality registries provide a particularly attractive opportunity for following up any group on whom baseline information has been collected, even when there is no effort to follow the cohort in person. An excellent example is the follow-up of the 360,000 men whose coronary risk factors were screened during the recruitment phase of the MRFIT. This analysis, which was not envisioned until years after the baseline data were collected, produced some of the most important findings in the whole study. The enormous size of the cohort permitted new conclusions on, for example, the risk relationships between serum cholesterol and mortality from cancer (29).

Sometimes it is even possible to use secondary data in the equivalent of a randomized experiment. In a **natural experiment,** people have received a random or nearly random assignment in the past (such as adoption, medical provider, or job assignment) for reasons unrelated to research, and a data base is available with which to assess an outcome that might have been affected by this assignment. We recently studied the effect of the 1970–1972 draft lottery (involving 5,200,000 20-year-old men assigned randomly by date of birth) on delayed mortality (assessed by state death certificate registries) (30). The predictor variable in this study (date of birth) was a proxy for military service during the Vietnam era. Men randomized to be eligible for the draft had significantly higher mortality from suicide and motor vehicle accidents in the 10 years after they would have returned from the military. The study was done for less than $2000 (not including the investigators' time), yet it was a more unbiased approach to examining the delayed effect of military service on specific causes of death than other studies of this topic with much larger budgets (31).

TERTIARY DATA ANALYSIS

Tertiary analysis refers to the combination and reanalysis of previously reported data, all relating to the same research question, from multiple sources. **Pooling projects** of this type may be particularly useful when the published studies on a topic have yielded conflicting findings or have each been too small to produce conclusive results. A compilation of nine previous randomized studies of diuretic treatment during pregnancy for example, found that diuretics produce a significant reduction in preeclampsia (32). This finding contrasted with the general opinion of most obstetricians that such treatment is not helpful, an opinion that resulted from many small studies, no one of which conclusively demonstrated any benefits from diuretics.

The process of pooling data from several randomized trials has been criticized by some authors (33), who have expressed concern over the appropriateness of combining data collected in different ways from different populations. We take the alternative view set forth by Yusuf et al. (34): the large sample size that results often makes pooling worthwhile, provided that the differences among the studies in interventions and populations are not so large that they would be likely to produce "qualitative interactions"—entirely different conclusions. This is often a reasonable presumption, and we encourage the reader to look up examples of tertiary analysis (32,35) that illustrate the usefulness of this approach to research and its accessibility to the young investigator.

SUMMARY

1. *Secondary data analysis* has the advantage of greatly reducing the time and cost needed for doing research, and the disadvantage of leaving the investigator with little or no control over his data.

2. One good source of data for secondary analysis is an *existing project* at the investigator's institution; another is the large number of *computerized data bases* now available in remote locations. Although individual data are preferable, aggregate data can also sometimes be useful for ecological analysis.

3. Investigators may begin either by looking for research questions to fit an existing data base or by looking for a data base that can help to answer a particular research question. In practice, a combination of both approaches may be most productive.

4. Any type of study design can be carried out with secondary data: cross-sectional, case-control, cohort, or experimental. A type of analysis unique to secondary data involves combining and reanalyzing data from several published studies of a single research question; this is called *tertiary data analysis*.

5. The use of secondary data is an excellent way for new investigators to get started in research and can increase the productivity of established investigators. Time or money spent locating or gaining access to the right data set is well worth the investment.

REFERENCES

1. Svendsen KH, Kuller LH, Martin MJ, et al: Effects of passive smoking in the Multiple Risk Factor Intervention Trial (MRFIT) *Am J Epidemiol* 126: 783–795, 1987.
2. Connor MJ, Gillings D: An empiric study of ecological inference. *Am J Public Health* 74(6): 555–559, 1984.
3. Keys A: Atherosclerosis: a problem in newer public health. *J Mt Sinai Hosp* 20:118–134 1953.
4. United Nations: *1984 Demographic Yearbook.* New York, United Nations, 1986.
5. United Nations: *1982 Statistical Yearbook.* New York, United Nations, 1985.
6. U.S. Bureau of the Census: *Statistical Abstract of the United States 1985*, ed 105. Washington, DC, U.S. Bureau of the Census, 1984.

7. Shin EH: Economic and social correlates of infant mortality: a cross-sectional and longitudinal analysis of 63 selected countries. *Social Biol* 22(4): 315–325, 1975.
8. National Center for Health Statistics: *Vital Statistics of the United States 1977.* DHHS Pub. No. (PHS) 80-1102, Public Health Service. Washington, DC, U.S. Government Printing Office, 1980.
9. California Health Facilities Commission Discharge Data Program: *1983 Discharge Data Tape Format Documentation.* Sacramento, California Health Facilities Commission, 1985.
10. National Center for Health Statistics (Schoenborn CA, ed): An inventory of alcohol, drug, and mental health data available from the National Center for Health Statistics. *Vital and Health Statistics,* Series 1, No. 17. DHHS Pub. No. (PHS) 85-1319, Public Health Service. Washington, DC, U.S. Government Printing Office, 1985.
11. Wilke JW, Haber S (eds): *Statistical Abstract of Latin America* Los Angeles: UCLA Latin American Center Publications, 1983, vol. 22.
12. Centers for Disease Control: *CDC Surveillance Summaries* 35 (No. 1SS), 1986, (Published four times a year.)
13. Bureau of the Census: *1980 Census of Population.* Washington, DC, Department of Commerce, 1983.
14. National Center for Health Statistics: *User's Manual: The National Death Index.* DHHS Publication No. (PHS) 81-1148, Public Health Service. Washington, DC, U.S. Government Printing Office, 1981.
15. National Center for Health Statistics: *Plan and Operation of the Health and Nutrition Examination Survey.* DHEW Publication No. (HRA) 76-1310. Rockville, MD, U.S. Department of Health, Education, and Welfare, 1973.
16. Biometry Branch Division of Cancer Prevention and Control, National Cancer Institute: *SEER Program: Cancer Incidence and Mortality in the United States 1973-1981.* NIH Pub. No 85-1837. Bethesda, MD, National Institute of Health, 1984.
17. McDonald, CJ, Tierney WM: Research uses of computer-stored practice records in general medicine. *J Gen Intern Med* 1:S19–S24, 1986.
18. Goldman L, Mushlin AI, Lee KL: Using medical databases for clinical research. *J Gen Intern Med* 1:525–530, 1986.
19. Mullner RM, Byre CS, Killingsworth CL: An inventory of U.S. health care data bases. *Rev Public Data Use* 11(2):85–192, 1983.
20. Zarozny S, Horner M: *The Federal Data Base Finder.* Potomac, MD, Information USA, Inc., 1984.
21. Coronary Drug Project Research Group: Clofibrate and niacin in coronary heart disease. *JAMA* 231:360–381, 1975.
22. Canner PL: Mortality in CDP patients during a nine-year post-treatment period. *J Am Coll Cardiol* 8:1245–55, 1986.
23. Wentworth DN, Neaton JD, Rasmussen WL: An evaluation of the SSA Master Beneficiary Record File and the National Death Index in the ascertainment of Vital Status. *Am J Public Health* 73: 1270–1274, 1983.
24. Williams RL, Marinko JA, Shields ML: An automated vital statistics system. *In Proceedings of the*

19th National Meeting of the Public Health Conference on Records and Statistics. Rockville, MD, National Center for Health Statistics, 1983.

25. *Community and Organization Research Institute: AVSS User's Guide.* Santa Barbara, Regents of the University of California, 1983.

26. Winkelstein W, Sacks ST, Ernster VL, et al: Correlation of the incidence rates for selected cancers in the nine areas of the Third National Cancer Survey. *Am J Epidemiol* 109:107–419, 1977.

27. Winkelstein W, Shillitoe EJ, Brand R, Johnson KK: Further comments on cancer of the uterine cervix, smoking, and herpes virus infection. *Am J Epidemiol* 119(1):1–8, 1984.

28. Simopoulos AP, Van Itallie TB: Body weight, health, and longevity. *Ann Intern Med* 100:285–295, 1984.

29. Sherwin RW, Wentworth DN, Cutter JA, et al: Serum cholesterol and cancer; mortality in the 361,662 men screened for the MRFIT. *JAMA* 257:943–948, 1987.

30. Hearst N, Newman TB, Hulley SB: Delayed effects of the military draft on mortality: a randomized natural experiment. *N Engl J Med* 314:620–624, 1986.

31. Center for Disease Control: *Protocol for Epidemiologic Studies of the Health of Vietnam Veterans.* Atlanta, GA, Centers for Disease Control, 1983.

32. Collins R, Yusuf S, Peto R: Overview of randomized trials of diuretics in pregnancy. *Br Med J* 290:17–23, 1985.

33. Goldman L, Feinstein AR: Anticoagulants and myocardial infarction: the problems of pooling, drowning, and floating. *Ann Intern Med* 90:92–94, 1979.

34. Yusuf S, Collins R, Peto R: Why do we need some large, simple randomized trials? *Stat Med* 3:409–420, 1984.

35. May GS, Eberlein KA, Furberg CD, et al: Secondary prevention after myocardial infarction: review of long-term trials. *Prog Cardiovas Dis* 24:331–352, 1982.

ADDITIONAL READINGS

Connor MJ, Gillings D: An empiric study of ecological inference. *Am J Public Health* 74(6):555–559. (*A good review of some of the problems with ecological studies, including illustrative examples.*)

Kelsey JL, Thompson WD, Evans AS: *Methods in Observational Epidemiology.* New York, Oxford University Press, 1986, pp 46–76. (*A useful draft on sources of routinely collected data on disease occurrence.*)

Mullner RM, Byre CS, Killingsworth CL. An inventory of U.S. health care data bases. *Review of Public Data Use* 1983; 11(2):85–192. (*Probably the most thorough listing of health-related data bases available.*)

National Center for Health Statistics, Schoenborn, CA. An inventory of alcohol, drug, and mental health data available from the National Center for Health Statistics. Vital and Health Statistics. Series 1, No. 17. DHHS Pub. No. (PHS) 85-1319. Public Health Service. Washington. U.S. Government Printing Office, 1985. (*Descriptions of the major national surveys conducted by NCHS and the information collected in each.*)

Public Health Service: *Promoting Health/Preventing Disease: Objectives for the Nation.* Washington, DC, U.S. Government Printing Office, 1980. (*Information on data bases available for assessing numerous health indicators on the national and local levels.*)

CHAPTER 7

Designing a New Study: I. Cohort Studies

Steven R. Cummings, Virginia Ernster, and Stephen B. Hulley

INTRODUCTION 63

PROSPECTIVE COHORT STUDIES 63
Structure
Strengths
Weaknesses

RETROSPECTIVE COHORT STUDIES 65
Structure
Strengths
Weaknesses

NESTED CASE-CONTROL STUDIES 67
Structure
Strengths
Weaknesses

DOUBLE-COHORT STUDIES AND EXTERNAL
CONTROLS 68
Structure
Strengths
Weaknesses

STEPS IN PLANNING A COHORT STUDY 69
When to use a cohort design
Choosing among cohort designs
Selecting subjects
Measuring predictor and confounding variables
Following subjects and measuring outcomes
Analysing cohort studies: incidence and relative
risk

SUMMARY 73

REFERENCES 74

ADDITIONAL READINGS 74

INTRODUCTION

Cohort studies involve following groups of subjects over time. There are two primary purposes: **descriptive**, that is, to describe the incidence of certain outcomes over time; and **analytic**, that is, to analyze associations between risk factors and those outcomes. Two basic variations of this design are possible: **Prospective** studies, in which the investigator defines the sample and measures predictor variables before any outcomes have occurred; and **retrospective** studies, in which the investigator defines the sample and collects data about predictor variables after the outcomes have occurred.

PROSPECTIVE COHORT STUDIES

Structure

The word cohort was the ancient Roman term for a group of soldiers that marched together into battle. In clinical research, a cohort means a group of subjects followed together over time. In a prospective cohort study, the investigator chooses or defines a sample of subjects who do not yet have the outcome of interest, such as heart disease. He measures factors in each subject, such as exercise habits, that might predict the subsequent outcome. He follows these subjects with periodic surveys or examinations to detect the outcome(s) of interest (Fig. 7.1).

Following the cohort over a period of time allows the investigator to describe the incidence of the outcomes (such as death from coronary disease) in the cohort. If the purpose of the study is simply to describe the incidence of certain events in a group, this may be sufficient. However, most cohort studies are done to find out whether the incidence of certain conditions, such as myocardial infarction, is different in people who have different levels of a predictor variable, such as sedentary or active life-styles. This is accomplished by comparing the incidence of the condition in those with the predictor of interest with the incidence in those who do not have the predictor or who have a different level of the predictor. In single cohort studies, these comparisons involve "internal controls;" comparisons are made between groups within one cohort. Alternatively, a second cohort is used as an "external" control group.

Example 7.1.
To determine whether exercise protects against coronary heart disease (CHD), Paffenbarger and colleagues (1) undertook a prospective cohort study. The three basic steps in performing the study were to:

1. *Assemble the cohort*: In 1962 the investigators identified 16,936 Harvard alumni.
2. *Measure predictor variables*: They administered a questionnaire about activity and other potential risk factors and collected data from college records.
3. *Follow-up the cohort and measure outcomes*: 10 years later they sent a follow-up questionnaire about CHD and collected data about CHD from death certificates for those who died.

Those with sedentary habits had an incidence of 24 deaths due to CHD per 10,000 person-years of follow-up whereas those with regular exercise had an incidence of 16 deaths per 10,000 person-years: The relative risk is the ratio of these rates, or 24/16=1.5.

Strengths

The prospective cohort design is a powerful strategy for defining the incidence and investigating the potential causes of a condition. Because potential causative factors are measured before the outcome occurs, a cohort study can establish that they preceded the outcome. This time sequence strengthens the inference that the factor may be a cause of the outcome.

A prospective study gives the investigator an opportunity to measure important variables completely and accurately. This may be particularly important for studies of certain types of predictors, such as exercise habits, that are difficult for a subject to remember accurately. Measuring current levels of the predictor variable before the outcome occurs will generally produce more accurate data than attempts to reconstruct past exposures after the outcome has already happened. This also prevents measurements from being biased by knowledge of the outcome.

Prospective cohort studies are especially valuable for studying the antecedents of fatal diseases. When fatal diseases are studied retrospectively, it is necessary to reconstruct past predictor variables from medical records or friends and relatives of the deceased. Histories that come from surviving relatives, such as spouses, may be reasonably accurate for classifying subjects by

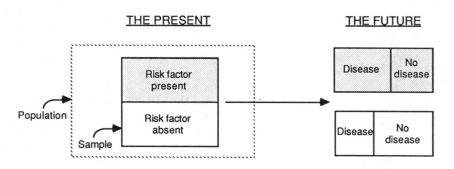

Steps:
1. Select a sample from the population
2. Measure predictor variables (risk factor present or absent)
3. Follow-up the cohort
4. Measure outcome variables (disease present or absent)

Figure 7.1.   Prospective cohort design

prominent personal characteristics, such as whether or not they smoked, but are much less accurate for quantifying variables, such as number of cigarettes smoked per day (2).

Weaknesses

The prospective cohort design is an expensive and inefficient way to study risk factors for the occurrence of a disease and this type of design cannot be used for studying rare diseases. Even common diseases, such as CHD, happen so infrequently (less than 1% per year in Harvard alumni) that large numbers of subjects must be followed for long periods of time in order to observe enough outcomes to produce meaningful results.

Prospective cohort designs become more efficient as the outcomes become more common. About 20% percent of patients die within a year after a heart attack. Therefore, a prospective cohort study of risk factors for death in men who have had a heart attack would be much less costly and less time-consuming than a prospective cohort study of risk factors for the occurrence of heart attacks in healthy men.

Associations found in cohort studies can sometimes be misleading if they are due to the effects of **confounding variables**. A confounding variable is one that is associated with both the predictor and outcome variables of interest. For instance, cigarette smoking might confound the association between exercise and CHD in example 7.1. If smokers exercise less than non smokers and also have a higher incidence of CHD, then the apparent association between less exercise and a higher incidence of CHD might really be due to the confounding variable, cigarette smoking.

Inferences about cause and effect can be strengthened by measuring all potential confounding variables and adjusting for their effects in statistical analyses (see Chapter 10). Cigarette smoking, for example, was measured in Harvard Alumni and, in statistical analyses, did not account for the lower incidence of CHD among those who exercised more. It is possible, however, that associations of modest strength found in observational studies might be due to an unrecognized confounding factor. This possibility can

only be addressed by a randomized trial (see Chapter 11).

By excluding subjects who are known to have the outcomes of interest, the investigator assumes that the predictor variables that are measured at the beginning of the study have not been influenced by the outcomes. However, some conditions, like CHD, can be present before the patient or physician knows that they are present. In these cases, some predictor variables, such as physical activity, can be influenced by the outcome. Consider, for example, the possibility that some Harvard alumni had CHD at the start of the study, but were not conscious of it. If these alumni exercised less because of vague symptoms produced by their "silent" CHD, they would report less exercise and would have a higher rate of subsequent CHD. This would mislead the investigator to conclude that lack of exercise causes CHD when, in fact, it was a consequence.

If the condition being studied has a long preclinical phase, this potential problem might be minimized in two ways: First, very sensitive tests might be used to screen and exclude all potential subjects who have "subclinical" forms of the disease of interest (e.g., a treadmill test for CHD). Second, the investigator might increase the follow-up time so that the period from measurement of the predictor variable to the occurrence of the outcome is longer than the silent preclinical phase of the disease. If the association persists well beyond the likely duration of the preclinical phase, this supports a causal association.

RETROSPECTIVE COHORT STUDIES

Structure

The design of a retrospective cohort study is essentially the same as that of a prospective cohort study: a group of subjects is followed over time with measurements of potential predictor variables at the beginning and then ascertainment of subsequent outcomes (Fig. 7.2). The difference is that the assembly of the cohort, baseline measurements, follow-up, and outcomes all happened in the past. This type of study is only possible if adequate data about the risk factors and outcomes are available on a cohort of subjects which has been assembled for other purposes.

Example 7.2.

To determine the prognosis of mitral valve prolapse, Nishimura (3) conducted a retrospective cohort study. The three basic steps in performing the study were to:

1. *Identify a suitable cohort*: The investigators identified 343 patients who were found to have mitral-valve prolapse on echocardiograms performed at the Mayo Clinic between 1975 and 1979.
2. *Collect data about predictor variables*: They collected data from the medical records and made measurements of the "redundancy" of the mitral valves on the original echocardiograms.
3. *Collect data about outcomes at a later time*: In 1984 they collected data about sudden death, cerebral embolus and endocarditis from records of subsequent office visits and from questionnaires to or telephone interviews with the patients.

The investigators found that 10% of those with redundant valves and 0.7% of those with nonredundant valves died suddenly or suffered a cerebral embolus or endocarditis, a relative risk of $10/0.7 = 14$.

Strengths

Like prospective cohort studies, retrospective cohort studies can establish that predictor variables preceded the outcomes. Because measurements were collected before the outcomes were known, this type of study can also guarantee that the measurement of predictor variables was not biased by knowledge of which subjects had the outcome of interest.

Retrospective cohort studies are much less costly and time-consuming than prospective ones. In retrospective studies, the subjects are already assembled, baseline measurements, have already been made and the follow-up period has already taken place. Retrospective cohort studies have the advantage over case-control studies that all of the subjects who developed the outcome (cases) and all those who did not (controls) come from the same population. This minimizes the potential for bias that may arise from selecting cases and controls from different sources (see Chapter 8).

Weaknesses

In a retrospective cohort study, the investigator has no control over the nature and the quality of the measurements that were made. The existing data may not include information that is important to answering the research question. The study of exercise and CHD in Harvard alumni (1), for example, did not collect information about social supports and, therefore, could not be used to study whether alumni with more social sup-

Steps:
1. Identify a cohort that has been assembled in the past
2. Collect data on predictor variables (measured in the past)
3. Follow-up the cohort
4. Collect data on outcome variables (measured in past or present)

Figure 7.2. Retrospective cohort design

port have lower mortality rates. Even if the existing data include information about key variables, they may be incomplete, inaccurate, or measured in ways that are not ideal for answering the research question.

NESTED CASE-CONTROL STUDIES

Structure

A nested case-control design literally has a case-control study "nested" within a prospective or retrospective cohort study. It is an excellent design for predictor variables that are expensive, and that can be measured at the *end* of the study.

The investigator begins by identifying a suitable cohort of subjects with enough cases to provide adequate statistical power to answer the research question. The investigator describes the criteria that define the outcome of interest and then identifies all of the individuals in the cohort who have developed the outcome (the cases). Next, the investigator selects a probability sample of subjects who were also part of the cohort but who have not developed the outcome of interest (the controls). The investigator then retrieves samples or records that were taken before the outcomes had occurred, measures the predic-

tor variables for cases and controls, and compares levels of the risk factor in cases to the levels in the sample of controls.

Example 7.3

To determine whether low levels of vitamins A and E and carotenoids increase the risk of cancer, Willett and colleagues (4) conducted a nested case-control study: The basic steps in performing this study were to:

1. *Identify a cohort with adequate samples*: The investigators obtained permisssion to study 10,940 subjects from the Hypertension Detection and Follow-up Program (HDFP) study who had serum drawn during their baseline examination and put into frozen storage.
2. *Identify cases at the end of follow-up*: Based on a review of hospital records and death certificates, the investigators identified 111 subjects who had developed cancer during the 20 year follow-up.
3. *Select controls*: The investigators drew a sample of 210 controls who matched the cases by age, race and sex.
4. *Measure predictors on baseline samples from cases and controls*: Levels of vitamins A and E and caretenoids were measured in the samples of frozen serum from the baseline examination of cases and controls.

There were no significant differences in the concentrations of these vitamins between the groups, suggesting that reduced serum concentrations of

Steps:

    1. Identify a cohort with a bank of specimens collected at baseline
    2. Identify those who develop the disease during followup (the cases)
    3. Select a sample of the rest (the controls)
    4. Measure predictor variable in the baseline bank of specimens

Figure 7.3. Nested case-control design

these vitamins do not play a role in the occurrence of cancer.

Strengths

Nested case-control studies are most useful for costly analyses of specimens, like biochemical analyses of serum samples, that are taken at the beginning of the study and then preserved for later analysis. Making expensive measurements on cases and only a sample of controls is much less costly than making those measurements on the entire cohort. For example, in the study described in Example 7.3, measuring vitamin levels in 111 cases and 210 controls was far less expensive than measuring those levels in the entire cohort of 11,000. When data are available for the entire cohort at no additional cost, then nothing is gained by studying only a sample of controls; the analysis should be conducted on the whole cohort.

This design preserves all the advantages of cohort studies that result from collecting predictor variables before the outcomes have happened. In addition, if the cases are a complete sample of cases in that cohort, including fatal cases, this design avoids the potential biases of other case-control designs that cannot include fatal cases. Because all controls are drawn from the same cohort, this design can also minimize the problems that can arise in other types of case-control studies where cases and control subjects are taken from different populations (Chapter 8).

Controls selected for nested studies should be a probability sample of all members of the cohort who did not develop the outcome (see Chapter 3). However, if subjects have been followed for different lengths of time, for each case it may be best to select a control that entered the study at approximately the same time (5). In certain situations, matching controls to selected characteristics of cases, as was done in the study of vitamins and cancer, might also improve the statistical power of this design, but the decision to match should be considered cautiously because matching makes it impossible to analyze the factors that have been used to match the groups and it may also have other undesirable effects (Chapter 10).

Weaknesses

Opportunities for nested case-control studies are limited to research questions that involve expensive measurements that can be carried out on baseline samples preserved until the outcomes are known. This design has been used less often than it could be, however. Investigators who are planning large prospective studies should consider preserving biologic samples (e.g., creating banks of frozen sera) or storing voluminous records for subsequent nested case-control analyses.

Opportunities for *retrospective* nested case-control studies are limited because existing cohort or experimental studies may not have preserved samples that are adequate to answer the investigator's research question. Additionally, samples or records may have been lost or deteriorated with time.

The investigator may decide to collect new samples or new information from the cases and the sample of controls. For example, in Example 7.3, the investigator could also interview cases and controls about their past dietary intake of foods rich in vitamins A or E. This has the advantage that cases and controls are all from the same cohort. Because the data are collected after the outcomes are known, however, the design forfeits the advantages of prospective collection of data: one cannot be certain that the dietary habits actually preceded the cancers, and the recall of cases about their diets might be influenced by knowing that they have cancer.

This design shares certain disadvantages of other cohort designs: the possibilities that observed associations are due to the effect of confounding variables and (in studies of slowly progresssive diseases) that some baseline measurements may be affected by silent preclinical disease.

DOUBLE-COHORT STUDIES AND EXTERNAL CONTROLS

Structure

Double-cohort studies have two distinct samples of subjects: one group with exposure to a potential risk factor and a second group of controls that have no exposure or a lower level of exposure (Fig. 7.4). After defining suitable cohorts that have an adequate number of subjects or outcomes, the investigator proceeds to measure predictor variables (the exposure and the potential confounding variables) and to assess outcomes, either prospectively or retrospectively, as in any other type of cohort study.

Although the double-cohort design uses two different samples of subjects, it should not be confused with the case-control design (Chapter 8). The samples in a double-cohort study are chosen on the basis of having different *exposures* to a potential risk factor. In contrast, in a case-control study the cases have the *outcome* of interest and controls do not.

The double-cohort design is used in occupational and environmental medicine where, for example, two separate groups may have different levels of exposure to a certain factor and differences in subsequent outcomes are used to assess the effect of the exposure.

Example 7.4.

To determine whether physicians who were exposed to radiation had higher mortality rates, Matanoski and colleagues (6) undertook a *triple* cohort study. The basic steps in performing the study were to:

1. *Identify cohorts with different exposures*: The investigators obtained the membership lists for the Radiological Society of North America, the American College of Physicians, and the American Academy of Opthalmology and Otolaryngology; the lists included all who had joined since 1920.
2. *Determine outcomes*: The investigators determined the vital status for all members of these societies as of 1969, including year and cause of death for those who had died.

Radiologists had a higher mortality rate than the members of the other two societies, supporting the hypothesis that exposure to radiation increased mortality rates.

A variant of the double-cohort design is to compare the outcomes of members of a study cohort to data from a census or registry, which take the place of a second cohort. For example, to determine whether uranium miners had an increased incidence of lung cancer, Wagoner and colleagues (7) compared the incidence of respiratory cancer in 3415 uranium miners with that of white men who lived in the same states. The increased incidence of lung cancer observed in the miners helped establish occupational exposure to ionizing radiation as an important cause of lung cancer.

Strengths

The double-cohort design may be the only feasible approach for studying rare exposures, and exposures to potential occupational and environmental hazards. Using data from a census or registry as the external control group has the additional advantage of being population-based and economical. Otherwise, the strengths of this design are similar to those of other cohort studies.

Weaknesses

The problem of confounding is often accentuated in a double cohort study. The cohorts may be different in other important ways, besides exposure to the predictor variable, that could influence the outcomes. Some of these potentially confounding differences may be measurable, others may be unknown or impossible to measure. Similarly, population groups that are used as external controls may be different in important ways from the subjects enrolled in a cohort study. Although some of these differences, such as age and race, may be known, other important data about the control population may not be available.

Double-cohort studies that are done retrospectively share a shortcoming common to other retrospective cohort studies. The data may not have been collected for research purposes (e.g., medical records kept by an industrial clinic) or may have been collected for very different research purposes. Thus, important data may be imprecisely recorded, incomplete, or non-existent.

STEPS IN PLANNING A COHORT STUDY

When to use a cohort design

There are several reasons for choosing a cohort design over less expensive and less time

<u>**Steps:**</u>

1. Select samples from populations with different levels of the predictor
2. Follow-up the cohorts
3. Measure outcome variables

Figure 7.4. Prospective double-cohort design (double-cohort studies can also be conducted retrospectively).

consuming designs. *First,* this is the best design for accurately describing the incidence and natural history of a condition. *Second,* cohort studies are often the only way to establish the temporal sequence of predictor and outcome variables. Low concentrations of vitamin A and E in the serum of cases with cancer, for example, could be an effect of the cancer rather than its cause. To be certain that the lower concentrations of vitamins really came first, it is essential to measure them long before the cancer is diagnosed. *Third,* cohort studies are the only way to study certain rapidly fatal diseases. To study whether exercise protects against cardiac arrest, for example, an investigator might interview survivors of cardiac arrests about their previous exercise habits. However, excluding those whose cardiac arrest was fatal may distort the results. Avoiding this **survivor bias** generally requires a cohort design. *Fourth,* cohort studies permit the investigator to study numerous outcome variables (e.g., all of the health consequences of smoking) whereas a case-control study is limited to a single outcome. And *finally,* as the follow-up of a cohort continues and more events accumulate, a cohort study gains power to study an ever-increasing number of health outcomes. The advent of the National Death Index (Chapter 6) has

made long term mortality follow-up a cheap and easy option for any cohort study.

Choosing among cohort designs

If the research question can be answered with data that already exist, then a **retrospective cohort design** is by far the most economical and quickest approach. An investigator should search for studies and sources of data on exisiting cohorts or stored biological samples from cohorts that might be suitable for answering the question (see Chapter 6).

If the research question involves outcomes that occur very frequently, such as discharge to a nursing home after hospitalization for a hip fracture, then a **prospective cohort design** may be relatively inexpensive and has many advantages. If the outcomes are less common, such as the occurrence of hip fractures in healthy older women, then a prospective cohort study will be much more expensive and will require many years of follow-up. In this case, a prospective cohort study should be done only if the questions are important to public health. In general, a prospective cohort study should be undertaken when less expensive approaches fail to answer the important questions satisfactorily, when good case-control studies have produced results that conflict, or when certain key measurements must be made before the outcome occurs.

Selecting subjects

The hallmark of a cohort study is the definition of a group of subjects at the beginning of a period of follow-up (Fig. 7.1). As in any study, subjects should be selected who are appropriate to the research question (Chapter 3). No subject should be included who cannot develop the outcome of interest. This means that a study of risk factors for cervical cancer, for example, should exclude women who have had a hysterectomy. If a condition can recur, it may be reasonable to include subjects who have had the outcome of interest once before in order to study the risk of recurrence. A study of risk factors for hip fracture, for example, may include patients with a previous hip fracture because they are at risk for fractures of the other hip or recurrent fractures in the same hip.

To minimize the size, duration, and expense of the study, it may be important to select samples that have a relatively high incidence of the outcomes of interest. For example, a study of predictors of hip fracture might include only elderly white women because they have the highest incidence of such fractures.

Selection of subjects for a cohort study also depends on whether the primary purpose of the study is descriptive or analytic. If the primary aim is *descriptive*, to estimate of the incidence or natural history of a condition, then the sample must closely resemble the target population to which the results will be applied. If the primary purpose is *analytic*, to analyze potential relationships between predictor variables and outcomes, the most important consideration is that the sample contain enough subjects with the major predictor characteristics and a sufficient number of outcomes during the study to allow meaningful analyses of the results. Ideally, the subjects for any cohort study would be a probability sample of the target population for whom the research question is important. But such samples are rarely assembled because they are difficult and expensive to recruit into a study.

Double-cohort studies select subjects based on their exposure to potential risk factors. To help control confounding in these studies, subjects selected for the comparison group are sometimes "matched" to subjects in the exposed group on the basis of characteristics such as age or race. However, matching often has disadvantages that outweigh the advantages (see Chapter 10).

Measuring predictor and confounding variables

The quality of the results of the study will depend on the quality of the measurement of the main predictor and outcome variables. The ability to draw inferences about cause and effect will also depend on how completely and accurately the investigator has measured potential important confounders (see Chapter 10).

Some predictor variables may change during the study; people may change their exercise habits, for example. If a variable tends to change, then a single measurement taken at entry into a long-term study will provide a less complete and less accurate picture of the predictor variable than measurements that are repeated during the period of follow-up. However, having subjects return for periodic measurements is an expensive and sometimes difficult strategy. Whether and how frequently measurements should be repeated depends on these practical considerations and on the nature of the characteristic to be measured. A subject's use of medications may change from year to year, and require yearly updates. In contrast, serum cholesterol levels tend to remain stable from year to year, so that a single baseline measurement may suffice.

Following subjects and measuring outcomes

Complete follow-up of subjects is particularly important to cohort studies that aim to describe the incidence of relatively uncommon outcomes such as CHD in healthy Harvard alumni. Even a small loss of subjects who developed CHD could cause the study to seriously underestimate the true incidence of CHD.

Loss of subjects can be minimized in several ways (Table 7.1). Subjects who plan to move out of reach during the study or who will be very difficult to follow for other reasons should be excluded. At entry to the study, the investigator should collect information that will allow the subjects to be found if they move or die, such as the names, addresses, and telephone numbers of their personal physician and of one or two close friends or relatives who do not live with them. It is important to obtain the subjects' social security and (for those over 65) Medicare numbers. This information will allow the investigator to determine the vital status of subjects who are lost to follow-up using the National Death Index and to obtain hospital discharge information from the Social Security Administration for subjects who receive Medicare. Periodic contact with the subjects during the study helps keep track of them and may improve the timeliness and accuracy of recording the outcomes of interest. Finding subjects for follow-up assessments sometimes requires persistent and repeated efforts by mail, telephone, or even personal visits.

Outcomes should be assessed using standardized criteria and blindly—without awareness of the values of the predictor variables. If an investigator knew the exercise habits of the subjects, for example, he might be more aggressive in looking for CHD among those who were more sedentary, or more permissive in classifying clinical findings as due to CHD. This bias could create a spurious association between sedentary lifestyle and the risk of CHD.

Table 7.1.
Strategies for Minimizing Losses during Follow-up

During design and enrollment

1. Exclude those likely to be lost
   a. Planning to move
   b. Unwilling to return
2. Obtain information to allow future tracking
   a. Complete address and telephone number(s) from subject
   b. Address and telephone for one or two close friends or relatives who do not live with the subject
   c. Name, address, and telephone number of primary physician
   d. Social security (and Medicare) numbers

During follow-up

1. Periodic contact with subjects
   a. By telephone: multiple attempts, including calls during weekends and evenings
   b. By mail: repeated mailings with stamped, self-addressed return cards or envelopes
2. For those who are not reached by phone or mail:
   a. Contact friends, relatives, or physicians
   b. Request forwarding addresses from postal service
   c. Determine vital status from National Death Registry
   d. (for subjects receiving Medicare) Collect data about hospital discharges from Social Security Administration
   e. Seek address through other sources, such as telephone directories and voter registration, drivers license, and credit bureau listings

Analyzing cohort studies: incidence and relative risk

Cohort studies describe the change in a continuous outcome measure, or the incidence of a categorical outcome, over the period of observation. Descriptive statistics including means and proportions are accompanied by statistics describing the variability of the point estimates, such as standard deviations, ranges, and confidence intervals (see Chapter 15).

Associations between predictor and outcome variables in a cohort study are described using **relative risk** or similar statistics (8). Relative risk is the ratio of the risk of an outcome in persons with the factor of interest to the risk in those without the factor. It is calculated by dividing the rate of the outcome in exposed subjects by the rate in the unexposed subjects (see Example 7.1).

The choice of statistical tests and models for analysis of cohort studies depends on a number of factors, including 1) the type of predictor and outcome variables (categorical or continuous), 2) whether the distribution of data is appropriate for the test, and 3) whether subjects are followed for the same or different lengths of time until outcomes occur. The analysis of nested case-control studies must take into account the way the cases and controls were sampled (5). Approaches to controlling and analyzing the effects of confounding variables are discussed in Chapter 10. All of theses topics are discussed in more detail in the book on observational epidemiology by Kelsey (8).

SUMMARY

1. In *cohort studies*, subjects are followed over a period of time in order to *describe* the incidence or natural history of a condition and to *analyse* predictors (*risk factors*) for various outcomes.

2. *Prospective cohort studies* can provide strong evidence for cause-and-effect relationships because the predictor is measured before the outcome occurs; this establishes the sequence of events and helps control potential bias in measurement of predictor variables. When a disease is rapidly progressive or has common outcomes, the prospective cohort design is an especially efficient design.

3. Many cohort studies require large numbers of subjects followed for long periods of time. This disadvantage can sometimes be overcome by analyzing records or samples that have already been collected, using a *retrospective cohort design*.

4. Another cost effective variant is the *nested case-control design*; a bank of specimens is collected at baseline, and stored until the end of the study when measurements are made on the specimens for all subjects who have developed the disease and for a subset of those who have not.

5. The *double-cohort design*, which compares the incidence of outcomes in cohorts whose members have different levels of exposure to some factor, is a useful tool for studying the effects of rare and occupational exposures. A census or registry can provide an efficient *external control group*. These designs have the disadvantage that differences between the outcomes of the cohorts may be due to other differences between the groups besides exposure to the factor of interest.

6. In order to strengthen inferences about cause and effect, it is important to measure all important potential *confounding factors* that might explain the relationship between the predictor and outcome.

7. The strengths of a cohort design can be undermined by *incomplete follow-up* of subjects. These losses can be avoided by excluding subjects who are not likely to be available for follow-up, and by a system of periodic tracking and vigorous pursuit of all subjects.

8. To prevent biased assessment of outcomes, *measurement of outcomes should be carefully standardized*; whenever possible, those who ascertain the outcomes should be *blinded* to the values of predictor variables.

9. Cohort studies produce information about the *incidence of outcomes* and the

relative risk, the ratio of the incidence of disease in subjects exposed to a certain factor to the incidence in those who are not exposed.

REFERENCES

1. Paffenberger RS, Hyde RT, Wing AL, et al: A natural history of athleticism and cardiovascular health. *JAMA* 252:491–495, 1984.
2. Lerchen ML, Samet JM: An assessment of the validity of questionnaire responses provided by a surviving spouse. *Am J Epidemiol* 123:481–489, 1986.
3. Nishimura RA, McGoon MD, Shub C, Miller FA, Ilstrup DM, Tajik AJ: Echocardiographically documented mitral-valve prolapse. Long term follow-up of 237 patients. *N Engl J Med* 1985;313:1305–9.
4. Willett WC, Polk BF, Underwood BA: Relation of serum vitamins A and E and carotenoids to the risk of cancer. *N Engl J Med* 310: 430–434, 1984.
5. Flanders WD, Louv WC: The exposure odds ratio in nested case-control studies with competing risks. *Am J Epidemiol* 124: 684–692, 1986.
6. Matanoski GM, Seltser R, Sartwell PE, Elliot EA: The current mortality rates of radiologists and other physician specialists: deaths from all causes and from cancer. *Am J Epidemiol* 101:188–198, 1975.
7. Wagoner JK, Archer VE, Lundin FE, et al: Radiation as the cause of lung cancer among uranium miners. *N Engl J Med* 273:181–187, 1965.
8. Kelsey JL, Thompson WD, Evans AS: Methods in Observational Epidemiology. New York, Oxford University Press, New York, 1986, chapters 4–6.

ADDITIONAL READINGS

Doll R, Hill AB: Mortality in relation to smoking: ten years' observations of British doctors. *Br Med J* 1:1399–1410, 1964. (*A classic study that helped establish both the cohort method and the adverse effects of cigarette smoking.*)

Gracie WA, Ransohoff DF: The natural history of silent gallstones: the innocent gallstone is not a myth. *N Engl J Med* 307: 798–800, 1982. (*An example of a retrospective cohort study: the investigators took advantage of old records of "routine" oral cholecystograms taken on faculty at the University of Michigan to describe the natural history of gallstones.*)

Fletcher RH, Fletcher SW, Wagner EH: *Clinical Epidemiology—the Essentials*. Baltimore, Williams and Wilkins, 1988, chapter 7 (*Describes basic epidemiologic concepts fundamental to cohort studies.*)

Friedman GD: *Primer of Epidemiology*. New York, McGraw-Hill, 1974, pp 104–120. (*A review of the fundamentals of cohort studies.*)

Mendes MS, Comstock GW, Vuilleumier JP, et al: Serum beta-carotene, vitamins A and E, selenium, and the risk of lung cancer. *N Engl J Med* 315: 1250–4, 1986. (*This nested case-control study analysed samples of frozen serum from a 1974 population-based study. They found that subjects who subsequently developed lung cancer had lower levels of vitamin E and beta-carotene in 1974 than did the sample of controls.*)

Nelson KB, Ellenberg JH: Predictors of epilepsy in children who have experienced febrile seizures. *N Engl J Med* 295:1029–1033, 1976. (*A prospective cohort study that described the prognosis and analyzed predictors of recurrent epilepsy.*)

CHAPTER 8

Designing a New Study: II. Cross-sectional and Case-control Studies

Thomas B. Newman, Warren S. Browner,
Steven R. Cummings, and Stephen B. Hulley

INTRODUCTION 75

CROSS-SECTIONAL STUDIES 75
  Structure
  Designing a cross-sectional study
  Strengths and weaknesses of cross-sectional
    studies

SERIAL SURVEYS 78

CASE-CONTROL STUDIES 78
  Structure
  Designing a case-control study
  Strengths of case-control studies
  Weaknesses of case-control studies

CHOOSING AMONG OBSERVATIONAL
  DESIGNS 84

SUMMARY 84

REFERENCES 86

ADDITIONAL READINGS 86

APPENDIX 8.A. Calculating measures of
  association 204

APPENDIX 8.B. Why the odds ratio is a proxy
  for relative risk 206

INTRODUCTION

Chapter 7 dealt with cohort studies, in which the sequence of making the measurements is the same as the chronology of cause and effect: first the predictor, then (after an interval of follow-up) the outcome. In this chapter we turn to two kinds of observational studies in which causal inference is not guided by this logical sequence.

In a **cross-sectional (prevalence)** study, the investigator makes all of his measurements on a single occasion. He draws a sample from the population and looks at distributions of variables within that sample; he may then infer cause and effect from associations between variables he decides (using information from various sources) to designate as predictor and outcome. In a **case-control** study, the investigator works backward; he begins with the outcome, choosing one sample from a population of patients with the disease (the cases) and another from a population without it (the controls). He then compares the levels of the predictor variables in the two samples to see which ones are associated with the disease outcome.

CROSS-SECTIONAL STUDIES

Structure

The structure of a cross-sectional study is similar to that of a cohort study except that all the measurements are made at once, with no follow-up period (Fig. 8.1). Cross-sectional designs are very well suited to the goal of **describing variables** and their distribution patterns; in the Health and Nutrition Examination Survey (HANES), for example, a sample carefully selected to represent the U.S. population was interviewed and examined (1). The HANES is a major source of information about the health and habits of the U.S. population, providing estimates of such things as the prevalence of hypertension and the average daily fat intake.

Cross-sectional studies can also be used

THE PRESENT

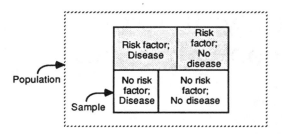

Steps:

1. Select a sample from the population
2. Measure predictor and outcome variables

Figure 8.1. Cross-sectional design

for **examining associations**, although the choice of which variables to label as predictors and which as outcomes depends on the cause and effect hypotheses of the investigator, rather than on the study design. This choice is easy for constitutional factors such as age and race; these cannot usually be altered by other variables and therefore are generally predictors. For most variables, however, the choice is more difficult. The cross-sectional finding of an association between blood lead level and childhood hyperactivity could either occur if children who eat peeling chips of lead paint become hyperactive, or if hyperactive children are more likely to eat paint chips. One solution to this problem is to collect historic information on the time course—did the child have a history of chewing on painted objects before he became hyperactive?

Designing a cross-sectional study

The approach to designing a cross-sectional study follows the general pattern established in Chapters 1–4 and spelled out for cohort studies in Chapter 7. The first step is to settle on the research question. Next the investigator must specify criteria for the target and accessible populations and establish the design for drawing the sample. Then he decides what phenomena to study in this sample, and defines the approach to measuring appropriate variables.

Example 8.1 presents a cross-sectional

study of the risk factors for sexually transmitted disease among women attending a venereal disease clinic. The investigator asks each woman about past oral contraceptive use, and sends a cervical swab to the lab for chlamydia culture. Note that there are several time elements in this study: the predictor variable addresses the use of oral contraceptives over the past year, the outcome variable is not available until several days later, and the investigator takes 6 months to examine all the women. The study is still cross-sectional, however, because the investigator makes all the measurements for each subject on a single occasion.

Example 8.1
The research questions are: What is the prevalence of chlamydia in the population, and is it associated with the use of oral contraceptives? In a cross-sectional study to answer these questions, the investigator might:

1. *Select a sample* of 100 women attending a venereal disease clinic.
2. *Measure the predictor and outcome variables* by taking a history of oral contraceptive use and sending a cervical swab to the lab for chlamydia culture.

Suppose the findings are that 50 of the women report taking oral contraceptives, and that 10 of these women have positive cultures, compared with 5 of the 50 women not taking oral contraceptives. Then, the overall prevalence of chlamydia infection in this sample of venereal disease clinic users (who may not represent the general popoulation) is 15 in 100 (15%) and there is an association between oral contraceptive use and chlamydia that has a relative prevalence of $10/5=2.0$.

Example 8.1 reveals an important *descriptive statistic* obtained from all cross-sectional studies, the **prevalence**. (In fact, such studies are often called "prevalence studies.") Prevalence is the proportion of the population who *have* a disease *at one point in time,* and is distinguished from incidence (the statistic obtained from a cohort study) which is the proportion who *get* the disease *over a period of time* (Table 8.1). Although the term is often applied to a disease, it can be used broadly, so that prevalence of risk factors or any other attribute can be studied. Prevalence is useful to the health planner who wants to know how many people have

Table 8.1.
Statistics for expressing disease frequency in observational studies

Type of Study	Statistic	Definition
Cross-sectional	Prevalence	$\dfrac{\text{Number of people who have the disease at one point in time}}{\text{Number of people at risk at that point}}$
Cohort	Incidence	$\dfrac{\text{Number of new cases of disease over a period of time}}{\text{Number of people at risk during that period}}$

certain diseases so that he can allocate enough resources to care for them, and it is useful to the clinician who must estimate the likelihood that the patient sitting in his office has a particular disease. Other important descriptive data obtained from cross-sectional studies include means, proportions, and other statistics for describing individual variables.

Example 8.1 also gives an example of an *analytic statistic* obtained from cross-sectional studies, the **relative prevalence**. This is the ratio of the prevalence of an outcome in subjects classified by their level of a predictor variable. It is a measure of association, the cross-sectional analogue of relative risk, and in fact a good approximation of relative risk if the risk factor does not affect the *duration* of the outcome (see prevalence/incidence bias, page 78).

Strengths and weaknesses of cross-sectional studies

A major **strength** of cross-sectional studies over cohort studies (and experiments) is that there is no waiting to see who will get the disease. This makes them relatively fast and inexpensive, and it means that there is no problem with loss to follow-up. The cross-sectional design is the only one to give the prevalence of a disease or risk factor. Cross-sectional studies are convenient for examining networks of causal links; in Example 8.1, the investigator could examine age as a predictor of the outcome oral contraceptive use, and then examine oral contraceptive use as a predictor of the outcome chlamydia infection.

Cross-sectional designs can be included as the first step in a cohort study or experiment at little or no added cost. The results define the demographic and clinical charac-

teristics of the study group at baseline, and can sometimes reveal cross-sectional associations of interest. A report on the cross-sectional association between alcohol intake and HDL-cholesterol level (2), for example, was one of the earliest demonstrations of a relationship that was later shown in cohort studies and experiments to represent cause and effect (3).

A **weakness** of cross-sectional studies is the difficulty of establishing causal relationships from data collected in a cross-sectional time frame. (Strategies to establish the causal link are discussed in Chapter 10.) Cross-sectional studies are also impractical for the study of rare diseases if the design involves collecting data on a sample of individuals from the general population. A cross-sectional study of stomach cancer in 45–59 year old men, for example, would need about 10,000 subjects to find just one case.

Cross-sectional studies *can* be done on rare diseases if the sample is drawn from a population of diseased patients rather than from the general population. A **case series** of this sort is better suited to describing the characteristics of the disease than to analyzing differences between these patients and healthy people, although informal comparisons with prior experience can sometimes identify very strong risk factors. Of the first 1000 patients with AIDS, for example, 727 were homosexual or bisexual males and 236 were i.v. drug abusers (4). It did not require a formal control group to conclude that these groups were at increased risk. Furthermore, within a sample of patients with a disease there may be associations of interest, for example, the higher risk of Kaposi sarcoma among AIDS patients who are homosexual than among those who are i.v. drug abusers.

The fact that cross-sectional studies can only measure prevalence, and not incidence, limits the information they can produce on prognosis and natural history. Morover, they are susceptible to **prevalence/incidence bias** in which effects of a risk factor on disease duration are mistaken for effects on disease occurrence. For example, an initial report of a high frequency of the A2 human lymphocyte antigen (HLA-A2) among children with acute lymphocytic leukemia suggested that children with this HLA type were at increased risk of acquiring this disease (5). Subsequent studies, however, showed that HLA-A2 was not a risk factor for the incidence of leukemia—it was actually associated with an *improved* prognosis, and the longer lifespan of leukemic children with HLA-A2 made them more likely to be included in a cross-sectional study than children with other HLA types (6).

SERIAL SURVEYS

A series of cross-sectional studies of a single population observed at several points in time is sometimes used to draw inferences about changing patterns over time. A good example is the use of census data to characterize changes in the age structure of the U.S. population from one decade to the next. This is not a cohort design because it does not follow a single group of people over time—there are changes in the population through birth, death, and migration into and out of the U.S.

The **serial survey** design is also useful when the investigator wants to characterize changes in a population over time, but is concerned that in a cohort design the initial examination will produce a learning effect, influencing the responses to follow-up examinations. An example is the Stanford Five-City Project, which sampled the populations of five California cities over a number of years to observe trends in the prevalence of CHD risk factors. Two kinds of samples were drawn in each city, one a true cohort of individuals in whom the factors predicting within-individual changes could be observed, and the other a series of independent samples of new individuals who had not

been contaminated by the health education effect of a prior examination (7).

CASE-CONTROL STUDIES

Structure

To investigate the causes of all but the most common diseases, both cohort and cross-sectional studies are expensive: each would require thousands of subjects to identify risk factors for a rare disease like stomach cancer. We have seen that a case series of patients with the disease can identify an obvious risk factor (such as homosexuality for AIDS), using prior knowledge of the prevalence of the risk factor in the general population. For most risk factors, however, it is necessary to assemble a reference group, so that the prevalence of the risk factor in subjects with the disease (cases) can be compared with the prevalence in subjects without the disease (controls).

The structure of a case-control study is shown in Figure 8.2. Whereas cohort studies begin with people at risk and follow them forward in time to see who gets the disease, and cross-sectional studies look at a single point in time, case-control studies are generally **retrospective**. They identify groups of subjects with and without the disease, then look backward in time to find differences in predictor variables that may explain why the cases got the disease and the controls did not[a].

Case-control studies are the "house red" on the research design wine list: more mod-

---

[a] Two notes on the terminology used in this chapter:

(1) Case-control studies are most commonly used to compare people who have a disease to those who do not, but the design works equally well for comparing any two populations. For example, to identify predictors of successful smoking cessation, the "cases" could be successful quitters, and the "controls" could be patients who continued to smoke.

(2) The terms "predictor" and "outcome" variable can be confusing in a case-control study. From a statistical viewpoint, the search for associations in these studies uses the presence or absence of the disease as the predictor and the level of various risk factors as the outcome. However, this reverses the biologic meaning of these terms, and we have elected to continue the convention of using predictors and outcomes to reflect the putative cause and effect relationships.

Steps:

1. Select a sample from a population of people with the disease (cases)
2. Select a sample from a population at risk that is free of the disease (controls)
3. Measure predictor variables

Figure 8.2. Case-control design.

est and a little riskier than the other selections, but much less expensive and sometimes surprisingly good. The design of a case-control study is challenging because of the increased opportunities for bias, but there are many examples of well-designed studies that have yielded important results, such as the links between vaginal cancer and diethylstilbestrol (8), Reye's syndrome and aspirin (9), and toxic shock syndrome and Rely® tampons (10,11).

Designing a case-control study

The approach to designing a case-control study (Example 8.2) begins, as usual, with the research question. Next the investigator specifies criteria, first for the target and accessible populations of subjects who have the disease (the cases) and then for the target and accessible populations of subjects who do not have it (the controls); he also establishes designs for drawing samples from these populations. Finally he defines the variables and measurement approaches, and establishes the hypotheses to be tested. These steps are challenging, particularly the selection of study subjects and the blinding of predictor variable measurements, and we shall discuss them at length in the sections below.

Example 8.2.
The research question is whether there is an association between use of aspirin and the development of Reye's syndrome, a rare but serious childhood illness. In a case-control study to answer this question the investigator might:

1. *Draw the sample of cases*—all 30 patients with Reye's syndrome who are accessible to him for study;
2. *Draw the sample of controls*—60 patients drawn from the much larger population of accessible patients who have had minor viral illnesses without Reye's syndrome; and
3. *Measure the predictor variables*—ask the subjects in both groups about their use of aspirin.

Suppose the findings are that 28 of the 30 cases reported taking aspirin during the viral illness that preceded the Reye's syndrome, whereas only 35 of the 60 controls took aspirin. The prevalence and incidence of Reye's syndrome cannot be estimated, but the relative risk associated with aspirin can be approximated by the odds ratio, which is computed to be 10.0 (see Appendix 8.A for the calculation).

Case-control studies cannot yield estimates of the incidence or prevalence of a disease, because the proportion of study subjects who have the disease is determined by how many cases and how many controls the investigator chooses to sample, rather than by their proportions in the population.

What case-control studies do provide is some descriptive information on the characteristics of the cases and, more important, an estimate of the strength of the association between each predictor variable and the presence or absence of the disease. These estimates are in the form of the **odds ratio**, which approximates the relative risk if the prevalence of the disease is not too high (Appendix 8.B.)

Strengths of Case-Control Studies

Efficiency for rare outcomes: One of the major strengths of case-control studies is their high yield of information from relatively few subjects. Consider a study of the effect of circumcision on subsequent carcinoma of the penis. This cancer is very rare in circumcised men, but is also rare in uncircumcised men: their lifetime cumulative incidence is about 0.16% (12). To do a cohort study with a reasonable chance (80%) of detecting even a very strong risk factor (say a relative risk of 50) would require more than 6000 men, assuming that roughly equal proportions were circumcised and uncircumcised. A randomized clinical trial of circumcision at birth would require the same sample size, but the cases would occur at a median of 67 years after entry into the study. It would take three generations of epidemiologists to follow the subjects! Now consider a case-control study of the same question. For the same chance of detecting the same relative risk, only 16 cases and 16 controls (and not much investigator time) would be required. For diseases that are either rare, or have long latent periods between exposure and disease, case-control studies are far more efficient than the other designs. In fact, they are often the only feasible option.

Usefulness for generating hypotheses: The retrospective approach of case-control studies, and their ability to examine a large number of predictor variables, makes them useful for generating hypotheses about the causes of a new outbreak of disease. An epidemic simulating neonatal sepsis (but with negative cultures) recently occurred in a Toronto neonatal intensive care unit (13). Investigators assembled the 16 cases and

compared them with 17 control babies who were in the nursery at the same time but did not become ill. The surprising finding, which emerged because the investigators measured everything they could think of, was that cases were much more likely to have received oral vitamin supplements. This led to the discovery of a medication error: epinephrine had been substituted for Vitamin E, the bottles being nearly identical. This hypothesis was then confirmed by examining previously collected gastric aspirates from the cases and finding high levels of epinephrine.

Weaknesses of case-control studies

Case control studies are a cheap and practical way to investigate risk factors for rare diseases, or to generate hypotheses about new diseases or unusual outbreaks. These are great strengths, but they are achieved at a considerable cost. The information available in case-control studies is limited: there is no direct way to estimate the incidence or prevalence of the disease, nor the attributable or excess risk. There is also the problem that only one outcome can be studied (the presence or absence of the disease that was the criterion for drawing the two samples), whereas cohort and cross-sectional studies (and experiments) can study any number of outcome variables. But the biggest weakness of case-control studies is their *increased susceptibility to bias.* This bias comes chiefly from two sources: the separate sampling of the cases and controls, and the retrospective measurement of the predictor variables. These two problems, and the strategies for dealing with them, are the topic of the next two sections.

Sampling bias, and how to control it: The sampling in a case-control study begins with the cases. Ideally, the sample of cases would be a random sample of everyone who has the disease under study. An immediate problem comes up, however. How do we know who has the disease and who does not? In cross-sectional and cohort studies the disease is systematically sought in all the study participants, but in case-control studies the cases must be sampled from patients in whom the disease has already been diagnosed, and who are available for study. This sample is not representative of all patients with the disease because those who are undiagnosed, misdiagnosed, or dead are less likely to be included (Fig. 8.3).

In general, sampling bias is important when the sample of cases is unrepresentative *with respect to the risk factor being studied*. Diseases that almost always require hospitalization and are relatively easy to diagnose, such as anencephaly and traumatic amputations, can be safely sampled from diagnosed and accessible cases. On the other hand, conditions that may not come to medical attention are not well suited to retrospective studies because of the selection that precedes diagnosis. For example, women seen in a gynecology clinic with first-trimester spontaneous abortions would probably differ from the entire population of women experiencing spontaneous abortions because those with greater access to gynecologic care would be over-represented. If a predictor variable of interest is associated with gynecologic care in the population (such as past use of an intrauterine device) sampling from the clinic could be an important source of bias. If, on the other hand, a predictor is unrelated to gynecologic care (such as blood type) there would be less likelihood of sampling bias.

Although it is important to think about these issues, in actual practice the **selection of cases** is often straightforward because the accessible sources of subjects are limited. The sample of cases may not be entirely representative, but it is all there is. The more difficult decisions faced by an investigator designing a case-control study usually relate to the more open-ended task of **selecting the controls**. The general goal is to find an accessible population of people at risk of the disease who otherwise represent the same population as the cases, and there are four main strategies for achieving this goal.

1.   Sampling the cases and controls in the same way: One strategy is to choose a control group that *compensates* for an unrepresentative sample of cases by being unrepresentative in the same way. For example, in the study of past use of an intrauterine device (IUD) as a risk factor for spontaneous abortion, the problem that sampling from a gynecology clinic might yield cases who were unrepresentative because of greater access to gynecologic care could be avoided by selecting controls from a population of women seeking care for vaginitis at the same gynecology clinic. These controls would also represent the population of women with ready access to gynecologic care.

However, selection of an unrepresentative sample of controls to compensate for an unrepresentative sample of cases is a strategy fraught with difficulty (14). If use of an IUD increased the risk of vaginitis, for example, there would be an excess of IUD users among the controls, hiding a possible real association between IUD use and spontaneous abortion. On the other hand, women with more sexual partners, who are at

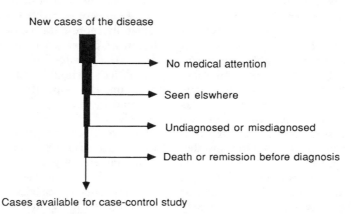

New cases of the disease

→ No medical attention

→ Seen elswhere

→ Undiagnosed or misdiagnosed

→ Death or remission before diagnosis

Cases available for case-control study

Figure 8.3.   Reasons that the cases in a case-control study may not be representative of all cases of the disease.

greater risk of vaginitis, are poor candidates for an IUD because of their greater risk of pelvic infection. This could cause a low prevalence of IUD use in controls, and a spurious association.

Because hospital-based and clinic-based control subjects are usually unwell, and because their diseases may be positively or negatively associated with the risk factors being studied, the use of hospital- or clinic-based controls is not always successful in compensating for an unrepresentative sample of cases. Such control groups are often used, however, because of another consideration in selecting controls: *convenience.* Investigators work in clinics and hospitals, and the populations of control subjects most readily accessible to them are those that are in the hospital or clinic for other reasons. What the investigator must decide is whether the added convenience of hospital- or clinic-based controls is worth the possible threat to the validity of the study.

2. Matching: Matching is a simple method of ensuring that cases and controls are comparable with respect to major factors that are related to the disease but not of interest to the investigator. So many risk factors and diseases are related to age and sex, for example, that the study results may be meaningless unless the cases and controls are made comparable with regard to these two variables. A case-control study of whether hypertension is a risk factor for prostatic cancer in which the cases had higher blood pressures but were also older than the controls would hardly be convincing.

One approach to avoiding this problem is to choose controls that match the cases on constitutional predictor variables related to the outcome such as age, sex, and race. Matching does have its costs, however, particularly when modifiable predictors such as income or serum cholesterol level are matched. The reasons for this, and the general costs and benefits of matching, are discussed in Chapter 10.

3. Using two or more control groups: Because selection of a control group can be so tricky, particularly when the cases may not be a representative sample, it is sometimes advisable to use two or more control groups selected in different ways. The Public Health Service study on Reye's syndrome and medications (9), for example, used four types of controls: emergency room controls (seen in the same emergency room as the case), inpatient controls (admitted to the same hospital as the case), school controls (attending the same school or day care center as the case), and community controls (identified by random-digit dialing). The odds ratios for salicylate use in cases compared to each of these control groups (in the order listed above) were 49.4, 57.5, 9.5, and 12.6, and each was statistically significant. The consistent finding of a strong association using control groups that would have a variety of sampling biases makes a convincing case for the inference that there is a real association in the population.

What happens if the control groups give conflicting results (15)? Luckily, this happens less often than one might expect, and when it does it is helpful, revealing some inherent fragility to the case-control method for the research question at hand. It is much better to have inconsistent results and conclude that the answer is not known than to have just one control group and draw the wrong conclusion.

4. Using a population-based sample: Population-based case-control studies are now possible for many diseases, because of a rapid increase in the use of disease registries. In the San Francisco Bay Area, for example, there are registries of all new cases of cancer, birth defects, and sudden infant death. Because cases obtained from such registries are generally representative of the general population of patients in the area with the disease, the choice of a control group is simplified: it should be a representative sample from the population living in the area covered by the registry. Such a sample can be selected by door-to-door household sampling. A more economic alternative is random-digit dialing; this can include a matching strategy by repeatedly dialing the same prefix as the case (thereby matching roughly on city district) until an age- and sex-matched individual is reached.

As the disease registry approaches completeness and the population it covers approaches complete stability (i.e., no migration in or out), the population-based case-control study approaches a nested case-control cohort study (Chapter 7). This design has the potential for *eliminating* sampling bias, because both cases and controls are selected from the same population. When designing the sampling approach for a case-control study, the nested case-control cohort design is useful to keep in mind as the model to emulate.

Differential measurement bias, and how to control it: The second particular problem of case-control studies is bias that affects one group more than the other caused by the retrospective approach to measuring the predictor variables. Case-control studies of birth defects, for example, are hampered by *differential* recall bias: parents of babies with birth defects may be more likely to recall drug exposures than parents of normal babies, because they will already have been worrying about what caused the defect. Differential recall bias cannot occur in a cohort study, because the parents are asked about exposures before the baby is born.

In addition to the strategies set out in Chapter 4 for controlling biased measurements (standardizing the operational definitions of variables, choosing objective approaches, supplementing key variables with data from several sources, etc.) there are two specific strategies for avoiding bias in measuring risk factors in case-control studies.

1. Use of data recorded before the outcome occurred: It may be possible, for example, to examine the prenatal records in a case-control study of birth defects. This excellent strategy is limited to the extent that recorded information about the risk factor of interest is available and of satisfactory reliability. Bias can still occur, however, if the investigator searches the medical records for evidence of past habits more vigorously in the cases than in the controls. This bias can be controlled by blinding.

2. Blinding: The general approach to blinding was discussed in Chapter 4, but there are some issues that are specific to designing interviews in case-control studies. Because both observers and study subjects could conceivably be blinded both to the case/control status of each subject and to the risk factor being studied, four types of blinding are possible (Table 8.2).

Ideally, neither the study subjects nor the investigators should know which subjects are cases and which are controls. If this can be done successfully, differential bias in measuring the predictor variable can be eliminated. In practice, this is often difficult. The subjects know whether they are sick or well, so they can be blinded to case-control status only if controls are drawn from patients who are also ill, with diseases that could plausibly be related to the risk factors being studied. Efforts to blind the investigators are hampered by the obvious nature of some diseases (an interviewer can hardly help noticing if the patient is jaundiced or has had a laryngectomy), and by the clues that interviewers may discern in the patient's responses.

Table 8.2.
Approaches to blinding interview questions in a case-control study

Person blinded	Blinding case/control status	Blinding specific risk factor being studied
Subject	Possible if both cases and controls have diseases that could plausibly be related to the risk factor.	Include "dummy" risk factors, and be suspicious if they differ between cases and controls. May not work if the risk factor for the disease has already been publicized.
Observer	Possible if cases are not externally distinguishable from controls, but subtle signs and statements volunteered by the subjects make it difficult	Possible if interviewer is not the investigator, but unblinding due to "leaks" or to interviewer noticing trends in the data is hard to stop.

Blinding to the specific risk factor being studied is usually easier than blinding as to case-control status. Both the study subjects and the interviewer can be kept in the dark about the study hypotheses by including "dummy" questions about plausible risk factors not associated with the disease. For example, if the specific hypothesis to be tested is whether honey intake is associated with increased risk of infant botulism, equally detailed questions about jelly, yogurt, and bananas could be included in the interview. This type of blinding does not actually prevent differential bias, but it allows an estimate of whether it is a problem: If the cases report more exposure to honey, but no increase in the other foods, then differential measurement bias is less likely. This strategy would not work if the association between infant botulism and honey had previously been widely publicized, or if some of the dummy risk factors turned out to be real risk factors. In addition, it is hard to keep someone working on a study from hearing about the study's hypotheses, or from generating his own hypotheses during the data collection.

Blinding the observer to the case-control status of the study subject is a particularly good strategy for laboratory measurements such as blood tests and x-rays. Blinding under these circumstances is easy—someone other than the individual who will make the measurement simply applies coded identification labels to each specimen—and it should always be done. Its importance is illustrated by the 15 case-control studies comparing measurements of bone mass between hip fracture patients and controls; much larger differences were formed in the studies that used unblinded measurements than in the blinded studies (16).

CHOOSING AMONG OBSERVATIONAL DESIGNS

The pros and cons of the chief observational designs presented in the last two chapters are summarized in Table 8.3. We have already described these issues in detail, and will make only one final point here. Among all these designs, none is best and none is worst; each has its place and purpose, depending on the research question and the circumstances.

SUMMARY

1. In a *cross-sectional study*, all the variables are measured at a single point in time, with no structural distinction between predictors and outcomes. Cross-sectional studies are valuable for providing descriptive information about *disease prevalence and its correlates*; they also have the advantage of avoiding the time, expense, and dropout problems of a follow-up design.

2. Cross-sectional studies yield *weaker evidence for causality* than cohort studies, however, because the predictor variable is not shown to precede the outcome. A further weakness is the need for a large sample size (compared with that of a case-control study) when studying the prevalence of uncommon diseases and variables in the general population. The cross-sectional design can be used for an uncommon disease in a case series of patients with that disease, however, and it often serves as the *first step of a cohort study or experiment*.

3. In a *case-control* study, the prevalence of risk factors in a sample of subjects who have a disease (the cases) is compared with that in a sample who do not (the controls). This design, in which people with and without the disease are sampled separately, is relatively *inexpensive and uniquely efficient for studying rare diseases*.

4. One problem with case-control studies is their *susceptibility to sampling bias*. The likelihood of sampling bias depends on both the disease and risk factor in question. Four antidotes are to sample controls and cases in the same (admittedly unrepresentative) way, to match the cases and controls, to use several control groups sampled from disparate populations, and to do a population-based study in which all cases in a given region are compared with a random sample of everyone else.

Table 8.3.
Advantages and disadvantages of the major observational design

Design	Advantages	Disadvantages*
COHORT	Establishes sequence of events Avoids bias in measuring predictors Avoids survival bias Can study several outcomes Number of outcome events grows over time Yields incidence, relative risk, excess risk	Often requires large sample sizes Not feasible for rare outcomes
•Prospective	More control over selection of subjects More control over measurements	More expensive Longer duration
•Retrospective	Less expensive Shorter duration	Less control over selection of subjects Less control over measurements
•Double cohort	Useful when distinct cohorts have different or rare exposures	Potential bias from sampling two populations
CROSS-SECTIONAL	May study several outcomes Control over selection of subjects Control over measurements Relatively short duration A good first step for a cohort study Yields prevalence, relative prevalence	Does not establish sequence of events Potential bias in measuring predictors Potential survivor bias Not feasible for rare conditions Does not yield incidence or true relative risk
CASE-CONTROL	Useful for studying rare conditions Short duration Relatively inexpensive Relatively small Yields odds ratio (usually a good approximation of relative risk)	Potential bias from sampling two populations Does not establish sequence of events Potential bias in measuring predictors Potential survivor bias Limited to one outcome variable Does not yield prevalence, incidence or excess risk
NESTED CASE-CONTROL (prospective or retrospective)	Scientific advantages of cohort design Relatively inexpensive	Requires bank of samples stored until outcomes occur

*All of these observational designs have the disadvantage (compared to experiments) of being susceptible to the influence of confounding variables.

5. The other major problem with case-control studies is their *retrospective design*, which makes them susceptible to *differential bias* (between cases and controls) *in measuring the predictor variables*. Such bias can be reduced by obtaining past measurements of the predictor variable, and by blinding the subjects and observers.

REFERENCES

1. National Center for Health Statistics: Plan and operation of the HANES. *Vital and Health Statistics*, Series 1, Nos 10a and 10b. DHEW Pub No (HSM) 73–130. Washington, DC, U.S. Government Printing Office, 1973.
2. Castelli WP, Doyle JT, Gordon T, et al: Alcohol and blood lipids: the Cooperative Lipoprotein Phenotyping Study. *Lancet* 2:153, 1977.
3. Hulley SB, Gordon S: Alcohol and HDL cholesterol: causal inference from diverse study designs. *Circulation* 64:III57–III63, 1981.
4. Jaffe HW, Bregman DJ, Selik RM: Acquired Immune Deficiency in the U.S.: the first 1000 cases. *J Inf Dis* 148:339–345, 1983.
5. Rogentine GN, Yankee RA, Gart JJ, et al: HL-A antigens and disease. Acute lymphocytic leukemia. *J Clin Invest* 51:2420–2428, 1972.
6. Rogentine GN, Trapani RJ, Henderson ES. HL-A antigens and acute lymphocytic leukemia: the nature of the HL-A2 association. *Tissue Antigens* 3:470–476, 1973.
7. Farquhar JW, Fortmann SP, Maccoby N, et al: The Stanford Five-City Project: Design and methods. *Am J Epidemiol* 122:323–334,1985.
8. Herbst AL, Ulfelder H, Poskanzer DC. Adenocarcinoma of the vagina. Association of maternal stilbestrol therapy with tumor appearance in young women. *N Engl J Med* 248:995–1001, 1971.
9. Hurwitz ES, Barrett MJ, Bregman D, et al: Public Health Service study on Reye's syndrome and medications. *N Engl J Med* 313:849–857, 1985.
10. Anon: Follow-up on toxic-shock syndrome. *MMWR* 29:441–445, 1980.
11. Schlech WF, Shands KN, Reingold AL, et al: Risk factors for the development of toxic shock syndrome: association with tampon brand. *JAMA* 248:839, 1982.
12. Kochen M, McCurdy S: Circumcision and the risk of cancer of the penis: a life-table analysis. *Am J Dis Child* 134:484–486, 1980.
13. Wallace EM, Ford-Jones EL, Baker WM, et al: Medication errors with inhalant epinephrine mimicking an epidemic of neonatal sepsis. *N Engl J Med* 310:166–170, 1984.
14. Hutchison GB, Rothman KJ: Correcting a bias? *N Engl J Med* 299:1129–1130, 1978.
15. West DW, Schuman KL, Lyon JL et al: Differences in risk estimations from a hospital and a population-based case-control study. *Int J Epidemiol* 13:235–239, 1984.
16. Cummings SR: Are patients with hip fractures more osteoporotic? *Amer J Med* 78:487–494, 1985.

ADDITIONAL READINGS

Cole P: The evolving case-control study. *J Chron Dis* 32:15–27, 1979. (*A clear discussion of some of the major issues in case-control research.*)

Feinstein AR: Experimental requirements and scientific principles in case-control studies. *J Chron Dis* 38:127–133, 1985. (*Raises some interesting and important issues.*)

Fletcher R, Fletcher S, Wagner E: *Clinical Epidemiology.* Baltimore, Williams & Wilkins, 1988, Ch 10. (*A very clear description; highly recommended.*)

Hayden GF, Kramer MS, Horwitz RI: The case-control study: a practical review for the clinician. *JAMA* 247:326–331, 1982. (*A well-written review.*)

Shlesselman JJ: *Case-Control Studies: Design, Conduct, Analysis.* New York, Oxford University Press, 1982. (*The definitive reference on case-control studies, advanced but clearly and carefully written.*)

Spitzer WO: Ideas and words: two dimensions for debates on case controlling. *J Chron Dis* 38:541–542, 1985. (*Introductory comments on a recent series of reports discussing controversies in methodology and terminology.*)

CHAPTER 9

Designing a New Study: III. Diagnostic Tests

Warren S. Browner, Thomas B. Newman, and Steven R. Cummings

INTRODUCTION **87**

BASIC PRINCIPLES **87**

STRUCTURE **88**
  The test result as the predictor variable
  The disease as the outcome variable

ANALYSIS **88**
  Sensitivity and specificity
  Choice of a cutoff point
  Receiver operator characteristic (ROC) curves
  Prevalence, prior probability, and predictive
    value
  Likelihood ratios

LIMITATIONS AND STRATEGIES **92**
  Random error
  Systematic error

STEPS IN PLANNING A STUDY OF A
  DIAGNOSTIC TEST **95**

SUMMARY **96**

REFERENCES **96**

ADDITIONAL READINGS **97**

— — — — — — — — — — —

INTRODUCTION

Clinical research often involves the evaluation of diagnostic tests *(Among patients with hypertension, is a serum renin level useful in the diagnosis of renovascular disease?).* Diagnostic test studies use designs that resemble those described for other observational studies (Chapters 7 and 8), but their goals and statistics are different. In this chapter, we point out these differences, show how they influence the general approach to this type of study,

and discuss how to design and analyze studies of these sorts of tests.

Studies of prognostic tests *(Does a ten-point scale of trauma severity predict which patients are likely to survive?)* share many features with diagnostic test studies. The main difference between them is the type of outcome variable: diagnostic tests predict the *presence* of a disease; prognostic tests predict the *outcome* of a disease. Although we concentrate on studies of diagnostic tests, readers planning to study a prognostic test can usually just substitute the word "outcome" for the word "disease" when reading this chapter.

BASIC PRINCIPLES

The ideal diagnostic test would always give the right answer—a positive result in everyone with the disease, and a negative result in everyone else—and would be quick, safe, simple, painless, reliable, and inexpensive. But few, if any, tests are ideal; thus there is a need for clinically useful substitutes.

It is helpful to keep two models in mind when designing studies to evaluate the clinical usefulness of diagnostic tests. The first is the **randomized blinded trial**: If patients were randomly assigned to receive the new test (versus the usual diagnostic workup), would the recipients of the new test have a better outcome? Would they have shorter hospital stays, or a longer life expectancy? Or would they just end up with bigger bills?

The second is **usual clinical practice:** Will the test be studied in the same way it would be used in a clinical setting? Demonstrating that a test can separate the very sick from the very healthy does not mean that it will be useful in distinguishing patients with mild cases of the disease from others with similar symptoms. A biochemical test that differentiates skid row alcoholics from teetotalers would not be very helpful, since most people can make that distinction from across a room.

STRUCTURE

Studies of diagnostic tests have a straightforward structure, similar to other types of observational studies. They have a **predictor variable** (the test result) and an **outcome variable** (the presence or absence of the disease).

The test result as the predictor variable

Just like predictor variables in other observational studies, a diagnostic test can have dichotomous, categorical, or continuous values. It is simplest to think about those that have dichotomous results: such tests are either positive or negative. But if categorical or continuous predictors are an option, the investigator should consider their use because they usually contain more information. Consider, for example, a study of whether glycosuria is useful in the diagnosis of pheochromocytoma: the test could give dichotomous (positive, negative), categorical (++++, +++, ++, +, −) or even continuous (milligrams of glucose per deciliter) results.

The disease as the outcome variable

The outcome variable in a diagnostic study is the presence or absence of the disease, as determined with a **gold standard.** A gold standard is always positive in patients with the disease, and negative in those without the disease. Sometimes, however, it is easier to rule in a disease with a gold standard than to rule one out. Suppose an investigator is studying whether a new serum protein is useful in the diagnosis of multiple myeloma. All patients in whom the test is performed must be classified as either having myeloma or not. Although the disease can be definitively diagnosed with a bone marrow aspiration and biopsy, it is not necessarily ruled out in those who have a single bone marrow aspiration and biopsy free of myeloma cells. Serial bone marrow biopsies may not be feasible or ethical. Instead, a reasonable substitute, such as remaining free of evidence of the disease for several years, may be used to "rule out" a disease.

When studying a prognostic test, the outcome variable is the outcome of a disease, such as hospitalization or death. It may be difficult to choose a gold standard for such outcomes. Consider a study of whether respiratory rate in asthmatic patients in an emergency room predicts the need for hospitalization, for example. How should a patient who was not admitted to the hospital ward, but who returned to the emergency room on two more occasions, be classified? Did she "need" hospitalization or not? When facing this type of dilemma, the best solution is usually to redefine the outcome by avoiding one that is ambiguous, such as "needed hospitalization," in favor of one that is indisputable, such as "admitted to the hospital or returned to an emergency room within 2 days."

ANALYSIS

Although the structure of studies of diagnostic (and prognostic) tests resembles that of other observational studies, there is an important difference in how the results are usually analyzed. Most observational studies are designed to provide information about the etiology of a disease, by showing that there is an association between a predictor variable and the disease. Diagnostic test studies, on the other hand, are designed to determine how well a test can discriminate between the diseased and the non-diseased; just showing that there is an association between the test result and the disease is not sufficient.

As an example, consider a test for cancer in women with solitary breast masses (Table 9.1): of 100 patients with biopsy-proven breast cancer, 65 have a positive test; of 100 patients with benign masses, only 30 have a positive test. Statistically, a positive test result is highly associated (P <0.001) with the presence of breast cancer. Nevertheless, the test would not be very useful. More than one in three patients with breast cancer has a negative result, hardly good enough to obviate the need for biopsies in women with negative tests. Furthermore, treating 30% of women with benign breast disease for cancer is not acceptable.

Table 9.1.
Results of a diagnostic test for breast cancer

| Test result | Disease status* | |
	Breast cancer	Benign nodule
Positive	65	30
Negative	35	70

*Of 100 women with breast cancer, 65 have a positive test; of 100 women without breast cancer, 70 have a negative test.

Sensitivity and specificity

When evaluating a diagnostic test (Table 9.2), four situations are possible: (a) a **true-positive** (TP) result: the test is positive and the patient has the disease; (b) a **false-positive** (FP) result: the test is positive but the patient does not have the disease; (c) a **false-negative** (FN) result: the test is negative but the patient has the disease; and (d) a **true-negative** (TN) result: the test is negative and the patient does not have the disease. The best diagnostic tests are those with few false-positives and false-negatives.

Table 9.2.
Determining sensitivity and specificity*

| Test result | Disease status | |
	Present	Absent
Positive	True-positive (TP)	False-positive (FP)
Negative	False-negative (FN)	True-negative (TN)
	TP + FN	FP + TN

*Sensitivity equals TP/(TP+FN). Specificity equals TN/(FP+TN).

In general, diagnostic tests are evaluated by calculating their sensitivity and specificity. **Sensitivity**—the proportion of subjects with the disease who have a positive test—indicates how good a test is at identifying the diseased. It equals TP/(TP+FN). The breast cancer test in the example had a sensitivity of 65%: out of 100 women with breast cancer, 65 had positive tests. **Specificity**—the proportion of subjects without the disease who have a negative test—indicates how good a test is at identifying the nondiseased. It equals TN/(TN+FP). The breast cancer test had a specificity of 70%: of 100 women with benign nodules, 70 had a negative result on the test.

Choice of a cutoff point

Many diagnostic tests, such as a serum alanine aminotransferase (ALT) in the diagnosis of hepatitis, yield continuous results (Fig. 9.1). With such tests, a decision must be made as to what will constitute a positive test, a value called the **cutoff point**. This decision requires trading an increase in sensitivity for a decrease in specificity, or vice versa. Calling an ALT greater than 400 U/liter "positive" would make the test very specific: just about everyone with values that high has hepatitis. But it would also have a low sensitivity, since many patients with hepatitis do not have ALT levels that high. On the other hand, setting the cutoff at 20 U/liter identifies virtually all patients with hepatitis (sensitivity is high), but many patients without hepatitis would also have positive test results (specificity is therefore low).

The investigator must weigh the relative importance of the sensitivity and specificity of the diagnostic test, and set the cutoff point accordingly. One way to do this is to consider the implications of the two possible errors. If false-positive results must be avoided (such as the test result being used to determine whether a patient undergoes dangerous surgery), then the cutoff point might be set to maximize the test's specificity. If false-negative results must be avoided (as with screening for neonatal phenylketonuria), then the cutoff should be set to ensure a high test sensitivity. These principles are covered in greater detail in the texts by

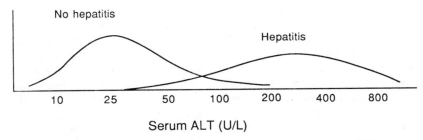

Serum ALT (U/L)

Figure 9.1. Hypothetical distribution of serum alanine aminotransferase (ALT) among patients with and without hepatitis.

Fletcher, Fletcher and Wagner (1), and Sackett, Haynes and Tugwell (2).

Receiver operator characteristic (ROC) curves

Another way to set the cutoff point is to use receiver operator characteristic (ROC) curves. Originally used in electronics, ROC curves are a graphic way of portraying the trade-offs involved between improving either a test's sensitivity or its specificity (Fig. 9.2). The investigator selects several cutoff points, and determines the sensitivity and specificity at each point. She then graphs sensitivity as a function of [1-specificity]; this latter quantity is sometimes called the false-positive rate. The values of the test itself can be written along this curve. An ideal

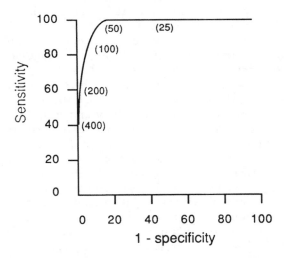

Figure 9.2. ROC curve for serum ALT in the diagnosis of hepatitis, based on the distributions in Fig. 9.1. The ALT values of chosen cutpoints are in parentheses.

test is one that reaches the upper left corner of the graph (100% sensitivity and 100% specificity). A worthless test follows the diagonal from the lower left to the upper right corners: each incremental gain in sensitivity is matched by an equal loss in specificity.

Most ROC curves have a very steep section, in which the sensitivity increases a great deal while the false-positive rate hardly changes. It makes little sense to choose the cut-off point in this section, since moving up the curve will increase sensitivity without substantially reducing specificity. Similarly, selecting the cutoff point in the flat region, in which the sensitivity stays about the same while the false-positive rate increases, is unwise. Usually, the best cutoff point is where the ROC curve "turns the corner," in this case, when the ALT is about 50 U/liter. An important advantage of ROC curves is that the curves for different diagnostic tests can be compared; the better a test, the closer its curve is to the upper left corner.

Prevalence, prior probability and predictive value

The value of a diagnostic test depends not only on its sensitivity and specificity, but also on the **prevalence** of the disease in the population being tested. As the prevalence of a disease decreases it becomes less likely that someone with a positive test actually has the disease, and more likely that the test represents a false-positive. Thus the rarer a disease (such as colon cancer in asymptomatic adults), the more specific a test must be in order to be clinically useful.

Conversely, if a disease is common (such as coronary artery disease among middle-aged smokers with typical angina), a test must be very sensitive to be useful to clinicians. Otherwise, a negative test is likely to represent a false-negative.

In a single patient, the "prevalence" of the disease is usually called the **prior probability.** It is the probability, based on demographic and clinical characteristics, that a particular patient has the disease, as estimated *before* performing the test. The prior probability of coronary artery disease (CAD) would be very low, say 1%, in a young, asymptomatic military recruit, but much higher, say 90%, in a middle-aged smoker with typical angina.

The relationship between the sensitivity and specificity of a test and the prior probability of the disease, can be expressed more formally through the use of Bayes' theorem (3). The **predictive value of a positive test** (PV+) is the probability that a person with a positive result actually has the disease. It equals the likelihood of having a true-positive test divided by the chance of either a true-positive or a false-positive test.

$$PV+ = \frac{\text{Likelihood of a true-positive}}{\text{Likelihood of a true-positive} + \text{Likelihood of a false-positive}}$$

or

$$PV+ = \frac{\text{Sensitivity} \times \text{Prior probability}}{[\text{Sensitivity} \times \text{Prior probability}] + [(1- \text{specificity}) \times (1 - \text{Prior probability})]}$$

Similarly, the **predictive value of a negative test** (PV-) is the probability that a person with a negative result does not have the disease. It equals the likelihood of having a true-negative test divided by the likelihood of either a true-negative or a false-negative test.

$$PV- = \frac{\text{Likelihood of a true-negative}}{\text{Likelihood of a true-negative} + \text{Likelihood of a false-negative}}$$

or

$$PV- = \frac{\text{Specificity} \times (1-\text{Prior probability})}{[\text{Specificity} \times (1 - \text{Prior probability})] + [(1- \text{sensitivity}) \times \text{Prior probability}]}$$

Predictive value is sometimes called the **posterior probability,** since it is determined *after* knowing the test results.

Because it incorporates information on both the test and the population being tested, predictive value is a good measure of overall clinical usefulness. As an example, consider thallium-201 exercise treadmill tests in the diagnosis of CAD (Table 9.3). (Assume that this test has a sensitivity and specificity of about 90% for CAD.) The meaning of a positive test depends on the prior probability of CAD in the person being tested. If the prior probability of CAD is 1%, as in the military recruit, the predictive value of a positive test is only 8%: more than likely, the test had a false-positive result. If the prior probability of CAD is 90%, as in the man with angina, the likelihood of CAD is very high, about 99%. On the other hand, even a negative test would not rule out CAD in the man with angina, who would still have a 50% chance of having CAD.

Likelihood ratios

There is another approach to analyzing the results of a diagnostic test study that is especially useful when a test result is categorical or continuous. This strategy involves determining **likelihood ratios** for the possible test results. A likelihood ratio is simply the likelihood that a person with a disease would have a particular test result divided by the likelihood that a person without the disease would have that result. For example, suppose that an investigator measures asparagine kinase (AK) values in 100 patients with known myocardial infarction (MI), and in 200 patients in whom myocardial infarction has been ruled out (Table 9.4). The likelihood that a patient with an MI would have an AK value less than 100 IU/dl is 15% (15/100), whereas the likelihood that a patient without an MI would have an AK value in this range is 75% (150/200). Thus the likelihood ratio for the diagnosis of MI in patients with AK values less than 100 IU/dl is 1:5 (15% ÷ 75%). Similarly, the likelihood ratio for an AK value between 100 and 199 IU/dl is 5:4, and the likelihood ratio for an AK value of 200 or greater is 12:1.

When combined with information on the prior probability of a disease, likelihood ra-

Table 9.3.
The predictive value of a test with sensitivity of 90% and specificity of 90% at various prior probabilities of disease

Prior probability of disease	Predictive value of a positive test	Predictive value of a negative test
0.001	0.01	0.9999
0.01	0.08	0.999
0.05	0.32	0.994
0.10	0.50	0.99
0.20	0.69	0.97
0.50	0.90	0.90
0.80	0.97	0.69
0.90	0.99	0.50
0.95	0.994	0.32
0.99	0.999	0.08
0.999	0.9999	0.01

tios can be used to determine the predictive value of a particular test result. This requires expressing the prior probability of a disease as the **prior odds** of that disease. The odds of a disease are simply the ratio of the proportion of persons with the disease to the proportion without the disease. If, for example, the prior probability of a disease is 50%, then the prior odds of the disease are 1:1 (50% ÷ 50%); if the prior probability is 25%, then the prior odds are 1:3 (25% ÷ 75%). In general, if the probability of a disease is p, then the odds of the disease are **p:(1-p)**. Conversely, if the odds of a disease are x:y, the probability of the disease is x ÷ (x+y).

The prior odds of the disease are multiplied by the likelihood ratio for the test result to determine the posterior odds of the disease. Suppose, for example, the prior odds of a myocardial infarction in a 45 year old man complaining of an hour of substernal chest pain are 4:1 (i.e, a prior probability of 80%), and the AK value is 150 IU/dl. Multiplying the prior odds (4:1) by the likelihood ratio for

MI with this result (5:4 in Table 9.4) yields the posterior odds of 20:4, or 5:1, a posterior probability of about 83% (5 ÷ 6).

One important advantage of likelihood ratios is that they are a convenient way to express a test's characteristics at a variety of different cutoff points. In addition, likelihood ratios for a sequence of different tests can be multiplied together if the tests are independent, thereby yielding an overall likelihood ratio for a given set of test result (2).

LIMITATIONS AND STRATEGIES

Just like other types of observational research, studies of diagnostic tests are susceptible to errors due to chance and to bias. Design phase (and to a lesser extent, analysis phase) strategies are available to deal with these errors.

Random error

Studies of diagnostic tests are susceptible to random error: by chance alone, some patients with a disease will have normal results

Table 9.4.
Use of likelihood ratios

Aparagine kinase level (IU/dl)	Patients with myocardial infarction	Patients without myocardial infarction	Likelihood ratio
0-99	15	150	15/100 ÷ 150/200 = **1:5**
100-199	25	40	25/100 ÷ 40/200 = **5:4**
>200	60	10	60/100 ÷ 10/200 = **12:1**
Total	100	200	

on a diagnostic test. Although random error is unavoidable, it is quantifiable. The most informative way to quantify random error is to construct **confidence intervals** for the sensitivity and the specificity of the test. Confidence intervals allow the reader to see the range of values consistent with the reported results, and compare that range with other tests. For example, consider an existing diagnostic test, tested in hundreds of patients, that is 80% sensitive and 70% specific. A new diagnostic test is reported to be positive in 5 out of 5 patients with the disease (100% sensitive), and negative in 9 out of 10 without the disease (specificity of 90%). Although impressive, these results are based on just a few subjects. In fact, the 95% confidence interval for the new test's sensitivity runs from about 57% to 100%; for the specificity, it runs from 60% to 98%. Both of these intervals overlap the values for the old test. Thus it is not at all clear that the new test is an improvement; it may even be worse.

To avoid this problem, sample size for a diagnostic study can be estimated based on constructing confidence intervals of a given size around the desired sensitivity and specificity of the test. These calculations will indicate the approximate number of "diseased" and "nondiseased" subjects that are needed. Suppose, for example that an investigator wishes to design her study to be large enough to determine the 95% confidence intervals for the sensitivity and specificity (within ± 5%) of a new diagnostic test. She anticipates that the test will have a sensitivity of about 80%, and a specificity of about 90%. This requires calculating two separate sample sizes: one to estimate the number of subjects with the disease (80% of whom are expected to have a positive test), and another for the nondiseased (90% of whom are expected to have a negative test). Chapter 13 gives an example (13.7) of how to go about making these estimates.

A special type of random error can occur when an investigator is studying whether the results of a series of tests can be used to predict an outcome. In this type of study, the predictor variable consists of a summary measure of several tests (4). For example,

consider a study of whether a few simple variables can predict which patients with right lower quadrant tenderness have appendicitis. An investigator might measure twenty or thirty variables in the hopes of finding a combination of two or three—such as vomiting, fever and leukocytosis—that discriminate between patients with appendicitis and those without the disease. If, as is often the case, the investigator defines what constitutes a positive test *after* the study is completed, the play of chance usually leads one or another combination of variables to separate diseased and nondiseased subjects quite well. The result is that the test's apparent sensitivity and specificity will be higher than their actual values in clinical practice (5-7).

A summary measure is most meaningful if its components are chosen before the study is analyzed, rather than if the investigator waits until she has looked at the data to decide which variables to include. Usually, this requires a two-stage design. First, in the **test phase**, the investigator determines what will constitute a positive test result. Second, in the **validation phase**, she measures the test's sensitivity and specificity in a new sample of subjects.

Systematic error

In general, diagnostic studies are subject to the same biases as other observational studies (Chapters 7 and 8). The most common ones are sampling bias, measurement bias, and reporting bias.

Sampling bias. Often, the study sample is not representative of the target population in which the test will eventually be used (8). Subjects with a disease may have been selected from a referral center, for example. Such cases are likely to be severe and therefore to have more abnormal test results than subtle cases of the disease. This overestimates the test's sensitivity (ability to identify the diseased) in actual practice. Similarly, if the nondiseased were selected from volunteers, they are likely to be healthier than symptomatic but disease-free patients in a clinician's office. In this situation, the test's specificity (ability to identify the nondiseased) may be exaggerated.

The best strategy for dealing with this problem is to study a sample similar to the population in which the test will actually be used. For example, if a test will be used to differentiate patients with lung cancer from those without this diagnosis, then patients in whom lung cancer is being considered clinically (such as those who present with a solitary pulmonary nodule) should be studied. It would be misleading to use a sample of volunteers with normal chest radiographs to represent the nondiseased.·

There is a second effect of sampling bias: because the prevalence of disease among subjects selected for studying a diagnostic test is almost always higher than the prior probability of the disease that clinicians encounter, the investigator tends to overestimate the predictive value of a test. (Often, for example, the investigator studies an equal number of subjects with and without the disease; in her sample, therefore, the prior probability of the disease is 50%.) The investigator can avoid this trap when she publishes her findings by presenting the positive and negative predictive values of the test at various prior probabilities of the disease that are likely to be encountered in clinical practice, as in Table 9-3. Such calculations will enable a clinician reading the study to assess how useful the test will be in her own practice.

This type of selection bias can be especially troublesome in prognostic studies, since the prognosis of a disease depends a great deal on disease severity, and severe cases of a disease tend to be treated at referral centers. The likelihood that a febrile seizure in childhood will be followed by subsequent epilepsy, for example, is much greater if the sample of children is selected at

---

· It may, however, be appropriate to *begin* the evaluation of a new diagnostic test with a pilot study using a sample of patients at a referral center and normal volunteers. If the test fails to reliably differentiate between the very sick and the asymptomatic well, it probably will not differentiate between the not-so-sick and the sick-with-another-disease, and the investigator will have saved much time and effort. If the new test succeeds in the pilot study, then a study that is more representative clinically should be undertaken.

a referral hospital than if the sample is community-based (9).

Measurement bias. Studies of diagnostic tests are susceptible to several types of measurement bias. As with other observational studies, the risk of bias increases if the outcome is known to the person measuring the predictor. It is easy to imagine how knowing whether the patient has the disease can influence the determination of whether a diagnostic test is positive. Suppose the person interpreting the results of a new diagnostic test for pulmonary embolism has access to the patient's pulmonary angiogram. Even the most objective scientist will have difficulty ignoring this information. Bias is even possible if the predictor is measured first: If a pathologist reading a cytology slide knows that a new (and promising) diagnostic test was positive for malignancy, she may be influenced in her interpretation, especially if the slide was otherwise difficult to classify.

Another type of bias can arise when classifying the results of a new diagnostic test. Such tests often have "technically unsatisfactory" or "borderline" results (10). The investigator should decide in advance how to treat these results. Disregarding them when estimating the test's sensitivity and specificity can be misleading, since that makes the test look better than it will actually be (especially if borderline results are common in patients with "borderline" disease, who often present the most difficult diagnostic dilemmas).

The best strategy for dealing with all types of measurement bias is to have separate, blinded determinations of the results of the diagnostic test and the outcome. Prior to the study (or at least before looking at the data), the investigator should determine the criteria for a positive diagnostic test and for a case of the disease. If the investigator has chosen the cutoff point after analyzing the data, she should discuss the possibility that random variation in the data may have overestimated the true usefulness of the test. (To a lesser extent, because of random variation in the distribution of test results, measurement bias applies whenever the cutoff point for a positive test is defined after the study's results have been analyzed, such as when an ROC curve is used.)

Reporting bias. Studies of diagnostic tests that do not show promise usually go unreported. When another investigator (by chance, perhaps) finds the same test to be more promising, the results are likely to be reported. Thus the literature is biased in favor of successes and away from diagnostic failures. To lessen this problem, the investigator should design her study with a large enough sample so that negative results will be meaningful, and (try to) publish them. This is generally preferable to the alternative, which is intentionally not to publish some positive results!

STEPS IN PLANNING A STUDY OF A DIAGNOSTIC TEST

There are several steps that most studies of diagnostic tests should follow (Table 9.5). First, the investigator should *determine whether there is a need* for a new diagnostic test. In what ways are available tests inadequate, and does the new test address these deficiencies? Will patients benefit from the introduction of the new test?

Second, the investigator should *describe the way in which the subjects will be selected* (Chapter 3). Suppose that an investigator is interested in determining whether a new diagnostic test (an elevated serum lipase isoenzyme) can distinguish patients with early pancreatic cancer from those with similar symptoms but who are free of the disease. In this example, the investigator should define sampling criteria that include subjects in whom early pancreatic cancer was a diagnostic possibility (such as patients with vague abdominal pain or unexplained depression) and exclude those with advanced cases of the disease.

Third, the investigator should have a *reasonable gold standard* with which the results of the test can be compared, and she should be certain that it will be feasible, ethical, and affordable to apply both the diagnostic test and the gold standard to all potential subjects. In this example, she must be sure that all patients presenting with the relevant symptoms have an isoenzyme determination, and that they either have a histo-

logic diagnosis of pancreatic cancer or a sufficient (perhaps 2-year) follow-up without manifesting the disease.

Fourth, the investigator must assure that the gold standard and the diagnostic test of interest can be applied to all subjects in a *standardized and blinded fashion.* This generally means that at least two persons must be involved: one to perform the diagnostic test, and the other to ascertain disease status based on the gold standard. Neither person can be aware of the results of the other person's determination. Another option is to perform the diagnostic tests on coded samples. In the example, the investigator might store and freeze serum from each subject, and assign each sample a number. After determining disease status based on histology and/or follow-up, the investigator could thaw and process the sera, blinded to whether any individual sample came from a subject with pancreatic cancer or not.

Fifth, the investigator should *estimate the sample size* required to achieve 95% confidence limits for the test's sensitivity and specificity that are reasonably precise (e.g., ±5%). She should aim for a sensitivity and a specificity that are at least as good as current tests (unless the new test has other important advantages, such as lower cost or greater safety).

Sixth, the investigator must *find a sufficient number of willing subjects* to satisfy both the sample size estimate and the sampling criteria. When planning the study, a review of medical records or even a small pretest provides that best assurance that the number of subjects will be adequate. If there were only 15 cases of early pancreatic cancer in the past 3 years at the investigator's institution, for example, she can anticipate that there will be a similar number in the future, and should look elsewhere for additional subjects.

Finally, the investigator should plan to *report the results of the study in terms of sensitivity and specificity,* as well as the test's potential positive and negative predictive value at different prior probabilities of the disease. If the test is categorical or continuous, the investigator should consider using ROC curves or likelihood ratios to describe the test's performance.

SUMMARY

1. A diagnostic test study determines the usefulness of a test in the diagnosis of a disease. Good tests are those that distinguish the diseased from the nondiseased, and are *safe, quick, simple, painless, reliable,* and *inexpensive.* When designing a study of a diagnostic test, it is useful to keep in mind the randomized blinded trail and usual clinical practice as models.

2. The structure of diagnostic test studies resembles that of other observational studies: there is a *predictor variable* (the test result) and an *outcome variable* (the disease, determined by a gold standard). The difference is that the goal is not to determine whether an association is present, but to describe how strong the association is, in terms of its sensitivity and specificity.

3. The *sensitivity* of a test is the proportion of patients with the disease who have a positive test. The *specificity* of a test is the proportion of patients without the disease who have a negative test. The investigator must determine the appropriate *cutoff point* for calling a result "positive." This can involve estimating the costs of false-positive and false-negative results, or the use of *ROC curves.*

4. The investigator should determine the *predictive value of a positive test* (the likelihood that someone with a positive result actually has the disease) and the *predictive value of a negative test* (the likelihood that someone with a negative result actually is free of the disease). This involves combining the *prevalence* or *prior probability* of the disease with the sensitivity and specificity of the test. Alternatively, *likelihood ratios* can be presented.

5. Studies of diagnostic tests are subject to several biases; the most important are sampling bias, measurement bias, and reporting bias. Studying a sample as similar as possible to the population of clinical interest can reduce the problem of *sampling bias.* Separate, blinded determinations of the results of the diagnostic test and disease status should be made to avoid *measurement bias.* Attention to having an adequate sample size can alleviate some of the problems of *reporting bias.*

6. There are seven steps in planning a diagnostic test study: (a) determine that there is a need for the test; (b) set the sampling criteria; (c) define the test and the gold standard; (d) design a way to apply the test and the gold standard blindly; (e) calculate the sample size; (f) ensure that enough subjects are available; and (g) report the results in terms of sensitivity, specificity and predictive value.

REFERENCES

1. Fletcher RH, Fletcher SW, Wagner EH: *Clinical Epidemiology—The Essentials.* Baltimore, Williams & Wilkins, 1987.
2. Sackett DL, Haynes RB, Tugwell P: *Clinical Epidemiology: A Basic Science for Clinical Medicine.* Boston, Little, Brown and Company, 1985.
3. Diamond GA, Forrester JS: Analysis of probability as an aid in the clinical diagnosis of coronary-artery disease. N Engl J Med 300:1350–1358, 1979.
4. Wasson JH, Sox HC, Neff RK, Goldman L: Clinical prediction rules: applications and methodologic standards. N Engl J Med 313: 793–799, 1985.
5. Fischl MA, Pitchenik A, Gardner LB: An index predicting relapse and need for hospitalization in patients with acute bronchial asthma. N Engl J Med 305:783–789, 1981.
6. Rose CC, Murphy JG, Schwartz JS: Performance of an index predicting the response of patients with acute bronchial asthma to intensive emergency department treatment. N Engl J Med 310:573–577, 1984.
7. Centor RM, Yarbrough B, Wood JP:. Inability to predict relapse in asthma. N Engl J Med 310: 577–580, 1984
8. Ransohoff DF, Feinstein AR: Problems of spectrum and bias in evaluating the efficacy of diagnostic tests. N Engl J Med 299:926–930, 1978.
9. Ellenberg JH, Nelson KB: Sample selection and the natural history of disease: studies of febrile seizures. JAMA 243:1337–1340, 1980.
10. Philbrick T, Horwitz RJ, Feinstein AR, Langou RA, Chandler JP.: The limited spectrum of patients studied in exercise test research: analyzing the tip of the iceberg. JAMA 248:2467–2470, 1982.

ADDITIONAL READINGS

Boyd JC, Marr JJ: Decreasing reliability of acid-fast smear techniques for detection of tuberculosis. Ann Intern Med 82:489–492, 1975.

Cummings SR, Papadakis M, Melnick J, Gooding GAW, Tierney LM: The predictive value of physical examination for ascites. West J Med 142:633–636, 1985.

Eddy DM: *Screening for Cancer: Theory, Analysis, and Design.* Englewood Cliffs, New Jersey, Prentice-Hall, Inc., 1980.

Griner PF, Mayewski RJ, Mushlin AI, Greenland P: Selection and interpretation of diagnostic tests and procedures. Principles and applications. Ann Intern Med 94:553–600, 1981.

Lilienfeld AM, Lilienfeld DE; *Foundations of Epidemi-ology,* ed 2. New York, Oxford University Press, 1980.

McNeil BJ, Hanley JA. Statistical approaches to the analysis of receiver operating characteristic (ROC) curves. Med Decis Making 4:137–150, 1984. *(How to compare ROC curves.)*

Morrison AS: *Screening in Chronic Disease.* New York: Oxford University Press, 1985. *(Includes a discussion of the effects of early treatment, lead time, and prognostic selection.)*

Sox HC Jr, Liang MH: The erythrocyte sedimentation rate: guidelines for rational use. Ann Intern Med 104:515–523, 1986.

Vecchio TJ: Predictive value of a single diagnostic test in unselected populations. N Engl J Med 274:1171–1173, 1966. *(Seminal article.)*

CHAPTER 10

Enhancing Causal Inference in Observational Studies

Thomas B. Newman, Warren S. Browner, and Stephen B. Hulley

INTRODUCTION **98**

SPURIOUS ASSOCIATIONS **98**

Ruling out spurious associations due to chance
Ruling out spurious associations due to bias

REAL ASSOCIATIONS OTHER THAN CAUSE-
EFFECT **101**

Effect-cause
Effect-effect (confounding)

COPING WITH CONFOUNDERS IN THE DESIGN
PHASE **102**

Specification
Matching

COPING WITH CONFOUNDERS IN THE
ANALYSIS PHASE **106**

Stratification
Adjustment

CHOOSING A STRATEGY **107**

Positive evidence for causality

SUMMARY **108**

REFERENCES **109**

APPENDIX 10.A.   A Numerical Example of
Confounding **207**

APPENDIX 10.B.   A Simplified Example of
Adjustment **208**

— — — — — — — — — — —

INTRODUCTION

One of the most important aspects of clinical research is the inference that an association represents a **cause-effect relationship.** In this chapter we discuss ways to strengthen causal inferences based on associations in observational studies. We begin with a discussion of how to avoid spurious associations and then concentrate on ruling out real associations that do not represent cause-effect, especially those due to confounding.

Suppose that a study reveals an association between coffee drinking and myocardial infarction (MI). One possibility is that coffee drinking is a cause of MI. Before reaching this conclusion, however, four rival explanations must be considered (Table 10.1). The first two of these, **chance** (random error) and **bias** (systematic error), represent **spurious associations:** coffee drinking and MI are not really associated in the population, only in the study findings.

Even if the association is real, however, it may not represent a cause-effect relationship. Two rival explanations must be considered. One is the possibility of an **effect-cause** relationship—that having an MI makes people drink more coffee (this is just cause and effect in reverse). The other is the possibility of an **effect-effect** relationship (confounding)—that coffee drinking and MI are both caused by some third factor like anxiety.

SPURIOUS ASSOCIATIONS

Ruling out spurious associations due to chance

Imagine that 60% of the entire population of MI patients are coffee drinkers. If we were to select a random sample of 20 MI patients we would expect about 12 of them to drink coffee. But by chance alone, we might happen to get 19 coffee drinkers in a sample of 20 MI patients. In that case a spurious association between coffee consumption and MI might be observed. Such an association due to ran-

Table 10.1.
The five explanations when an association between coffee drinking and myocardial infarction (MI) is observed in a sample

Explanation	Type of association	Basis for association	What's really going on in the population	Causal model
1. Chance	Spurious	Random error	Coffee drinking and MI are not related	
2. Bias	Spurious	Systematic error	Coffee drinking and MI are not related	
3. Effect-cause	Real	Cart before the horse	MI is a cause of coffee drinking	Coffee drinking ← MI
4. Effect-effect	Real	Confounding	Coffee drinking and MI are both caused by a third, extrinsic factor	Factor X ↙ ↘ Coffee drinking MI
5. Cause-effect	Real	Cause and effect	Coffee drinking is a cause of MI	Coffee drinking → MI

dom error (chance) is called a **Type I error** (see Chapter 12).

Strategies for minimizing random errors are available in both the design and analysis phases of research (Table 10.2). The *design strategy of increasing the sample size* is an important way to reduce random error; this and other strategies are discussed in Chapters 4 and 13. The *analysis strategy of testing the statistical significance* of the association is a well known strategy that is actually more complicated than is generally recognized, a topic discussed in Appendix 18.

Ruling out spurious associations due to bias

Associations that are spurious because of bias are a trickier matter. To understand bias it is important to distinguish between the research question and the actual study (Chapter 1). The research question is the uncertainty in the universe the investigator really wishes to settle, and the actual study is the operationalized counterpart addressed by the study plan. Bias can be thought of as a *systematic difference between the research*

Table 10.2.
Strengthening the inference that an association has a cause-effect basis: ruling out spurious associations

Type of spurious association	Design phase (How to prevent the rival explanation)	Analysis phase (How to evaluate the rival explanation)
Chance (due to random error)	Increase sample size and other strategies (see Chapters 4 and 13)	Interpret p value in context of prior evidence (see Appendix 18)
Bias (due to systematic error)	Carefully consider the potential consequences of each difference between the research question and the study plan: Subjects Predictor Outcome	Obtain additional data to see if potential biases have actually occurred. Check consistency with other studies (especially those using different methods).

question and the actual question answered by the study that causes the study to give the wrong answer. Strategies for minimizing these systematic errors are available in both the design and analysis phases of research (Table 10.2).

Design Phase: Many kinds of bias have been identified (1), and dealing with some of these has been a major topic of this book. To the specific strategies noted in Chapters 3, 4, 7, and 8 we now add a general approach to minimizing sources of bias. Write down the research question and the study plan side by side as in Figure 10.1. Then carefully think through the following three concerns:

1. Do the study subjects accurately represent the target population?

2. Does the measurement of the predictor accurately represent the predictor variable of interest?
3. Does the measurement of the outcome accurately represent the outcome variable of interest?

For each question answered "No" or "Maybe not," consider whether the bias is large enough that the study could give the wrong answer.

To illustrate this with our coffee and MI example, consider the implications of drawing the sample of control subjects from a population of clinic patients. If many of these have chronic illnesses that have caused them to reduce their coffee intake, the sample will not represent the general popula-

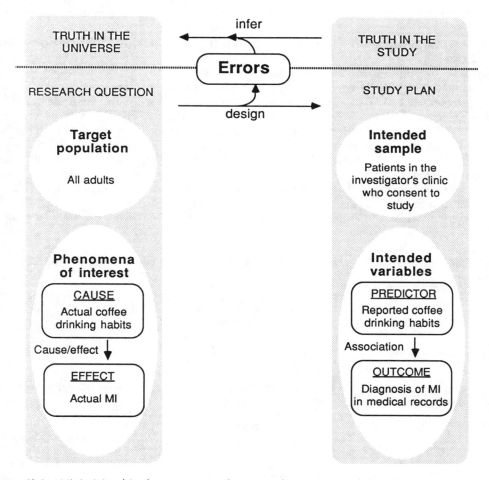

Figure 10.1.   Minimizing bias by comparing the research question and the study plan.

tion—there will be a shortage of coffee drinkers (2). Similarly, consider what might happen if coffee drinking is measured by an unblinded interviewer. If the questions are phrased differently to cases and controls, the predictor variable may not be accurately measured (3). Finally, what if esophageal spasm, which can be exacerbated by coffee, is misdiagnosed as MI? A spurious association between coffee and MI could be found because the measured outcome (diagnosis of MI) did not accurately represent the actual outcome (MI).

The next step is to think about possible strategies for preventing each potential bias. If the bias is easily preventable, revise the study plan and ask the three questions again. If the bias is not easily preventable, decide whether the study is still worth doing by making a judgment on the likelihood of the potential bias and the degree to which it will compromise the conclusions.

Analysis Phase: After the data have been collected, the investigator is often faced with one or more potential biases. Some may have been anticipated but too difficult to prevent, and others may not have occurred to the investigator until it was too late to avoid them.

In either situation, one solution is to consider obtaining **additional information** to estimate the magnitude of the potential bias. Suppose, for example, the investigator is concerned that the hospitalized control subjects have decreased their coffee intake because of chronic illness. The magnitude of this bias could be estimated by reviewing the

diagnoses of the control subjects and separating them into two groups: those with a chronic illness like peptic ulcer that might alter coffee habits, and those with an acute illness like hip fracture that would not (3). If both types of controls drank less coffee than the MI cases, then sampling bias would be a less likely explanation for the findings. Similarly, if the investigator is concerned that the interview responses were biased, she could assign a blinded interviewer to question the spouses of the cases and controls. Finally, if the outcome measure is in doubt the investigator could specify objective electrocardiographic and serum enzyme changes needed for the diagnosis.

The investigator can also look at the **results of other studies.** If the conclusions are consistent, the association is less likely to be due to bias. This is especially true if the other studies have used different methods, and are thus unlikely to share the same biases. In many cases, potential biases turn out not to be a major problem (4); the decision on how vigorously to pursue additional information and how best to discuss these issues in reporting the study are matters of judgment.

REAL ASSOCIATIONS OTHER THAN CAUSE-EFFECT

Once spurious associations have been made unlikely, the two types of associations that are real but do not represent cause-effect must be considered (Table 10.3).

Table 10.3.
Strengthening the inference that an association has a cause-effect basis: ruling out other real associations

Type of real association	Design phase (How to prevent the rival explanation)	Analysis phase (How to evaluate the rival explanation)
Effect-Cause (the outcome is actually the cause of the predictor	Do a longitudinal study Obtain data on the historic sequence of the variables	Consider biologic plausibility
Effect-Effect (confounding variable is a cause of both the predictor and the outcome)	See Table 10.4.	See Table 10.5.

Effect-cause

One possibility is that the cart has come before the horse—the outcome caused the predictor, rather than vice versa. Effect-cause is often a problem in cross-sectional and case-control studies, especially when the predictor variable is a laboratory test for which no previous values are available. Suppose, for example, that a study finds high serum triglyceride levels in men recovering from myocardial infarction; the MI may have caused the high triglyceride levels rather than vice versa.

Effect-cause is less commonly a problem in cohort studies, because risk factor measurements can be made in a group of patients who do not yet have the disease. Even in cohort studies, however, effect-cause is possible if the disease has a long latent period. A good example is the association between low serum cholesterol levels and excess cancer mortality that has been observed in many cohort studies (5). The observation that the excess cancer mortality was only present for the first 5 years after the cholesterol measurement (whereas the excess heart disease mortality in those with *high* cholesterol continued undiminished) suggested that preexisting but hidden cancer caused the low cholesterol level rather than vice versa (6).

This example illustrates a general approach to ruling out effect-cause—drawing inferences from assessments of the predictor variable at different points in time. In addition, effect-cause is often unlikely on the grounds of biologic implausibility. To most people outside of the Tobacco Institute, for example, it seems unlikely that predisposition to lung cancer causes cigarette smoking.

Effect-effect (confounding)

The other rival explanation in Table 10.3 is effect-effect, which occurs when there is a **confounding variable**, an extrinsic factor that is *associated with the predictor variable and a cause of the outcome variable.* Cigarette smoking is a likely confounder in the coffee and MI example: smoking is associated with coffee drinking and a cause of MI. Appendix 10.A gives a numerical example of

how cigarette smoking could cause an apparent association between coffee drinking and MI.

Setting aside concerns with bias, effect-effect is often the only likely alternative explanation to cause-effect and the most important one to try to rule out. It is also the most challenging; the rest of this chapter is devoted to discussing the available strategies.

COPING WITH CONFOUNDERS IN THE DESIGN PHASE

In observational studies, most strategies for coping with confounding variables require that an investigator be aware of and able to measure them. (This is not true of experiments, which offer the possibility of controlling unmeasured confounders by randomization—see Chapter 11.) The first step is to make a list of the variables that may be associated with the predictor variable of interest and that may also be a cause of the outcome. The investigator must then choose between the design and analysis strategies for controlling the influence of these potential confounding variables.

The two design-phase strategies (Table 10.4), **specification** and **matching**, involve changes in the sampling scheme. Cases and controls (in a case-control study) or exposed and unexposed subjects (in a cohort study) are sampled in such a way that they have the same value of the confounding variable. This removes the confounder as an explanation for any association that is observed between predictor and outcome.

Specification

The simplest strategy is to design inclusion criteria that *specify* a value of the potential confounding variable and exclude everyone with a different value. For example, the investigator studying coffee and MI could specify that only nonsmokers would be included in the study. If an association were then observed between coffee and MI, it obviously could not be due to smoking.

Specification is an effective strategy, but, as with all restrictions in the sampling

Table 10.4.
Design phase strategies for coping with confounders

Strategy	Advantages	Disadvantages
Specification	Easily understood	Limits generalizability
	Focuses the sample of subjects for the research question at hand	May make it difficult to acquire an adequate sample size
Matching	Can eliminate influence of strong constitutional confounders like age and sex	May be time consuming and expensive, less efficient than increasing the number of subjects (e.g.,the number of controls per case)
	Can eliminate influence of confounders that are difficult to measure	
		Decision to match must be made at outset of study and can have irreversible adverse effect on analysis and conclusions
	Can increase precision (power) by balancing the number of cases and controls in each stratum	
		Requires early decision about which variables are predictors and which confounders
	May be a sampling convenience, making it easier to select the controls in a case-control study	
		Removes option of studying matched variables as predictors or as intervening variables
		Requires matched analysis
		Creates the danger of overmatching (i.e., matching on a factor that is not a confounder, thereby reducing power)

scheme (see Chapter 3), it has disadvantages. First, even if coffee does not cause MI in nonsmokers, it may cause them in smokers. (This phenomenon—an effect of coffee on MI that is different in smokers than in non-smokers—is called an **interaction**.) Thus, specification limits the *quality* of information available from a study, in this instance compromising our ability to generalize to smokers. Second, if smoking is highly prevalent among the patients available for the study, the investigator may not be able to recruit a large enough sample of nonsmokers. Thus, specification may also limit the *quantity* of information that is available.

These problems can become serious if specification is used to control too many confounders or to control them too narrowly. Sample size and generalizability would be major problems if a study were restricted to lower income, nonsmoking, 70-75 year-old men.

Matching

In a case-control study, matching involves selecting for each case a control with the same value of the confounding variable. In the study of coffee as a predictor of MI, for example, the coffee drinking of a case (a patient with an MI) who smoked one pack-per-day would be compared with the coffee drinking of a control (a patient with no MI) who was also a one pack-per-day smoker. Matching and specification are both *sampling strategies* that prevent confounding by allowing comparison only of cases and controls who share the same level of the confounder. Matching differs from specification, however, in preserving generalizability: subjects at all levels of the confounder can still be studied.

Matching is most commonly used in case-control studies, but it can also be used with other designs. In a recently reported double-cohort study, for example, the research question was whether children with sickle cell trait have abnormal growth and development (7). Each of 50 babies with sickle cell trait detected on newborn screening was matched with a baby with normal hemoglobin who had the same birthdate, birth weight, gestational age, 5-minute Apgar score, race, sex, and welfare status. At 3-5 years of age the levels of physical and cognitive development were the same in the two groups. This study illustrates the use of matching when the research question is directed at one specific risk factor.

Advantages to matching: There are four main advantages to matching, the first three concerning the control of confounding variables, and the last a matter of logistics:

Matching is an effective way to *prevent confounding by constitutional factors like age and sex* that are strong determinants of outcome, are not susceptible to intervention, and are unlikely to be an intermediary in a causal pathway (see Appendix 10.A).

Matching can be used to *control confounders that cannot be measured* and controlled in any other way. For example, matching siblings (or, better yet, twins) with one another can control for a whole range of genetic and familial factors that would be impossible to measure, and matching for clinical center in a multicenter study can control for unspecified differences among the populations seen at the centers.

Matching may *increase the precision of comparisons* between groups (and thus the power of the study to find a real association) by balancing the number of cases and controls at each level of the confounder. This may be important if the available number of subjects is limited, or if the cost of studying subjects is high. However, the effect of matching on precision is modest and not always favorable (8-10). In general, the desire to enhance precision is a less important reason to match than the need to control confounding.

Matching may be used primarily as a *sampling convenience*, to narrow down an otherwise impossibly large number of potential controls. For example, in a nationwide study of toxic shock syndrome, victims were asked to identify friends to serve as controls (11). This convenience, however, runs the risk of "overmatching" (discussed below).

Disadvantages to matching: These advantages do not come without cost, and there are a number of disadvantages to matching (Table 10.4).

Matching sometimes requires *additional time and expense* to identify a match for each subject. In case-control studies, for example, the more matching criteria there are the larger the pool of controls that must be searched to match each case. Cases for which no match can be found will need to be discarded. The possible increase in statistical power from matching must thus be weighed against that which could be achieved at the same expense simply by keeping all of the cases and increasing the number of (nonmatched) controls per case (9).

Because matching is a sampling strategy, the decision to match must be made at the beginning of the study and is *irreversible*. This precludes further study of the effect of the matched variables on the outcome. It also can create a serious error if the matching variable is not a fixed (constitutional) variable like age or sex, but a modifiable one that may be influenced by the predictor of interest. Taking the research question of whether coffee is a cause of MI as an example, it might be a mistake to match on smoking even though the usual criteria for potential confounders are met (it is associated with coffee drinking and a likely cause of MI). The problem here is one that arises whenever the predictor of interest may also be a cause *of the potential confounder.*

Three causal models for the relationship between smoking and coffee are presented in Figure 10.2. Smoking is an apparent confounder in each model (a cause of MI and associated with coffee drinking), but each model has a different basis for the association with coffee drinking. In model #1, the smoking habit causes people to be more likely to drink coffee: here, matching the subjects for their smoking habits would do exactly what it is designed to do, prevent the investigator from observing an association between coffee and MI that does not represent cause-effect. (Matching would also, however, prevent the investigator from observing the cause-effect association between smoking and CHD in her study, a risk relationship that might be of interest.) In model #2, there is no direct relationship between coffee drinking and smoking, and both are consequences of a factor X (anxiety, for example). Here again, matching would be good, preventing the investigator from observing an association between coffee drinking and MI that does not represent cause-effect.

In model #3, however, coffee drinking causes people to be more likely to smoke cigarettes (because, for example, some of them have linked these habits so that every time they quit smoking they start again over an after-dinner cup of coffee). Here, matching would have the undesirable effect of preventing the investigator from observing the remote cause-effect association between coffee and MI, with smoking as the proximate and intermediary variable. She would fail to discover that coffee drinking, because of its effect on smoking, might be a suitable target for MI prevention advice to smokers.

Correct analysis of matched data requires *special analytic techniques* that compare each subject only with the individual(s)

with whom she has been matched, and not with subjects who have differing levels of confounders. The use of ordinary statistical analysis techniques on matched data can lead to incorrect results. This sometimes creates a problem because the appropriate matched analyses, especially multivariate techniques, are less readily available in packaged statistical programs than unmatched techniques (12).

A final disadvantage of matching is the possibility of *overmatching*, which occurs when the matching variable is not a confounder because it is not associated with the outcome. Overmatching can reduce the power of a case-control study, making it more difficult to find an association that really exists in the population (8). In the study of toxic shock syndrome that used friends for controls, for example, matching may have inappropriately controlled for regional differences in tampon marketing, making it more probable that cases and controls would use the same brand of tampon (13). It is important to note, however, that overmatching will not *distort* the estimated relative risk (provided that a matched analysis is used)—it will only reduce its statistical significance. Thus, when the findings of the study are statistically significant (as was the case in the toxic shock example (11)) overmatching is not a problem (14).

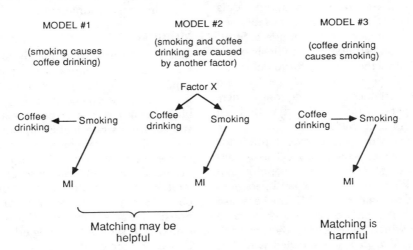

Figure 10.2. Three causal models to consider if smoking is associated with coffee drinking and is a cause of MI.

Table 10.5.
Analysis phase stratgegies for coping with confounders

Strategy	Advantages	Disadvantages
Stratification	Easily understood	Number of strata limited by sample size needed for each stratum:
	Flexible and reversible; can choose which variables to stratify upon after data collection	•Few covariables can be considered
		•Few strata per covariable leads to less complete control of confounding
		Relevant covariables must have been measured
Statistical adjustment	Multiple confounders can be controlled simultaneously	Model may not fit:
	Information in continuous variables can be fully used	•Incomplete control of confounding (if model does not fit confounder-outcome relationship)
	As flexible and reversible as stratification	•Inaccurate estimates of strength of effect (if model does not fit predictor-outcome relationship)
		Results are hard to understand
		Relevant covariables must have been measured

COPING WITH CONFOUNDERS IN THE ANALYSIS PHASE

Both design-phase strategies require deciding at the outset of the study which variables are predictors and which are confounders. **Stratification** and **adjustment,** two analysis-phase strategies, allow the investigator to defer that decision until she has looked at the data and seen which variables are in fact confounders (i.e., independently associated with both predictor and outcome).

Sometimes there are several predictor variables, each of which may act as a confounder to the others. For example, although coffee drinking, smoking, sex, and personality type are associated with MI, they are also associated with each other. The goal is to determine which of these predictors variables are *independently* associated with MI, and which are associated with MI only because they are associated with other (causal)

risk factors. In this section we discuss **multivariate analytic methods** for assessing the *independent* contribution of predictor variables in observational studies.

Stratification

Like specification and matching, stratification assures that only cases and controls (or exposed and unexposed subjects) with similar levels of a potential confounding variable are compared. It involves segregating the subjects into strata (subgroups) according to the level of the potential confounder, and then examining the relationship between the predictor and outcome separately in each stratum. Stratification is illustrated in Appendix 10.A. By considering smokers and nonsmokers separately ("stratifying on smoking"), the confounding effects of smoking can be removed.

Like matching, stratification is easily understood. An advantage is its flexibility: by performing several stratified analyses, the investigators can decide which variables are confounders, and ignore the remainder. (This is done most easily by determining whether the results of stratified analyses substantially differ from those of unstratified analyses.) No commitments need be made at the beginning of the study that might later be regretted.

The principal disadvantage of stratified analysis is the limited number of variables that can be controlled simultaneously. For example, possible confounders in the coffee and MI study might include age, systolic blood pressure, serum cholesterol, cigarette smoking, and alcohol intake. To stratify on these five variables, even if there were only three strata for each, would have required 3^5 (= 243) strata! With this many strata the number of subjects available for analysis in each stratum becomes too small.

On the other hand, if the strata are too broad, the confounder may not be adequately controlled. For example, if the above study stratified using only two age strata (e.g., age ≤ 50 and age > 50), confounding would still be possible if, *within each stratum*, the subjects drinking the most coffee were also the oldest and thus at highest risk of MI.

Adjustment

Confounders can also be controlled by one of several techniques available for statistical adjustment. These techniques **model** the nature of the associations among the variables in order to separate the effect of the confounder. For example, a study of the effect of lead ingestion on IQ in children might examine *parental* education as a potential confounder. Statistical adjustment might model the relationship between parents' years of schooling and the child's IQ as a straight line. The IQs of children with different lead levels could then be adjusted to remove the effect of parental education using the approach described in Appendix 10.B. Similar adjustments can be made for several confounders simultaneously using a multivariate analysis program on a computer.

One of the great **advantages** of multivariate adjustment techniques is the capacity to control the influence of many confounders simultaneously. Another advantage is their use of all the information in continuous variables. It is easy, for example, to adjust for a parent's education level in 1-year intervals, rather than stratifying into just two or three categories.

There are, however, two **disadvantages** of multivariate models. First, the model may not fit. Computerized statistical packages have made these models so accessible that the investigator may not stop to consider whether their use is appropriate to the particular study. Taking the example in Appendix 10.B, the investigator should plot the data to see whether the relationship between the parents' years of schooling and the child's IQ is actually linear. If not, then attempts to adjust IQ for parental education using a linear model will be imperfect, and the estimate of the independent effect of lead will be incorrect.

Second, even when the models do fit, the resulting highly derived statistics are difficult to understand. A p value that refers to the maximum likelihood estimate of a logistic regression coefficient divided by its standard error is substantially less meaningful to most of us than one that refers to a simple two-by-two table that presents the actual findings.

CHOOSING A STRATEGY

What general guidelines can be offered as to when to use each of these strategies? The use of specification to control confounding is most appropriate for situations in which the investigator is chiefly interested in specific subgroups of the population; this is really just a special form of the general process in every study of establishing criteria for selecting the study subjects (Chapter 3).

An important decision to make in the design phase of the study is whether to match. Matching is most appropriate when strong confounders are already known from previous studies, particularly fixed constitutional factors such as age, race, and sex. Matching is sometimes useful when the sample size is small compared with the number of strata necessary to control for known confounders, when the confounders are more easily matched than measured, and when there are advantages in efficiency or convenience. There are, however, some disadvantages to the strategy, the most serious being the irreversibility of the decision; matching can permanently compromise the investigator's ability to observe real associations. For this reason *matching should be used sparingly*, and in situations where it is clear that analysis-phase strategies are not as good.

The decision to stratify or adjust can wait until after the study is done and the investigator can analyze the data to see which factors are potential confounders (i.e., associated with both the predictor of interest and the outcome). However, it is important to consider which factors may be used for adjustment at the time the study is designed, because it helps with decisions on what variables to measure. Also, since these strategies for controlling the influence of a specific confounding variable can only succeed to the degree that the confounder is well-measured, it is important to design measurement approaches that have adequate precision and accuracy (Chapter 4).

Positive evidence for causality

The approach to enhancing causal inference has largely been a negative one so far— ruling out the four rival explanations in Table 10.1. A complementary strategy is to seek characteristics of associations that provide positive evidence for causality, of which the most important are the consistency and strength of the association, the presence of a dose-response relationship, and biologic plausibility (15).

When the results are **consistent** in studies of various designs, it is less likely that chance or bias is the cause of an association. Real but noncausal associations, however, will also be consistently observed. For example, if cigarette smokers drink more coffee and have more MI's in the population, studies will consistently observe an association between coffee drinking and MI.

The **strength** of the association is also important. For one thing, stronger associations give more significant p values, making

chance a less likely explanation. Stronger associations also provide better evidence for causality by reducing the likelihood of confounding (16). Associations due to confounding are indirect (i.e., via the confounder), and therefore are generally weaker than direct cause-effect associations. This is illustrated in Appendix 10.A: the very strong associations between coffee and smoking (odds ratio = 16), and between smoking and MI (odds ratio = 4), led to a much weaker association between coffee and MI (odds ratio = 2.25). Confounding is an unlikely explanation for associations with odds ratios that are greater than 2.5 (16).

A **dose-response relationship** provides positive evidence for causality. The association between cigarette smoking and lung cancer is an example: moderate smokers have higher rates of cancer than nonsmokers, and heavy smokers have even higher rates. Whenever possible, predictor variables should be measured continuously or in several categories, so that any dose-response relationship that is present can be observed.

Finally, **biologic plausibility** is an important consideration for drawing causal inference. The association between cigarette smoking and cervical cancer, for example, was initially thought to be noncausal because of biological implausibility (17, 18). Cause-effect has now been supported by identification of components of tobacco smoke in the cervical mucus and other body fluids of smokers (16, 19).

SUMMARY

1. Observational studies should be designed with a view to the problem of interpreting associations. The inference that the association represents a *cause-effect relationship* is strengthened by using either design or analysis strategies to reduce the likelihood of the four rival explanations (chance, bias, effect-cause, and effect-effect).

2. The role of *chance* can be minimized by designing a study with adequate sample size, and by using various strategies to improve precision. Once the study is

completed, the likelihood that chance is the basis of the association can be judged from the magnitude of the p value and the consistency of the results with previous evidence.

3. *Bias* arises from differences between the population and phenomena addressed by the research question and the actual subjects and measurements in the study. Bias can be avoided by basing design decisions on a careful assessment of whether these differences will lead to a wrong answer.

4. *Effect-cause* is made less likely by designing a study that permits assessment of temporal relationships, and by considering biologic plausibility.

5. *Effect-effect*, in which a *confounding variable* is responsible for the observation, is made less likely by the following strategies:

   a. *Specification* or *matching* in the **design phase,** which alters the sampling strategy to ensure that only groups with similar levels of the confounder are compared. These strategies are effective, but should be used carefully because they can irreversibly limit the information available from the study.

   b. *Stratification* or *adjustment* in the **analysis phase,** which accomplishes the same goal statistically. These are safer strategies, preserving more options for coping with confounders; adjustment permits multiple factors to be controlled simultaneously, but has the disadvantage that the data may not fit the statistical model.

6. Causal inference is further enhanced by positive evidence: the *consistency* and *strength* of the association, the presence of a *dose-response relationship*, and *biologic plausibility*.

REFERENCES

1. Sackett DL: Bias in analytic research. *J Chron Dis* 32:51–63, 1979.

2. Rosenberg L, Slone D, Shapiro S, et al: Case control studies on the acute effects of coffee upon the risk of myocardial infarction: problems in the selection of hospital control series. *Am J Epidemiol* 113:646–652, 1981.

3. Chalmers TC: Re: coffee and cancer of the pancreas (letter). *New Engl J Med* 304:1605, 1981.

4. Jick H: Re: coffee and myocardial infarction (letter). *Am J Epid* 113:103–4, 1981.

5. Rose G, Shipley MJ: Plasma lipids and mortality: A source of error. *Lancet* 1:523–6, 1980.

6. Sherwin RW, Wentworth DN, Cutler JA, et al: Serum cholesterol levels and cancer mortality in 361,662 men screened for the MRFIT. *JAMA* 257:943–948, 1987.

7. Kramer MS, Rooks V, Pearson HA: Growth and development in children with sickle cell trait. A prospective study of matched pairs. *New Engl J Med* 299:686–689; 1978.

8. Miettinen OS: Matching and design efficiency in retrospective studies. *Am J Epidemiol* 91:111–117, 1970.

9. Thompson WD, Kelsey JL, Walter SD: Cost and efficiency in the choice of matched and unmatched study designs. *Am J Epidemiol* 116:840–851, 1982.

10. McKinley SM: Pair matching—A reappraisal of a popular technique. *Biometrics* 33:725–735, 1977.

11. Shands KN, Schmid GP, Dan BB, et al: Toxic-shock syndrome in menstruating women: its association with tampon use and *staphylococcus aureus* and the clinical features in 52 cases. *New Engl J Med* 303:1436–1442, 1980.

12. Breslow NE, Day NE: *Statistical Methods in Cancer Research. Vol 1. The Analysis of Case-Control Studies.* Lyon. IARC Scientific Publ. 1980, p 253.

13. Shands KN, Schledr WF, Hargrett NT, et al. Toxic shock syndrome: case-controlled studies at the Centers for Disease Control. *Ann Int Med* 96:895–898, 1982.

14. Schlesselman JJ: *Case-Control Studies: Design, Conduct, Analysis.* New York, Oxford University Press, 1982. p 110.

15. Schlesselman JJ: *Case-Control Studies: Design, Conduct, Analysis.* New York, Oxford University Press, 1982. pp. 20–25.

16. Winkelstein W, Jr, Shillitoe EJ, Brand R, Johnson KK: Futher comments on cancer of the uterine cervix, smoking, and herpes virus infection. *Am J Epidemiol* 119:1–7, 1984.

17. Wright NH, Vessey MP, Kenward B, et al: Neoplasia and dysplasia of the cervix uteri and contrception: a possible protective effect of the diaphragm. *Br J Cancer* 38:273–279, 1978.

18. Harris RWC, Brinton LA, Cowdell RH, et al: Characteristics of women with dysplasia or carcinoma in situ of the cervix uteri. *Br J Cancer* 42:359–369, 1980.

19. Sasson IM, Haley NJ, Hoffman D, et al: Cigarette smoking and neoplasia of the uterine cervix: Smoke constituents in cervical mucus [letter]. *New Engl J Med* 312:315–316, 1985.

CHAPTER 11

Designing a New Study: IV. Experiments

Stephen B. Hulley, David Feigal, Michael Martin, and Steven R. Cummings

INTRODUCTION 110

   Types of experimental design

THE RANDOMIZED BLINDED TRIAL (RBT) 111

   Assembling the study cohort
   Measuring baseline variables
   Randomizing the study subjects
   Applying the intervention
   Measuring the outcome
   Analyzing the results

SPECIAL TYPES OF RANDOMIZED BLINDED DESIGNS 119

   Run-in design
   Factorial design
   Randomization of matched pairs
   Pre-randomization
   Group randomization

OTHER EXPERIMENTAL DESIGNS 121

   Nonrandomized between-group designs
   Nonblinded between-group designs
   Time series designs
   Other within-group designs
   Natural experiments

DECIDING TO DO AN EXPERIMENT 124

SUMMARY 124

REFERENCES 126

ADDITIONAL READINGS 127

APPENDIX 11.A. Randomization procedures for studies of small or moderate sample size 00

APPENDIX 11.B. Three analysis issues pertinent to designing an experiment 00

INTRODUCTION

Experiments are cohort studies in which the investigator *manipulates* the predictor variable (the intervention) and observes the effect on an outcome. The major advantage of an experiment over an observational study is the **strength of causal inference** it offers. It is the best design for controlling the influence of confounding variables.

Experiments are best reserved for relatively mature research questions—diseases for which observational studies have already revealed the basic descriptive characteristics (what, who, where, and when?), suggested etiology (why?), and pointed the way toward clinical and public health approaches to the problem (how prevent or treat?). At this stage experiments have the advantage over observational studies, not only in their ability to provide greater strength of causal inference, but also in their suitability for testing the efficacy of treatment programs.

Types of experimental design

Experiments examine the relationship between the predictor and outcome variables in a cohort of subjects followed over time. Causal inference is based on comparing the outcomes observed in subjects classified by the intervention (a form of predictor variable) they received.

Between-group designs compare the outcomes observed in two or more groups of subjects that receive different interventions, and **within-group designs** compare the outcomes observed in a single group before and after an intervention is applied. Between-group designs are the most widely used in clinical research, and one of them, the classic randomized control trial, is often held up as the optimal standard against which all other designs should be measured (1,2). However, the phrase "randomized control trial" does not specify whether the study includes blinding, a design feature as important to causal inference as randomization. We will use the phrase **randomized blinded trial (RBT)** for the ideal design to emulate.

This chapter presents detailed guidelines for designing the simplest form of the RBT prototype, and then goes on to consider some variations on this design.

THE RANDOMIZED BLINDED TRIAL (RBT)

There are five steps in designing an RBT (Fig. 11.1). The first tasks are to assemble the study cohort and make some baseline measurements. The investigator then randomizes the subjects into two or more study groups that receive blinded interventions. After a period of follow-up, she blindly as-certains the outcome and compares the findings between the study groups.

Assembling the study cohort

This task begins with deciding what kind of subjects to study and how to go about recruiting them. We have discussed in Chapter 3 how to specify inclusion and exclusion criteria defining target populations that are appropriate to the research question and accessible populations that are practical to study, how to design an efficient and scientific approach to sampling the accessible population in a representative way, and how to tackle the practical matter of recruitment. Here are some further points that are especially relevant to an experiment.

Define inclusion criteria that are appropriate to the research question: If the inclusion criteria are broad it will be easier to get study subjects and the findings may be generalizable to a relatively large and diverse target population. On the other hand, it is obviously not a good idea to include a mixture of subjects if some of them will produce qualitatively different findings. Many CHD prevention trials, for example,

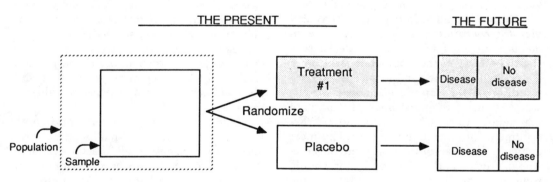

THE PRESENT   THE FUTURE

Treatment #1 / Randomize / Placebo / Disease / No disease / Population / Sample

Steps:
1. Select a sample from the population
2. Measure baseline variables
3. Randomize
4. Apply interventions (one should be a blinded placebo, if possible)
5. Followup the cohorts
6. Measure outcome variables (blindly, if possible)

Figure 11.1.   The randomized blinded trial (RBT), in this case of the efficacy of a treatment in preventing a disease.

have set an upper age limit of 60 years on the theory that elderly subjects might already have extensive atherosclerosis of their coronary arteries that would no longer be responsive to preventive efforts.

In designing the inclusion criteria, the investigator should consider the outcome of interest. If the outcome is a rare event like CHD incidence, subjects can be recruited from populations at high risk of developing the condition. The reason for selecting only men for the MRFIT, for example, was the fact that women have a much lower incidence of CHD.

Define exclusion criteria that will help control errors: It is a good idea to exclude subjects with extraneous conditions that will compete with the outcome of the study, for example an advanced cancer that may be fatal before the end of the follow-up period in a subject entering a CHD prevention study. It is also important to exclude subjects who have contraindications for the study intervention (like asthma in a study of treating hypertension with β-blockers), and those who may have difficulty complying with the intervention or the followup schedule, such as alcoholics, psychotic patients, and individuals planning to move to another state.

Design an adequate sample size and plan the recruitment accordingly: Experiments with too few subjects to detect substantial effects in the population have been distressingly common in the past (3), and estimating of the sample size needs of the study is one of the most important parts of planning a study (Chapters 12 and 13). Recruitment for an experiment is usually more difficult than recruitment for an observational study, and the investigator should plan a large accessible population and enough time and money to get the desired sample size when (as usually happens) the barriers to doing so turn out to be worse than expected.

Measuring baseline variables

Characterize the study cohort: The next step is to design measurements that will define the characteristics of the study subjects before they are randomized. The investigator should begin with basic identifying information, such as name, address, and hospital ID number. She should then include demographic and clinical factors such as age, sex, and diagnosis that will be used (when generalizing the findings) to characterize the target populations. These measurements also have the secondary purpose of providing a means for checking on the comparability of the study groups at baseline; the first table of the final report of an RBT typically compares the levels of baseline characteristics in the two study groups. The goal is to make sure that differences in these levels do not exceed what might be expected from the play of chance, which would suggest a technical error in carrying out the randomization.

Consider measuring the outcome variable: It is often useful to measure the outcome variable at the beginning of the study as well as at the end. In studies that have a dichotomous outcome—the incidence of CHD, for example—it may be important to demonstrate by history and electrocardiogram that the disease is not present at the outset. In studies that have a continuous outcome variable—a study of the effects of antihypertensive drugs, for example—it may be desirable to use the difference between the two groups in the degree of *change* in blood pressure over the course of the study. This approach controls for differences among the study subjects in their initial blood pressure levels and may offer more power than simply comparing the blood pressure values at the end.

Measure various predictors of outcome: Particularly in relatively small studies, it is a good idea to measure all baseline variables that are likely to be strong predictors of the outcome (smoking habits of the spouse in a test of a smoking intervention program, for example). This permits statistical adjustment of the results to reduce the effects of chance maldistributions of baseline factors between the two study groups, increasing the efficiency of the study. It also allows the investigator to examine these other predictors as a separate research question. There are fiscal advantages to the strategy of adding ancillary studies that involve a few additional measurements and do not interfere with the main objectives. The MRFIT Behavior Pattern Study (4) discussed in Chapter 4 was one of several observational cohort studies carried out in conjunction with the main clinical trial goal of the MRFIT: to test the effectiveness of risk factor intervention.

Be parsimonious: Having pointed out all these uses for baseline measurements, we should stress that the basic design of a randomized experiment does not require that *any* be measured, because randomization eliminates the problem of confounding by factors that are present at the outset. (Consider the draft lottery study (5) discussed in Chapter 6, in which the only baseline information other than birthdate was race and place of birth.) The disadvantage of making a lot of measurements is the expense and complexity they add. In a randomized study, time and money are usually better spent on things that are vital to the integrity of the study such as the sufficiency of the sample size, the success of efforts at blinding, and the completeness of follow-up. Yusuf et al. have written an excellent article on this topic entitled "Why Do We Need Some Large, Simple Randomized Trials?" (6).

Randomizing the study subjects

The third step in Figure 11.1 is to randomize the subjects into two or more study groups that will receive different interventions. The allocation to these groups serves as the main predictor variable of the study. In the simplest design, one group receives an active treatment and the other remains an untreated control group.

The random allocation of subjects to one or another of the study groups establishes the basis for testing the statistical significance of differences between these groups in the measured outcome. Randomization provides that age, sex, and other baseline characteristics that could confound an observed association will be distributed equally (except for chance variation) between the randomized groups. An important fact, not widely appreciated, is that the effects of any maldistributions that *do* occur as a result of chance (and on the average, 1 in every 20 baseline variables *will* differ at $P < .05$) are automatically included in the statistical tests

of the likelihood that chance is responsible for the overall difference in outcome between the randomly assigned groups.

Do a good job of randomizing: Because randomization is the cornerstone of an RBT, it is important that it be done correctly. The two most important features are (*a*) that a **true random allocation** procedure be designed, and (*b*) that the process of randomization be **tamperproof** so that neither intentional nor unintentional biases can influence the allocation process.

Ordinarily the participant completes the baseline examinations, is found eligible for inclusion, and gives consent to enter the study before starting the randomization process. She is then irreversibly randomized by applying a previously established algorithm to a set of random numbers. For example, if the design calls for an equal probability of assignment to each of three study groups, the algorithm could specify:

- Using the last digit of each number in a column of random numbers (Appendix 3),
- Representing the three study groups with 0, 1, and 2,
- Reading down each column in sequence,
- Skipping over the numbers 3-9 until the first 0, 1, or 2 is reached, and
- Assigning the participant to that group.

This manual approach is usually replaced in modern studies by an equivalent computerized system, but doing it by hand may be easier in a small study.

It is essential to design the randomization procedure so that members of the research team who have any contact with the study subjects cannot influence the allocation. A costly procedure appropriate for larger studies is to set up a separate randomization facility that the clinician contacts by telephone when she is ready to randomize a new subject. The clinician reads the name and study number of the new subject to a data manager at that facility, who records it and uses the specified randomization procedure to make the study group assignment.

If remote randomization is not feasible, random treatment assignments can be placed (in advance) in a set of sealed envelopes by someone who will not be involved in opening the envelopes. Each envelope must be numbered (so that all can be accounted for at the end of the study), opaque (to prevent transillumination by a strong light), and otherwise tamperproof. When a subject is randomized her name and the number of the next envelope are first recorded, then the envelope is opened. Elaborate precautions of this sort are needed because clinicians sometimes find themselves under intense pressure to influence the randomization process (e.g., for an individual who seems particularly suitable for an active treatment group in a placebo-controlled trial).

Consider special randomization techniques: In general, the greatest power results from randomizing *equal numbers* of participants to each group, but disproportionate allocation has been used in studies that have three or more groups, one serving as a control for each of the others (7). If no formal comparisons among the treatment groups are planned, the larger number of comparisons that involve the control group makes the precision of its outcome measure especially important and the investigator can consider assigning a larger proportion of subjects to the control group.[a] However there is no clear way to pick the best proportions to use, and disproportionate randomization in this and other situations can complicate the process of getting informed consent (1). Because the advantages are marginal (the effect of even a 2:1 disproportion on power is surprisingly modest (1)), the best decision is usually to assign equal numbers to each group.

Experiments of small to moderate size will have a small gain in power if special randomization procedures are used to balance the study groups in the numbers of subject they contain, and in the distribution of baseline variables known to predict the outcome. These procedures, which include blocked, stratified, and adaptive randomization, are described in Appendix 11.

Applying the intervention

In an experiment the investigator compares the outcome in groups of subjects that receive different interventions. Between-group designs always include an **experimental group** that receives a treatment to be tested, and a **control group** that receives either no active treatment or a standard comparison treatment. Sometimes there are also additional experimental groups that receive other treatments. There are a number of trade-offs to consider in choosing and applying these interventions.

Importance of blinding: Whenever possible the investigator should design the interventions in such a fashion that neither the study subjects, nor anybody who has any contact with them, has any knowledge of the study group assignment. Randomization only eliminates the influence of confounding variables that are present at the time of randomization; it does not protect the study from *confounding* by variables that develop *during the period of followup* (Table 11.1). In an unblinded study, for example, the investigator may give extra attention to patients she knows are receiving the active drug, and this **unintended intervention** (also known as a *co-intervention*) may be the actual cause of any difference in outcome that is observed between the groups. Unintended interventions can also affect the control group if, for example, subjects who discover that they are receiving placebo seek out other treatments that affect the difference in outcome between groups.

A partial solution to the problem of unintended interventions is to **specify and standardize the intervention.** An investigator who wishes to test the effect of vitamin C supplements for the common cold, for example, could specify in the operations manual the precise dose and frequency of taking vitamin C in the treated group, and she could prohibit the control subjects from taking these supplements. A much more effective strategy, however, is to conceal the na-

---

[a] This strategy is easy to implement by assigning more numbers to the control group in the algorithm that is applied to the table of random numbers. If the proportions in a control and two treatment groups are to be 42%, 29%, and 29%, for example, the last two digits of each number can be used, with the numbers 1-42 representing the control group, the numbers 43-71 one of the treatment groups, and the numbers 72-00 the other treatment group.

Table 11.1.
Randomization eliminates confounding by baseline variables and blinding eliminates confounding by unintended interventions. Thus, these two strategies rule out effect-effect as the basis for an association (see also Table 10.1.)

Explanation for association	Strategy to rule out rival explanation
1. Chance	Same as in observational studies
2. Bias	Same as in observational studies
3. Effect-cause	(Not a possible explanation in an experiment)

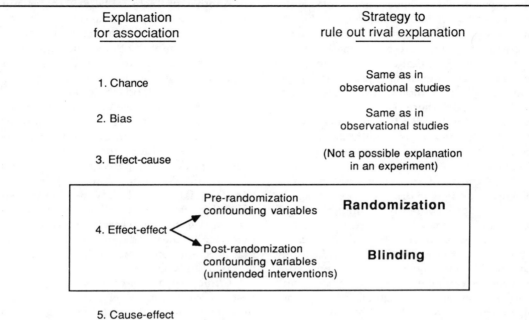

| 5. Cause-effect | |

ture of the study group assignment from both the investigator and the subjects by using identical capsules for the vitamin C or placebo. We have discussed the advantages of this **double-blind** approach (in which neither the investigator nor the subject knows the treatment assignment) in Chapters 4 and 10. When the double blind is technically successful, any unintended interventions that occur must affect all the study groups equally (with the exception, as for randomization, of chance maldistributions), and cannot alter the between-group comparison of outcomes.

Of the two main cornerstones of an RBT, randomization and blinding, the latter is by far the more difficult to carry out successfully. First there is the problem that many interventions cannot be blinded. For interventions such as a drug that can be blinded the logistic problems can be substantial. There is the need to get the manufacturer or pharmacy to prepare the identical capsules, and to develop foolproof systems for labeling and dispensing. In addition it may be necessary to

develop a 24-hour mechanism for unblinding in the event that the subject becomes acutely ill and her personal physician needs to know what drug she is taking (the hospital pharmacy will sometimes help to design and provide this service).

The other major difficulty in designing the system for blinding is assuring that neither the subjects nor the research team will be able to discern the treatment assignment. Telltale effects of the drugs on laboratory values (such as the effect of diuretics on serum potassium) may require setting up a system in which these results are reviewed by someone not involved in providing care to the subjects. After the study is over, it is a good idea to assess systematically whether the subjects and investigators can guess the treatment assignments; if a higher than expected proportion guesses correctly, the published discussion of the findings should include an assessment of the potential biases this partial unblinding may have caused.

Choice of experimental treatment: The scientific advantages of the double-blind approach can be an overriding consideration in the process of choosing an intervention. The best studies of whether lowering dietary fats prevents CHD have used cholesterol-lowering drugs (which are suitable for blinding) as a surrogate for diet (which is not). Unfortunately, many research questions address interventions that cannot be blinded in any fashion—surgical operations and psychotherapy are examples. Investigators who wish to study these issues must decide whether a non-blinded trial is a worthwhile undertaking, or whether additional observational and basic science designs will be more informative.

The choice of treatment often involves picking a particular drug or dose or health education procedure from among several promising options when there is no clear basis for knowing which is best. (If there *were* a clear basis, there would be no need for the study!) The investigator must use whatever evidence is available from prior research and pilot studies on the potential efficacy and side effects of each option. She may end up deciding to design two or more experimental groups in order to test each of several promising interventions. This is sometimes a reasonable strategy (for example the Coronary Drug Project tested four drugs for preventing CHD (7)), but it has its costs: a larger and more expensive study, and the complexity of dealing with multiple hypotheses (Chapter 12).

It is important to choose an intervention that will enhance generalizability through its relevance to the way medicine is practiced. A major criticism of the UGDP (University Group Diabetes Program) study of oral hypoglycemic agents for preventing CHD in mild diabetes (8) was the decision to use a single dose of tolbutamide in all patients assigned to this drug. When the study unexpectedly revealed a higher rate of CHD in these patients than in those who received no treatment, critics objected that this might not apply to the ordinary clinical situation in which dosage is individually tailored to the patient's blood sugar response. Choosing a relevant treatment can be especially difficult in studies that involve years of follow-up because a treatment that reflects current

practice at the outset of the study may have become outmoded by the end, transforming a pragmatic test into an academic exercise.

Another problem is the fact that many medical conditions are commonly addressed with combinations of treatments. It is possible to design the study to test such combinations, for example the MRFIT test of a program for eliminating smoking, hypertension, and high blood cholesterol (9), but there is the disadvantage that the outcome of such a study will not provide clear conclusions about any one intervention. (If a difference between study groups is observed, it is usually difficult to parcel out which parts of the intervention were responsible.) Clinical trials should only be undertaken when there is a *high likelihood of a conclusive answer* to the research question, and this usually means designing interventions that have only one major difference between any two study groups.

Choice of a comparison group: The best control groups receive *no active treatment in a way that can be blinded*, which usually means by identical placebo. This strategy compensates for any placebo effect of the active intervention (i.e., through suggestion and other nonpharmacologic mechanisms) so that any difference between study groups can be ascribed to a biologic effect.

Sometimes, however, it is not possible to withhold all treatment. Investigators in the MRFIT decided that it would be unethical to prohibit their control subjects from changing their CHD risk factors, and permitted usual care from sources outside the trial. The study was based on the assumption that the special intervention group would be much more successful in lowering their risk factor levels. Unfortunately, the difference between the two study groups in the extent of the risk factor reduction was diminished by the surprising efficacy of usual care in this setting (9), probably contributing to the failure of the study to detect a difference between the two groups in the CHD outcome.

A related problem is the test of a new treatment by comparing it with one already established as efficacious. Here the challenge is to establish the inference, if no significant difference is seen, that the two treatments are equivalent. **Tests of equivalence** involve a philosophic reversal of the usual circumstance that the investigator must show the experimental treatment to be better than the control, not just equivalent. There is the problem that a study which is too small or too biased to reveal a difference in outcome may appear to demonstrate that the new drug is as effective as the established one even though it is actually less effective. Statistical solutions to the problem of demonstrating equivalence involve testing whether the observed difference in outcomes between the two groups lies within some specified limits (10). A design solution, when feasible, is to add an untreated control group.

Assuring compliance: The effect of the intervention (and therefore the power of the study) is reduced to the degree that subjects fail to comply with the protocol. The first aspect of compliance in an outpatient study is **attending clinic visits** on schedule. The investigator can enhance this by discussing what is involved in the study before the consent is obtained, by scheduling the visits at a time that is convenient and with enough staff to prevent any waiting, by calling the subject the day before each visit, and by providing reimbursement for travel expenses and other out-of-pocket costs.

The other main aspect of compliance is **adhering to the intervention protocol.** The investigator should try to choose a study drug or behavioral intervention that will be well tolerated. Drugs that can be taken in a single daily dose are the easiest to remember and therefore preferable when there is a choice in the matter. These considerations also affect the generalizability of the study, since a drug like cholestyramine that requires several doses each day and is unpleasant to the taste may not be widely used in the population even though the study finds it to be effective (11). The operations manual should include provisions that will enhance compliance, such as instructing the subjects to take the pill at a standard point in the morning routine and giving them pill containers labeled with the day of the week.

There is also a need to consider how best to *measure* compliance, using such approaches as self-report, pill counts, and uri-

nary metabolite levels (12). This information can lead the investigator to bolster the intervention effort during the study in those subjects who are not complying, and it can help explain the finding if there is no difference between groups at the end.

Measuring the outcome

In choosing the outcome measure the investigator often needs to reach a judgment among competing considerations.

Appropriateness to the research question: The outcomes designed for studies are often surrogates for the actual phenomena of interest. In an experiment to determine the value of nutritional supplements in pregnant women, for example, the investigator might be interested in the effects of this intervention on the occurrence of congenital abnormalities. However, the rarity of this event would require an impossibly large study, and the investigator might decide to use low birth weight as a surrogate. This outcome is known to be associated with congenital abnormalities and can be studied with a reasonable sample size (see below); it has the disadvantage that a difference between study groups in birth weight would only suggest an effect on the outcomes of interest, not prove it.

Statistical characteristics: The outcome measure should be one that can be assessed *accurately and precisely.* An example of an outcome that meets these criteria is a newborn baby's weight; an example of one that does not is the presence or absence of a congenital learning deficit—a behavioral variable that represents the ill-defined end of a continuum.

Continuous outcome variables have the advantage over dichotomous ones of enhancing the power of the study, thus permitting a smaller sample size. In Chapter 13 we will see that a study with birth weight as a continuous outcome variable requires less than half the sample size needed for a study that looks at the proportion of newborns that weigh less than 2500 g. Unfortunately birth weight as a continuous variable is much less relevant to the research question (because differences in birth weight among those babies who weigh more than 2500—

about 90% of all babies—may not be related to congenital abnormalities).

If a dichotomous outcome is unavoidable, *power depends more on the number of events* than on the overall number of subjects (6). In the MRFIT, for example, the effective sample size was not the 12,866 men in the study, but the 239 who experienced the primary outcome, CHD death (9). A dichotomous outcome that was distributed more evenly—quitting smoking, which occurred in nearly half the smokers—could be tested with far more power.

Number of outcome variables: It is often desirable to have *several outcome variables* that measure different aspects of the phenomena of interest. In the MRFIT, CHD mortality was chosen as the primary end point, and two other end points—CHD incidence (including nonfatal heart attacks as well as CHD deaths), and all-cause mortality—were included to provide added information on the effects of the intervention program (9). (A single primary endpoint was preferred in order to avoid the problems of interpreting the results of testing multiple hypotheses [see Chapter 12]; CHD mortality was chosen despite its disadvantage of providing fewer events than either of the other two end points because it could be measured more completely and accurately than CHD incidence, and because it was a more specific measure of CHD than all-cause mortality.) In the end all three end points produced similar inferences about the effects of the intervention, strengthening the validity of the conclusions.

The investigator should usually design outcome measures that will detect the occurrence of specified **adverse effects** that may result from the intervention. Adverse effects may range from relatively minor symptoms like fatigue and anorexia to serious complications including death, and a surprising number of CHD prevention studies have revealed an unexpected increase in the number of deaths from drugs that seemed safe (13). Revealing whether the beneficial effects of an intervention outweigh the adverse ones is a major goal of most experiments, even those that test apparently innocuous treatments like a health education program. The

investigator should consider the problem that both the nature of the end point and the sample size requirements for detecting adverse effects may be different than those for detecting benefits. Unfortunately, rare side effects will usually be impossible to detect no matter how large the experiment, and can only be discovered with a case-control design after the drug has become widely used in the population.

Importance of blinding: The outcome variable should be one that can be measured without knowledge of the study group assignment. Use of a double-blind design is particularly important when the outcome requires judgment on the part of the observer: it prevents ascertainment bias from affecting one group more than the other. (The term **triple blind** is sometimes used to emphasize the need to conceal treatment assignment from three people— the subject, the person administering the intervention, and the person measuring the outcome.) Aspects of the outcome ascertainment can often be blinded even when the rest of the study is not; in the MRFIT, for example, cause of death was assigned by a panel of experts who reviewed clinical data pertaining to each death without knowing the study group assignment.

Completeness of follow-up: The strategies for achieving a high response rate are the same as those discussed for cohort studies (Chapter 7). The most important take place at the outset of the study: clearly informing the subject of the importance of follow-up to exclude those who will find this difficult, and recording the name, address and telephone number of one or two close acquaintances who will always know where the subject is. In addition to enhancing the investigator's ability to assess vital status, this may give her access to proxy outcome measures that can be obtained by telephone from those who absolutely refuse to come in at the end. In the MRFIT, only 92% of the men returned for their sixth annual visit, but information on hospitalization for possible heart attack was obtained in 96% and vital status was known in 99.8% (9).

Achieving nearly 100% follow-up can be essential when the outcome is uncommon and a possible cause of loss to follow-up. In the MRFIT, less than 2% of the men had the primary outcome of CHD death, so a loss of several percent could have had a profound effect on the outcome if death was one of the reasons for losing track of the men; for this reason the MRFIT investigators painstakingly tracked down the vital status of those who had dropped out. The need to achieve such a high follow-up percentage is less important if there is no reason to expect a substantially different outcome in those who were lost to follow-up. Outcome data that are 90% complete are often reported and provide valid conclusions in some situations.

Analyzing the results

The basic approach to testing the hypothesis of an RBT with dichotomous outcomes is to compare the proportions in the study groups using a chi-square test. When the outcome is continuous a t test may be used, or a nonparametric alternative if the outcome is not normally distributed. Lifetable methods are useful when there are differences in follow-up duration among study participants, and Cox regression analysis can be used to adjust for chance maldistributions of baseline confounding variables (increasing the power for any given sample size). The technical detail of when and how to use these methods is described in other books (1).

Three philosophical issues that should be considered in designing an experiment are the primacy of the **intention-to-treat** analytic approach, the ancillary role for **subgroup analyses**, and the question of whether to specify **early stopping rules**. These complex issues are important, and we highly recommend that the reader turn to Appendix 11.B where they are discussed.

SPECIAL TYPES OF RANDOMIZED BLINDED DESIGNS

There are five variations on the randomized blinded design that may be useful when the circumstances are right: the run-in design, the factorial design, randomization of matched pairs, prerandomization, and group randomization.

Run-in design

This is a useful design for increasing the proportion of study subjects who comply with the intervention and follow-up procedures. After identifying the study cohort and obtaining consent in the usual fashion, all subjects are placed on placebo. A specified time later (usually a few weeks) those who have complied with the intervention are randomized blindly to continue taking the placebo or to begin taking the active drug. Excluding the noncompliant subjects before randomization in this fashion increases the power of the study and permits a better estimate of the full effects of intervention.

A variant of this design shown in Figure 11.2 is the use of the active drug for the run-in period. Here the response of an **intermediary variable** (i.e., one that lies between the intervention and the outcome) to the treatment can be used as criterion for randomization. In a trial of an antiarrhythmic drug's effect on mortality, for example, the investigator might randomize only those subjects whose arrhythmias are satisfactorily suppressed without undue side effects. This design maximizes power by increasing the proportion of the intervention group that is responsive to the intervention. It also improves generalizability by mimicking the clinician's tendency to continue using a drug only when she sees evidence that it is working after a few weeks of trying it in a given patient. In reporting the findings from run-in design studies, it is important to note any differences in baseline characteristics between the sample that was randomized and the sample that was not.

Factorial design

This excellent design can answer two separate research questions in a single sample of subjects. A good example is the study illustrated in Figure 11.3 that was designed to test the effect of aspirin on myocardial infarction, and of β-carotene on cancer (14). The subjects have been randomized into four groups, but each of the two hypothesis can be tested by comparing two *halves* of the study cohort. First, all those on aspirin are compared with all those on aspirin placebo

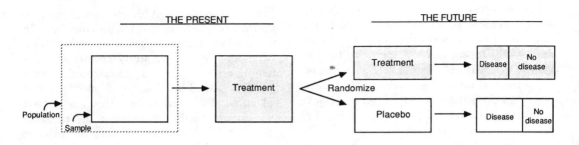

Steps:

1. Select a sample from the population
2. Measure baseline variables
3. Test a treatment in the whole cohort
4. Randomize
5. Apply interventions (one should be a blinded placebo, if possible)
6. Followup the cohorts
7. Measure outcome variables (blindly, if possible)

Figure 11.2.   An RBT preceded by a run-in period to test compliance.

(disregarding the fact that half of each of these groups received β-carotene); then, all those on β-carotene are compared with all those on β-carotene placebo (now disregarding the fact that half of each of these groups received aspirin). The investigator has two complete studies for the price of one.

The factorial design is an extremely efficient design, and it should be more widely used. The chief limitation is the problem of interactions between the two cause-and-effect relationships under study. In the example noted above, any influence of β-carotene on myocardial infarction would alter the outcome for half of the subjects receiving aspirin, reducing power and confusing interpetation. Factorial designs can actually be used to *study* such interactions, but large sample sizes are required and the results can be difficult to interpret. In clinical research, the best role for factorial designs is in studying two relatively independent research questions.

Randomization of matched pairs

One strategy for balancing baseline confounding variables involves selecting pairs of individuals who are matched on important factors like age and sex, then randomly as-

signing which member of each pair goes to which study group. A particularly attractive version of this design can be used when the circumstances permit a contrast of treatment and control effects in two parts of the same individual at the same time. In the Diabetic Retinopathy Study, for example, each subject had one eye randomly assigned to photocoagulation treatment while the other served as a control (15).

Pre-randomization

This design involves randomizing subjects who are found eligible for the study *before* obtaining informed consent. Consent is then requested using one or the other of two forms, each tailored to one of the study groups. This approach may increase the rate of enrollment by removing the psychologic barrier of uncertainty about study group assignment, but power is reduced to the degree that some participants will choose not to enroll but must still be analyzed to comply with intention-to-treat (see Appendix 11.B.). There is also an ethical problem with measuring outcome in these individuals, who have expressed the desire not to enter the study. The design is rarely used (16).

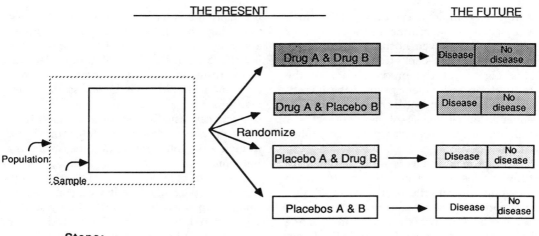

Steps:

1. Select a sample from the population
2. Measure baseline variables
3. Randomly assign two active interventions and their controls to four groups, as shown
4. Apply interventions blindly
5. Followup the cohorts
6. Measure outcome variables blindly

Figure 11.3.   A factorial design RBT, providing two studies for the price of one.

Group randomization

Instead of randomizing individuals, an investigator may choose to randomize naturally occurring clusters of subjects. A good example is the WHO study which enrolled 60 factories, randomly allocated half of them to receive intervention directed at CHD risk factors, and then observed a significantly lower incidence of CHD in these factories than in the remainder (17). Applying the intervention to groups of people may be more cost-effective than treating individuals one at a time, and it may better address research questions about the effects of public health programs in the population. Among the other advantages of this design over the usual individually randomized approach (18) is avoiding the problem that subjects who receive a transferrable intervention like dietary advice may discuss this advice with acquaintances in the same accessible population who have been assigned to the control group. A disadvantage of cluster randomization is the fact that sample size estimation and analysis are more complicated in cluster randomization (19).

OTHER EXPERIMENTAL DESIGNS

Nonrandomized between-group designs

Experiments that compare groups that have not been randomized are far less satisfactory than an RBT in controlling for the influence of confounding variables. Analytic methods can adjust for baseline factors that are observed to be unequally distributed between the two study groups, but this strategy does not deal with the problem of **unmeasured confounding variables** such as life-style. Chalmers has reviewed the findings of randomized and nonrandomized studies of the same research question (20); the apparent benefits of intervention were much greater in the nonrandomized studies, even after adjusting statistically for differences in baseline variables. This and other analyses (21) indicate that the problem of confounding in nonrandomized clinical studies can be serious, and that it cannot be fully removed by statistical adjustment.

Sometimes subjects are allocated to the study groups by a *pseudo* random mechanism. For example, every other subject may be assigned to the treatment group, or every subject with an even hospital record number. Such designs can offer minor logistic advantages, but the predictability of the study group assignment permits the investigator to tamper with it by manipulating the sequence or eligibility of new subjects. A fresh randomization is easy to accomplish and far safer.

Sometimes subjects are assigned to study groups by the investigator according to certain clinical criteria. For example, diabetic patients may be allocated to receive either insulin four times a day or long-acting insulin once a day according to their willingness to accept four daily injections. The problem is that even if the two groups of subjects appear identical in the severity of their disease, they may differ in important ways that have not been measured. Those willing to take four injections per day might be more compliant with other health advice, for example, and this might be the cause of any observed difference in the outcomes of the two treatment programs.

Nonrandomized designs are sometimes chosen in the mistaken belief that they are more ethical. In fact the randomized design has the advantage here as well, because studies are only ethical if they are designed well enough to have a reasonable likelihood of producing the correct answer to the research question, and randomized designs are more likely to lead to a conclusive result than nonrandomized designs. Moreover, the ethical basis for any experiment is the uncertainty as to whether the intervention will be beneficial or harmful, an uncertainty that must exist if the experiment needs to be done at all.

Nonblinded between-group designs

A randomized experiment in which the assignment to intervention and control groups is not double blind is also far less satisfactory than an RBT because of the susceptibility to confounding by unintended interventions, and to bias in the ascertainment of the outcome that affects one group more than the other.

When the circumstances do not permit the study to be fully blinded, **partial blinding** is usually possible. Some studies are designed to be single blind, to conceal the study group assignment from the subject but not from the investigator. This design does not protect the study from unintended interventions, however, and it should rarely be necessary—interventions that can be concealed from the subjects can usually also be concealed from those members of the research team involved in giving the intervention and measuring the outcome.

A more common form of partial blinding is the partially blinded outcome ascertainment process found in the many studies with open interventions. Such studies can produce useful conclusions, a good example being the CASS trial comparing medical versus surgical treatment for severe angina (22), but they are usually less conclusive than a blinded study. The open intervention can contribute to a negative result, as in the MRFIT example noted earlier, or to a positive result, as in the Hypertension Detection and Follow-up Program. In this study, the absence of blinding may have led subjects in the intervention group to receive unintended interventions above and beyond the antihypertensive treatment, perhaps contributing to the benefit that was observed (23).

Time series designs

Time series designs can be a useful option for some types of questions (Figure 11.4). Each subject serves as her own control during sequential treatment and control periods. This means that innate characteristics like age, sex, and genetic factors are not merely balanced (as they are in between group-studies) but actually *eliminated* as confounding variables. It also means that the sample size is doubled, in effect, because every subject provides both control and experimental observations.

The time series design is only useful in certain situations. These include studies of outcome variables that respond rapidly and reversibly to the intervention; the effect of alcohol intake on HDL-cholesterol level, for example, or the effect of insulin on blood sugar. Time series designs are also useful for certain long term experiments that cannot be randomized. In the Stanford Five City Proj-

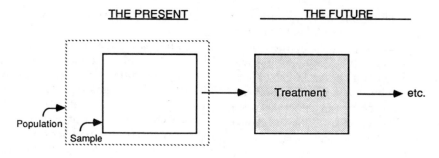

Steps:

1. Select a sample from the population
2. Measure baseline variables (including outcome variable)
3. Apply intervention to the whole cohort
4. Followup the cohort
5. Measure outcome variable again
6. (optional) Remove intervention and measure outcome variable again

Figure 11.4.   The time series design.

ect, the investigators provided CHD intervention to two entire cities using TV and other mass media, observing the CHD rates in each city before and after the onset of intervention (24). In addition to this within-group design, the investigators also studied three other cities, not randomly allocated, as controls. (Designs of this sort that lack a randomized control and have a mixture of within- and between-group comparisons are called "quasi-experimental" by Campbell and Stanley (25), but we do not favor this term; there is nothing quasi about the fact that an experiment is going on.)

The biggest disadvantage of within-group designs is the problem of **time dependent confounding** variables. One example is the **secular trend**, a change over time due to a factor like the season of the year that may affect the outcome differently in the second phase of the study than in the first. The other is the **carryover effect**, a residual influence of the intervention on the outcome during the period after it has been stopped (26). Blood pressure may not return to baseline levels for months after a course of diuretic treatment, for example. To reduce the carryover effect, the investigator can introduce an untreated "washout" period with the hope that the outcome variable will return to normal before starting the next inter-

vention, but it is difficult to know whether all carryover effects have been eliminated.

Another disadvantage occurs when the inclusion criteria specify a high value of the outcome variable. A study of the efficacy of treating hypertension, for example, might select subjects with a diastolic blood pressure > 90 mm Hg. Blood pressure would fall in some individuals during the period of observation purely because of the statistical phenomenon of regression to the mean (8), and in the absence of a concurrent control it would be difficult to distinguish this effect from a response to treatment.

Other within-group designs

The influence of time-dependent covariables can be controlled by a **crossover design** in which half of the participants are randomly assigned to start with the placebo and then switch to active treatment while the other half do the opposite. This approach (or an analog such as the latin square for more than two treatment groups (25)) permits between-group as well as within-group analyses. The advantages appear to be substantial: the control over time-dependent confounding of an RBT combined with the control over baseline confounding and effective doubling of sample size of a time series design. However the disadvantages are often even greater: a doubling of the duration of the study, and an added complexity of analysis and interpretation created by the elusive problem of carryover effects. Crossover studies are only a good choice when subjects are hard to come by, when there is good reason to believe that carryover effects will not be a problem, or when studying carryover effects is part of the research question.

Time series designs sometimes use the **repeated measures** strategy of repeatedly starting and stopping the treatment. If the onset and offset of the intervention produces matching patterns in the outcome, then the systematic influence of time-dependent confounding variables becomes less likely.

Natural experiments

In a natural experiment the investigator analyzes a situation in which someone else applies an intervention. For example, the relationship between the passage (and later recision) of laws requiring motorcycle helmets and the rate of serious injuries is a natural time-series experiment (27). Natural experiments actually resemble observational studies as much as experiments because the intervention is not manipulated by the investigator and the control over the influence of confounding variables is quite limited unless the experiment includes a randomization as in the draft lottery study (5) described in Chapter 6.

DECIDING TO DO AN EXPERIMENT

The reasons for undertaking an experiment are balanced by reasons for not doing so (Table 11.2). Experiments may be time consuming and expensive, particularly when the outcome is an infrequent event like CHD mortality. There are sometimes ethical barriers to applying or withholding interventions. Standardized interventations may be artificial, and experiments tend to restict the conclusions to a narrow research question with a yes/no answer. (This last disadvantage is partially neutralized, however, if the research question is expanded by carrying out observational studies within the study groups.)

The classic advantage of an experiment is its potential for controlling the influence of confounding variables, thus providing more conclusive answers. For some research questions an experiment is the only available approach. For others it may be faster and less expensive than observational studies, particularly when the outcome variable is continuous and rapidly responsive—it is difficult to demonstrate the relationship between dietary fat and serum cholesterol in an observational study (because of the large variation in the dietary variable) but relatively easy to do so in an experiment.

For many research questions, an experiment is a slow and costly approach, but it may nevertheless be worthwhile if the following three criteria are satisfied:

1. Strategies for answering the research question with observational studies have been exhausted.
2. The existing knowledge is not sufficient to determine clinical or public health policy.
3. An experiment is likely to provide an important extension of this knowledge.

The last criterion—the potential for a conclusive increment in knowledge—is particularly important. A clinical trial should not be undertaken when, because of the absence of randomization, blinding, or sufficient numbers of subjects, it is unlikely to provide a conclusive answer.

SUMMARY

1. The best experimental design is the classic *randomized blinded trial (RBT)*, which avoids three important sources of error in drawing inferences from the study sample to the population:

   a. **The randomization** eliminates bias due to *prerandomization confounding* variables.
   b. **Blinding the intervention** eliminates bias due to *unintended interventions.*
   c. **Blinding the outcome** measurement eliminates *ascertainment bias.*

Table 11.2.
The pros and cons of experimental design

Pros and Cons	Examples
Disadvantages	
Experiments are often costly in time and money	The MRFIT took 10 years and cost $120 million (9)
Many research questions are not suitable for experimental designs	
There may be ethical barriers	Drugs in pregnancy
The outcomes may be too rare	Unusual side effects like agranulocytosis due to chloramphenicol
Standardized interventions may be different from common practice (reducing generalizability)	Single fixed dose of orinase for treating diabetes in the UGDP (8)
Experiments tend to restrict the scope and narrow the study question	An experiment that tests whether a cholesterol-lowering drug prevents CHD focuses on that risk factor, whereas an analytic study can examine many risk factors
Advantages	
Experiments can produce the strongest evidence for cause and effect	The LRC study showing that cholestyramine prevents CHD (11)
Experiments can be the only possible design for some research questions	Studies of new synthetic drugs
Experiments can sometimes produce a faster and cheaper answer to the research question than observational studies	The effect of a low-fat diet on serum cholesterol is difficult to show in an observational study (because of the error in dietary assessments) but easy to show in an experiment

2. An RBT remains susceptible to three other errors, however: an investigator designing an experiment should think carefully about *generalizability* when choosing the study subjects and intervention, she should be sure that the *sample size* is adequate to control random sources of error, and she should take steps to prevent *technical errors*, particularly in the randomization procedure.

3. The best choice of *control* treatment in an experiment is usually a *placebo*. Studies that use an active treatment as the control group in an effort to establish the equivalence of another active treatment must be interpreted with caution.

4. There are several underutilized variations on the RBT design that can substantially increase efficiency under the right circumstance:

a. The *run-in-design* can enhance compliance and responsiveness to treatment before randomization.

b. The *factorial design* allows two independent experiments to be carried out for the price of one.

c. *Matched-pair randomization* ballances baseline confounding variables.

d. *Group-randomization* permits efficient studies of naturally occurring clusters.

5. *Nonrandomized* between-group designs are rarely a good choice. *Nonblinded* designs are acceptable in some situations—

for operations, procedures, and behavioral interventions that can neither be blinded nor studied as well as in any other way. In these circumstances it is often possible at least to blind the outcome measurement.

6. The *time series* design compares serial measurements of the outcome in a single group of subjects before and after an intervention is applied; this is efficient, but time-dependent confounding (especially *carryover effects*) can be a problem. *Crossover designs*, which combine the features of an RBT and a time series design, are occasionally useful when the number of subjects is limited.

7. In general, it is best to reserve experimental designs for relatively *mature research questions*—those that have already been examined by observational studies but require stronger evidence in order to establish health policy. Observational subgroup analyses can be included in experiment, as a hedge against a dull result in testing the main hypothesis and to increase the richness and variety of the study's conclusions.

8. The full potential of an RBT to eliminate the influence of baseline confounding variables is only realized when the results are examined by an *intention-to-treat* analysis, with all study subjects analyzed according to their random assignments (see Appendix 11.B.). Analyses on subgroups of the cohort classified by compliance and other postrandomization factors can also be carried out (cautiously) in a secondary effort to interpret the findings.

REFERENCES

1. Friedman LM, Furberg CD, DeMets DL: *Fundamental of Clinical Trials.* ed 2. Littleton, MA, PSG Publishing Co, 1985.
2. Horwitz RI, Feinstein AR: Improved observational method for studying therapeutic efficacy. *JAMA* 246:2455–2459, 1981.
3. Freiman JA, Chalmers TC, Smith H Jr, et al: The importance of beta, the Type II error and sample size in the design and interpretation of the randomized control trial: survey of 71 "negative" trials. *N Engl J Med* 299:690–694, 1978.
4. Shekelle RB, Hulley SB, Neaton JD, et al: The MRFIT Behavior Pattern Study: II. Type A behavior and the incidence of CHD. *Am J Epidemiol*, 122:550–570, 1985
5. Hearst N, Newman TB, Hulley SB: Delayed effects of the military draft on mortality: a randomized natural experiment. *N Engl J Med* 314:620–6244, 1986.
6. Yusuf S, Collins R, Peto R: Why do we need some large, simple randomized trials? *Statistics in Medicine* 3:409–420, 1984.
7. The CDP Research Group: Influence of adherence to treatment and response of cholesterol on mortality in the CDP. *N Engl J Med* 303:1038–1041, 1980.
8. Fletcher RH, Fletcher SW, Wagner EH: *Clinical Epidemiology—The Essentials.* Baltimore, Williams & Wilkins, 1988.
9. The MRFIT Group: The MRFIT: Coronary death, non-fatal MI and other clinical outcomes. *Am J Cardiol* 58;1–13, 1986.
10. Hauck WW, Anderson, S: A proposal for interpreting and reporting negative studies. *Statistics in Medicine* 5:203–209, 1986.
11. The LRC Group: The LRC Coronary Primary Prevention Trial. *JAMA* 251:351–364, 365–374, 1984.
12. Black DM, Brand RJ, Greenlick M, Hughes G, Smith J: Compliance to treatment for hypertension in the elderly: the SHEP Pilot Study. *J Geriat,* 42:552–557, 1987.
13. Oliver MF: Risks of correcting the risks of coronary disease and stroke with drugs. *N Engl J Med* 306:297–298, 1982.
14. Hennekins CH, Eberlein K: A randomized trial of aspirin and beta-carotene among U.S. physicians. *Prev Med* 14:165–168, 1985.
15. Diabetic Retinopathy Study Research Group: Preliminary report on effects of photocoagulation therapy. *Am J Ophthalmol* 81:383–396, 1976.
16. Ellenberg SS: Randomization designs in comparative clinical trials. *N Engl J Med* 310:1404–1408, 1984.
17. WHO European Collaborative Group: European collaborative trial of multifactorial prevention of CHD: Final report of the 6-year results. *Lancet,* 1:869–872, 1986.
18. Sherwin R: Controlled trials of the Diet-Heart Hypothesis: some comments on the experiment unit. *Am J Epidemiol* 108:92–99, 1978.
19. Donner A, Birkett N, and Buck C: Randomization by cluster: sample size requirements and analysis. *Am J Epidemiol* 114:906–914, 1981.
20. Chalmers TC, Celano P, Sacks HS, et al: Bias in treatment assignment in controlled clinical trials. *N Engl J Med* 309:1358–1361, 1983.
21. Pocock SJ: Current issues in the design and interpretation of clinical trials. *Brit Med J* 1985; 296:39–42.
22. CASS Principal Investigators: Coronary artery surgery study (CASS): a randomized trial of coronary artery bypass surgery. *Circulation* 68:939–950, 1983.
23. Hulley SB. The non-blinded usual care control: problems and solutions. *Institute for Health Policy Studies Discussion Paper,* University of California, San Francisco, 1983.
24. Farquhar JW, Fortmann SP, Maccoby N, et al: The Stanford Five-City Project: design and methods. *Am J Epidemiol* 122:323–334, 1985.

25. Cook TD, Campbell DT: *Quasi-experimentation: Design and Analysis Issues for Field Settings.* Boston, Houghton Mifflin Co., 1979.
26. Brown BW Jr: Statistical controversies in the design of clinical trials—some personal views. *Contr Clin Trials* 1:13–28, 1980.
27. Watson GS, Zador PL, Wilks A: Helmet use, helmet use laws, and motorcyclist fatalities. *Am J Public Health* 71:297–300.

ADDITIONAL READINGS

Bull JP: The historical development of clinical therapeutics. *J Chron Dis* 10:218–248, 1959. (*Fascinating discussion of the evolution of clinical trials over the past 2000 years.*)
Fredrickson DS: The field trial: some thoughts on the indispensible ordeal. *Bull NY Acad Med* 44:985–993, 1960. (*Literate and entertaining introduction to the era of large clinical trials.*)
Friedman LM, Furberg CD, DeMets DL: *Fundamental of Clinical Trials*, ed 2. Littleton, MA, PSG Publishing Co, 1985. (*An excellent book on clinical trials, with good examples and a special emphasis on large scale collaborative studies.*)
Kramer MS, Shapiro SH: Scientific challenges in the application of randomized trials. *JAMA* 252:2739–2745, 1984. (*A good discussion of six important issues in clinical trials.*)
Meinert C: *Clinical Trials.* New York, Oxford University Press, 1986. (*A comprehensive presentation of the philosophic and practical aspects of designing a clinical trial.*)
Pocock SJ: *Clinical Trials: A Practical Approach.* Chichester, England, John Wiley & Sons, 1983. (*A sound book on experiments.*)
Shapiro SH, Louis T: Clinical Trials: *Issues and Approaches.* New York, Marcel Dekker Inc., 1983. (*Useful essays by major figures in the field including Mosteller, Sackett, Armitage, Chalmers, and Meier.*)
Silverman WA: *Human Experimentation: A Guided Step into the Unknown.* Oxford, England, Oxford University Press, 1985. (*An extensive presentation of relevant historical events and the lessons we may learn from them.*)

CHAPTER 12

Getting Ready to Estimate Sample Size: Hypotheses and Underlying Principles

Warren S. Browner, Thomas B. Newman, Steven R. Cummings, and Stephen B. Hulley

INTRODUCTION   **128**

HYPOTHESES   **128**

   Characteristics of a good hypothesis
   Types of hypotheses

UNDERLYING STATISTICAL PRINCIPLES   **131**

   Type I and Type II errors
   Effect size
   α, β, and power
   P value
   Tails of the alternative hypothesis
   Type of statistical test

A FEW ADDITIONAL POINTS   **134**

   Variability
   Sampling unit
   Dropouts
   Confounding variables
   Multiple hypotheses
   Hypotheses generated by the study

SUMMARY   **137**

REFERENCES   **137**

— — — — — — — — — —

INTRODUCTION

After an investigator has decided who and what she is going to study, she must decide how many subjects to sample. Even the most rigorously executed study may fail to answer its research question if the sample size is too small. On the other hand, a study with too large a sample will be more difficult and costly than necessary. The goal of sample size planning is to estimate an appropriate number of subjects for a given study design.

Although a useful guide, sample size calculations give a deceptive impression of statistical objectivity. They are only as accurate as the data and estimates on which they are based, which are often just informed guesses. Sample size planning is best thought of as a scientific way of making a ballpark estimate. It often reveals that the research design is not feasible, or that different predictor or outcome variables are needed. Thus sample size should be estimated early in the design phase of a study, when changes can still be made.

Before setting out the specific cookbook approaches to calculating sample size for several common research designs in Chapter 13, we will spend some time considering the underlying principles. Readers who find some of these principles confusing will enjoy discovering that sample size planning does not require their total mastery. However, just as a recipe makes more sense if the cook is familiar with the ingredients, sample size calculations are easier if the investigator is acquainted with the basic concepts.

HYPOTHESES

In Chapter 1 we introduced the research question and discussed its transformation into an operational analog, the study plan. Many study questions undergo a further transformation into a final and most specific version, termed the hypothesis, that summarizes the elements of the study: the sample, the design, and the predictor and outcome variables. The primary purpose of the hypothesis is to establish the basis for tests of statistical significance.[a]

Hypotheses are not needed in descriptive studies that merely describe how characteristics are distributed in the population, such as a study of the prevalence of coffee drinking among patients with pancreatic cancer. Hypotheses are needed for studies that will use tests of statistical significance to compare findings among groups, such as a study of whether patients with pancreatic cancer report more coffee drinking than controls. Because most observational studies and all experiments do address research questions that involve making comparisons, most studies need to specify at least one hypothesis.

Characteristics of a good hypothesis

A good hypothesis must be based on a good research question. It should also be simple, specific, and stated in advance (Fig 12.1):

Simple versus complex: Whereas a simple hypothesis contains one predictor and one outcome variable, a complex hypothesis contains more than one predictor variable or more than one outcome variable (*The total average coffee intake and the habit of drinking coffee in the evening are associated with an increased incidence of pancreatic cancer*). Complex hypotheses like this one cannot be tested with a single statistical test, and should always be separated into two or more simple hypotheses.

Specific versus vague: A specific hypothesis leaves no ambiguity about the subjects and variables, or about how the test of statistical significance will be applied. It uses concise operational definitions that summarize the nature and source of the subjects and the approach to measuring variables (*The daily coffee intake 10 years ago reported by*

patients hospitalized for pancreatic cancer is greater than the intake reported by age-matched patients admitted for other diagnoses). This is a long sentence, but it communicates the nature of the study in a clear way that minimizes any opportunity for testing something a little different once the study findings have been looked at. It would be incorrect to substitute another predictor, such as all drinks that contain caffeine, without considering the issue of multiple hypothesis testing, a topic we discuss at the end of the chapter and in Appendix 18.

In advance versus after-the-fact: The hypothesis should be stated in writing at the outset of the study. This will help to keep the research effort focused on the primary objective, and create a stronger basis for interpreting the study's results than hypotheses that emerge as a result of inspecting the data. The original report of an association between coffee and pancreatic cancer (1) is an example of an after-the-fact hypothesis. Hypotheses that are first formulated after examination of the data are actually a form of multiple hypothesis testing, and have the same implications for tests of statistical significance.

Types of hypotheses

For the purpose of testing statistical significance, hypotheses are classified by the way they describe the expected difference between the study groups.

Null and alternative hypotheses: The **null hypothesis** states that there is no association between the predictor and outcome variables in the population (*There is no difference between the coffee-drinking habits of patients with pancreatic cancer and those of age- and sex-matched "control" patients hospitalized for other diagnoses*). The null hypothesis is the formal basis for testing statistical significance. By starting with the proposition that there is no association, statistical tests can estimate the probability that an observed association could be due to chance.

The proposition that there *is* an association—*that patients with pancreatic cancer will report different coffee-drinking habits from the controls*—is called the **alternative**

---

[a] The term "hypothesis" also has another meaning—an idea that the investigator has about the nature of the phenomena that she is studying. The diet-heart hypothesis, for example, specifies that dietary consumption of fat is a cause of coronary heart disease. In this book, however, we will not use hypothesis in this more general sense.

hypothesis. The alternative hypothesis cannot be tested directly: it is accepted by exclusion if the test of statistical significance rejects the null hypothesis (see below).

One- and two-tailed alternative hypotheses: A **one-tailed** (or one-sided) hypothesis specifies the direction of the association between the predictor and outcome variables. The prediction that patients with pancreatic cancer will have a higher rate of coffee drinking than control patients is a one-tailed hypothesis. A **two-tailed** hypothesis states only that an association exists; it does not specify the direction. The prediction that patients with pancreatic cancer will have a different rate of coffee drinking—either higher or lower—than control patients is a two-tailed hypothesis. (The word "tails" refers to the tail ends of the statistical distribution, such as the familiar bell-shaped normal curve, that is used to test a hypothesis. One tail represents a positive effect or association, the other a negative effect.)

A one-tailed hypothesis has the statistical advantage of permitting a smaller sample size than a two-tailed hypothesis. Unfortunately, one-tailed hypotheses are not always appropriate; in fact, some investigators believe that they should never be used. We disagree, believing that one-tailed hypotheses have been underused. They are clearly appropriate when only one direction for the

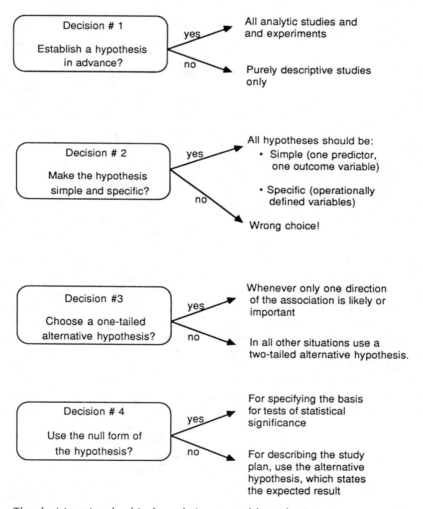

Figure 12.1. The decisions involved in formulating a good hypothesis.

association is important or biologically meaningful. An example is the one-sided hypothesis that a drug has a greater frequency of side effects than a placebo; the possibility that the drug has fewer side effects than the placebo is not usually worth testing. A one-tailed hypothesis may also be appropriate when there is good evidence from prior studies that an association is unlikely to occur in one of the two directions. An example is the Lipid Research Clinics experiment to test the efficacy of the cholesterol-lowering drug cholestyramine (2): Prior evidence that the drug was unlikely to increase the incidence of coronary heart disease justified the use of a one-tailed hypothesis. Further ramifications of this approach to interpreting statistical tests in the context of prior evidence are discussed in Appendix 18.

UNDERLYING STATISTICAL PRINCIPLES

A hypothesis, *(dietary carotene supplements are associated with a reduced incidence of co-*lon *cancer in middle-aged men)* is either true or false in the real world. Because an investigator cannot study all middle-aged men who are at risk for colon cancer, she must test the hypothesis in a sample of that target population. No matter how many data a researcher collects, she can never absolutely prove (or disprove) her hypothesis. As noted in Figure 1.7, there will always be a need to draw inferences about phenomena in the population from events observed in the sample.

In some ways, the investigator's problem is similar to that faced by a jury judging a defendant (Table 12.1). The absolute truth about whether the defendant committed the crime cannot be determined. Instead, the jury begins by presuming *innocence:* The defendant did not commit the crime. The jury must decide whether there is sufficient evidence to reject the presumed innocence of the defendant; the standard is known as *beyond a reasonable doubt.* A jury can err, however, by convicting a defendant who is innocent, or by failing to convict one who is actually guilty.

Table 12.1.
The analogy between jury decisions and statistical tests

Jury decision	Statistical test
Innocence: The defendant did not counterfeit money.	*Null hypothesis:* There is no association between dietary carotene and the incidence of colon cancer in the population.
Guilt: The defendant did counterfeit money.	*Alternative hypothesis:* There is an association between dietary carotene and the incidence of colon cancer.
Standard for rejecting innocence: Beyond a reasonable doubt.	*Standard for rejecting null hypothesis:* Level of statistical significance (α).
Correct judgment: Convict a counterfeiter.	*Correct inference:* Conclude that there is an association between dietary carotene and colon cancer when one does exist in the population.
Correct judgment: Acquit an innocent person.	*Correct inference:* Conclude that there is no association between carotene and colon cancer when one does not exist.
Incorrect judgment: Convict an innocent person.	*Incorrect inference (Type I):* Conclude that there is an association between dietary carotene and colon cancer when there actually is none.
Incorrect judgment: Acquit a counterfeiter.	*Incorrect inference (Type II):* Conclude that there is not an association between dietary carotene and colon cancer when there actually is one.

In similar fashion, the investigator starts by presuming the null hypothesis of no association between the predictor and outcome variables in the population. Based on the data collected in her *sample*, the investigator uses statistical tests to determine whether there is sufficient evidence to reject the null hypothesis in favor of the alternative hypothesis that there is an association in the *population*. The standard for these tests is known as the **level of statistical significance**.

Type I and Type II errors

Just like a jury, however, an investigator's conclusion may be wrong. Sometimes, by chance alone, a sample is not representative of the population. Thus the results in the sample do not reflect reality in the population, and the random error leads to an erroneous inference. A **Type I error** (false-positive) occurs if an investigator rejects a null hypothesis that is actually true in the population; a **Type II error** (false-negative) occurs if the investigator fails to reject a null hypothesis that is actually false in the population. Although Type I and II errors can never be avoided entirely, the investigator can reduce their likelihood by increasing the sample size (the larger the sample, the less likely that it will differ substantially from the population), or by manipulating the design or the measurements in other ways that will be discussed.

False-positive and false-negative results can also occur because of bias. (Errors due to bias, however, are not usually referred to as Type I and II errors.) Such errors are especially troublesome, since they may be difficult to detect and cannot usually be quantified. In this chapter and the next, we will deal only with ways to reduce random errors; see Chapters 1, 3, 4, and 7–11 for ways to reduce errors due to bias.

Effect size

The likelihood that a study will be able to detect an association between a predictor and an outcome variable depends, of course, on the actual magnitude of that association in the target population. If it is large (such as a 90% reduction in the incidence of colon cancer in men who use carotene supple-

ments), it will be easy to detect in the sample. Conversely, if the size of the association is small (such as a 2% reduction in cancer), it will be difficult to detect in the sample.

Unfortunately, the investigator does not usually know the actual magnitude of the association—one of the purposes of the study is to estimate it. Instead, the investigator must choose the size of the association that she would *like* to be able to detect in the sample. That quantity is known as the **effect size**. Selecting an appropriate effect size is the most difficult aspect of sample size planning. Sometime the investigator can use data from other studies or pilot tests to make an informed guess about a reasonable effect size. When there are no data with which to estimate it, she can choose the smallest effect size that would be clinically meaningful, for example, a 10% reduction in the incidence of colon cancer.

Of course, from the public health point of view, even a 1% reduction in colon cancer incidence would be important. Thus the choice of the effect size is always somewhat arbitrary, and considerations of feasibility are often paramount. When the number of available or affordable subjects is limited, the investigator may have to work backward (see Chapter 13) to determine whether the effect size that her study will be able to detect with that number of subjects is reasonable.

α, β, and power

After a study is completed, the investigator uses statistical tests to try to reject the null hypothesis in favor of its alternative (much in the same way that a prosecuting attorney tries to convince a jury to reject innocence in favor of guilt). Depending on whether the null hypothesis is true or false in the target population, and assuming that the study is free of bias, four situations are possible (Table 12.2). In two of these, the findings in the sample and reality in the population are concordant, and the investigator's inference will be correct. In the other two situations, either a Type I or Type II error has been made, and the inference will be incorrect.

The investigator establishes the maximum chance of making Type I and II errors

Table 12.2.
Truth in the population versus the results in the study sample: the four possibilities

		Truth in the population	
		Association between predictor and outcome	No association between predictor and outcome
Results in the study sample	Reject null hypothesis	CORRECT	TYPE I ERROR
	Fail to reject null hypothesis	TYPE II ERROR	CORRECT

in advance of the study. The probability of committing a Type I error (rejecting the null hypothesis when it is actually true) is called α (alpha). Another name for α is the **level of statistical significance.**

If a study of carotene and colon cancer is designed with $\alpha = 0.05$, for example, then the investigator has set 5% as the maximum chance of incorrectly rejecting the null hypothesis (and erroneously inferring that use of carotene supplements and colon cancer incidence are associated in the population). This is the level of reasonable doubt that the investigator is willing to accept when she uses statistical tests to analyze the data after the study is completed.

The probability of making a Type II error (failing to reject the null hypothesis when it is actually false) is called β (beta). The quantity $[1 - \beta]$ is called **power,** the probability of observing an effect in the sample if one of a specified effect size or greater exists in the population.

If β is set at 0.10, then the investigator has decided that she is willing to accept a 10% chance of missing an association of a given effect size between carotene and colon cancer. This represents a power of 0.90, i.e., a 90% chance of finding an association of that size. For example, suppose that there *really* would be a 30% reduction in colon cancer incidence if the entire population took carotene. Then 90 times out of 100 the investigator would observe an effect of that size or larger in her study. This does not mean, however, that the investigator will be absolutely unable to detect a smaller effect,

just that she will have less than 90% likelihood of doing so.

Ideally, α and β would be set at zero, eliminating the possibility of false-positive and false-negative results. In practice they are made as small as possible. Reducing them, however, usually requires increasing the sample size; other strategies are discussed in Chapter 13. Sample size planning aims at choosing a sufficient number of subjects to keep α and β at an acceptably low level without making the study unnecessarily expensive or difficult.

Many studies set α at 0.05, and β at 0.20 (a power of 0.80). These are somewhat arbitrary values, and others are sometimed used: the conventional range for α is between 0.01 and 0.10, and for β between 0.05 and 0.20. In general, the investigator should use a low α when the research question makes it particularly important to avoid a Type I (false-positive) error, and she should use a low β when it is especially important to avoid a Type II (false-negative) error.

P value

The null hypothesis acts like a straw man; it is assumed to be true in order to knock it down as false with a statistical test. When the data are analyzed, such tests determine the **P value,** the probability of obtaining the study results by chance if the null hypothesis is true. The null hypothesis is rejected in favor of its alternative if the P value is less than α, the predetermined level of statistical significance.

"Nonsignificant" results—those with P

values greater than α—do not imply that there is no association in the population; they only mean that the association observed in the sample is small compared with what could have occurred by chance alone. For example, an investigator might find that men with hypertension were twice as likely to develop prostate cancer as those with normal blood pressure, but with a P value of 0.09. This means that even if hypertension and prostatic carcinoma were not associated in the population, there was a 9% chance of finding such an association due to random error in the sample. If the investigator had set the significance level at 0.05, she would have to conclude that the association in the sample was "not statistically significant." It might be tempting for the investigator to change her mind about the level of statistical significance, and report "the results showed a statistically significant association (P < 0.10)." A better choice would be to report that "the results, although suggestive of an association, did not achieve statistical significance (P = 0.09)." This solution acknowledges that statistical significance is not an "all or none" situation (see Appendix 18 for a more complete discussion of this issue).

Tails of the alternative hypothesis

Recall that an alternative hypothesis actually has two **tails,** either or both of which can be tested in the sample by using one- or two-tailed statistical tests, respectively. When a two-tailed statistical test is used, the P value includes the probabilities of committing a Type I error in each of the two tails, which is twice as great as the probability in either tail alone. Thus it is easy to convert from a one-tailed P value to a two-tailed P value, and vice versa. A one-tailed P value of 0.05, for example, is identical to a two-tailed P value of 0.10.

When an investigator is only interested in one of the tails, and has so formulated the alternative hypothesis, sample size should be calculated accordingly. Although unnecessary use of two-tailed hypotheses needlessly increases the sample size, some statisticians and journal editors insist on their use in all situations. Thus, if the investigator has chosen a one-tailed alternative hypothesis and

an α of 0.05, a "significant" P value of 0.04 may be interpreted by critics as a "nonsignificant" two-tailed P value of 0.08. The investigator planning sample size to test a one-tailed hypothesis should be aware that she will have less power to test a two-tailed hypothesis should that eventually be required; she should therefore have a clear justification for her choice.

Type of statistical test

The formulas used to calculate sample size are based on certain mathematical assumptions, which differ for each statistical test. Thus before the sample size can be calculated, the investigator must decide on the statistical approach to analyzing the data. That choice depends mainly on the type of predictor and outcome variables in the study. Table 13-1 lists some common statistics used in data analysis, and Chapter 13 will provide simplified approaches to estimating sample size for studies that use these statistics.

A FEW ADDITIONAL POINTS

Variability

It is not simply the size of an effect that is important—its **variability** also matters. Statistical tests depend on being able to show a difference between the groups being compared. The greater the variability (or spread) in the outcome variable among the subjects, the more likely it is that the values in the groups will overlap, and the more difficult it will be to demonstrate an overall difference between them.

Consider a study of the effects of two diets (low-fiber and high-fiber) in achieving weight loss in 20 obese patients. If all those on the low-fiber diet lost about 5 kg and all those on the high-fiber diet failed to lose any weight (an effect size of 5 kg), it is likely that the low-fiber diet really is better (Figure 12.2A). On the other hand, suppose that although the average weight loss is 5 kg greater in the low-fiber group, there is a great deal of overlap between the two groups (the changes in weight vary from a loss of 8 kg to a gain of 8 kg). In this situation, even though the effect size is still 5 kg, it is less likely that the low-fiber diet would actually be better in the population (Figure 12.2B), and more likely that chance explains the results.

When the variables are dichotomous, variability is already included in other parameters entered into the sample size formulas and tables, and need not be specified. However, when one of the variables is continuous, the investigator will need to estimate its variability (see the section on the t test in Chapter 13 for details). For a more complete discussion of variability, see Lachin (3).

Sampling unit

Sample size techniques estimate the number of subjects required, with each individual subject representing one **sampling unit**. The sampling unit in clinical research is usually a single patient. Sometimes, however, particularly in health services research and in the evaluation of community-based interventions, the sampling unit is a group of individuals. In a study comparing the average duration of hospital stay among patients admitted to public hospitals with that in for-profit hospitals, the appropriate sampling unit is the hospital, not the patient.

The distinction is important: The unit used for sampling dictates the unit used for the analysis of the data, and influences the conclusions that can be drawn from the study. This means that comparing one or two public hospitals with one or two for-profit hospitals does not yield very secure inferences about public versus for-profit hospitals in general, even if the number of patients in each hospital is large. There is no easy solution; researchers planning such studies should be aware at the outset that it

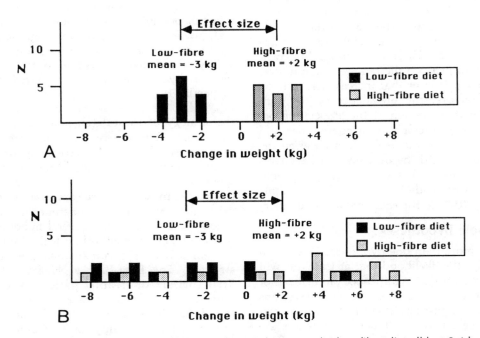

Figure 12.2.A.   Weight loss achieved by two diets. Subjects on the low-fiber diet all lost 2-4 kg, while those on the high-fiber diet all gained 1-3 kg; the effect size is 5 kg. Because there is no overlap between the two groups, it is reasonable to infer that the low-fiber diet really is better at achieving weight loss than the high-fiber diet.

Figure 12.2.B.   Weight loss achieved by two diets. There is a great deal of overlap between the two groups and some subjects in each group actually gained weight. Thus, even though the effect size is still 5 kg favoring the low-fiber diet, the study does not provide good evidence that the low-fiber diet really is better at achieving weight loss than the high-fiber diet.

may be difficult to assemble a sufficient sample size for hypothesis testing.

Investigators planning to use one of the more complex sampling schemes discussed in Chapter 3, such as cluster sampling, should consult one of the available references (4,5) when estimating sample size.

Dropouts

Each sampling unit must be available for analysis; thus subjects who are enrolled in a study but in whom outcome status cannot be ascertained (such as dropouts) do not count in the sample size. If the investigator anticipates that a substantial proportion of her subjects will not be available for follow-up, she should increase the size of the enrolled sample accordingly.

Confounding variables

Sometimes an investigator thinks that one or more variables will confound the association between the predictor and outcome (see Chapter 10), and wishes to plan her sample size accordingly. In general, analytic approaches that adjust for confounding variables will increase the required sample size. The magnitude of that increase depends on three factors: the prevalence of the confounder, the strength of the association between the predictor and the confounder, and the strength of the association between the confounder and the outcome. These effects are complex (6,7); a very rough approximation can be made by increasing the sample size by 10-20% for each major confounder.

Multiple hypotheses

When more than one hypothesis is tested in a study, the likelihood that at least one will achieve statistical significance on the basis of chance alone increases. Some statisticians advocate adjusting the level of statistical significance when simultaneous inferences are drawn from several hypotheses at once. This keeps the overall probability of accepting any one of the alternative hypotheses, when all the findings are due to chance, at the specified level. One approach, named after the mathematician **Bonferroni**, is to divide the significance level (say 0.05) by the number of hypotheses tested. If there were four hypotheses, for example, each would be tested at an α of 0.0125 (i.e., 0.05 divided by 4). This would require substantially increasing the sample size over that needed for testing each hypothesis at an α of 0.05.

Many statisticians believe that this type of approach is too stringent. Investigators do not adjust the significance levels of hypotheses tested in separate studies, and it is not clear that there is any more reason to do so when several unrelated hypotheses are tested in the same study. In our view, it is only mandatory to adjust α for multiple hypotheses when the hypotheses being tested are not fully independent of one another. An example would be a study in which two experimental treatment groups are compared with a single control group; if by chance the results in the control group are seriously distorted by random error, the comparison with each of the treatment groups would be affected, and the statistical analysis should take this possibility into account (8). In general, however, the issue of what significance level to use depends more on the prior probability of each hypothesis than on the number of hypotheses that are tested (see Appendix 18).

There are some definite advantages to the strategy of formulating more than one hypothesis. The use of multiple unrelated hypotheses increases the efficiency of the study, making it possible to answer more questions with a single research effort, and to discover more of the true associations that exist in the population. Sometimes it is also a good idea to formulate several hypotheses that are related to each other; if the findings are consistent, the conclusions are made stronger. The Beta-Blocker Heart Attack Trial (BHAT) of treating patients with β-blockers after a heart attack, for example, found that the drug reduced total mortality, cardiovascular mortality, and sudden death (9). Had only one of these hypotheses been tested, the inferences from the study would have been less conclusive.

A good rule is to establish in advance as many hypotheses as make sense, but specify one as the **primary hypothesis**. This helps to focus the study on its main objective, and provides a clear basis for the main sample size calculation. In addition, a single primary hypothesis can be tested statistically without argument about whether to adjust for multiple hypothesis testing.

Hypotheses generated by the study

Unanticipated associations that appear during collection and analysis of data are a rich source of interesting ideas and important research questions, and the common practice of going on hypothesis-generating ("fishing") expeditions is a good one (10). After all, the truth does not depend on whether a hypothesis is formulated in advance. On the other hand, the many informal comparisons made during data analysis are a form of multiple hypothesis testing, and significant P values for data-generated hypotheses are often due to chance. These P values should be regarded as "flags" that indicate potential associations, and as fertile source of research questions for future studies.

SUMMARY

1. *Sample size planning* is an important part of the design of both analytic and descriptive studies. The sample size should be estimated early in the process of developing the research design, so that appropriate modifications can be made.
2. Analytic studies and experiments need a *hypothesis* that specifies, for the purpose of subsequent *tests of significance*, the anticipated association between predictor and outcome variables. Purely descriptive studies, lacking the strategy of comparison, do not require a hypothesis.
3. Good hypotheses are *specific* (about how the population will be sampled and the variables measured), *simple* (there is only one predictor and one outcome variable), and formulated *in advance*.
4. The *null hypothesis*, which proposes that the predictor and outcome variables are not associated, is the basis for tests of statistical significance. The *alternative hypothesis* proposes that they are associated. Statistical tests attempt to reject the null hypothesis of no association in favor

of the alternative hypothesis that there is an association.
5. An alternative hypothesis is either *one-tailed* (only one direction of association will be tested) or *two-tailed* (both directions will be tested). One-tailed hypotheses can be used when only one direction of the association is likely or biologically meaningful; they offer more power for a given number of subjects.
6. For analytic studies and experiments, the *sample size is an estimate* of the number of subjects required to detect an association of a *given effect size* at a *specified likelihood* of making *Type I* (false-positive) and *Type II* (false-negative) *errors*. The maximum likelihood of making a Type I error is called α; that of making a Type II error, β. The quantity $(1 - \beta)$ is *power*, the chance of observing an association of a given size or greater in a sample if one is actually present in the population.
7. For some sample size calculations, the investigator must also determine the *variability* of the effect size, select the appropriate *sampling unit*, adjust for *loss to follow-up*, and/or consider the effect of *confounding* variables.
8. The more hypotheses tested in a study the greater the probability that one will achieve statistical significance on the basis of chance alone. To maximize the information that the study provides it is desirable to set up as *many hypotheses* in advance as make sense. To minimize problems of interpretation it is advantageous to specify one of these as the *primary hypothesis*. Unanticipated hypotheses emerging from the data are valuable as a source of new research questions.

REFERENCES

1. MacMahon B, Yen S, Trichopoulos, D, et al: Coffee and cancer of the pancreas. *N Engl J Med* 304:630–633, 1981.
2. Lipid Research Clinics Program: The LRC Coronary Primary Prevention Trial results: Reduction in incidence of coronary heart disease. *JAMA* 251:351–364, 1984.
3. Lachin JM: Introduction to sample size determination and power analysis for clinical trials. *Controlled Clin Trials* 2:93–114, 1981.

4. Donner A, Birkett N, Buck C: Randomization by cluster: sample size requirements and analysis. *Am J Epidemiol* 114:906–914, 1981.

5. Zar JH: *Biostatistical Analysis.* ed 2. Englewood Cliffs, NJ, Prentice-Hall, Inc., 1984.

6. Schlesselman JJ: *Case-Control Studies.* New York, Oxford University Press, 1982, pp 159–160.

7. Smith PG, Day NE: The design of case-control studies: the influence of confounding and interaction effects. *Int J Epidemiol* 13:356–365, 1984.

8. Glantz S: *Primer of Biostatistics.* New York, Mc-Graw-Hill, 1981, pp 84–89.

9. Beta-Blocker Heart Attack Trial Research Group: A randomized trial of propranolol in patients with acute myocardial infarction. I. Mortality results. *JAMA* 247:1707–1714, 1982.

10. Thomas DC, Siemiatycki J, Dewar R, et al: The problem of multiple inference in studies designed to generate hypotheses. *Am J Epidemiol* 122:1080–95, 1985.

See the end of Chapter 13 for additional readings.

Estimating Sample Size and Power

Warren S. Browner, Dennis Black, Thomas B. Newman,
and Stephen B. Hulley

INTRODUCTION **139**

SAMPLE SIZE TECHNIQUES FOR ANALYTIC
STUDIES AND EXPERIMENTS **139**

The *t* test
The *z* statistic
The correlation coefficient
Special situations

SAMPLE SIZE TECHNIQUES FOR DESCRIPTIVE
STUDIES **144**

Continuous variables
Dichotomous variables

WHAT TO DO WHEN SAMPLE SIZE IS
FIXED **145**

STRATEGIES FOR MINIMIZING SAMPLE
SIZE **146**

Use continuous variables
Use more precise variables
Use paired measurements
Use unequal group sizes
Use a more common outcome

HOW TO ESTIMATE SAMPLE SIZE WHEN THERE
IS INSUFFICIENT INFORMATION **149**

SUMMARY **150**

REFERENCES **150**

ADDITIONAL READINGS **150**

APPENDIX 13.A. Sample size required per group
when using the *t* test to compare means of
continuous variables **215**

APPENDIX 13.B. Sample size required per group
when using the *z* statistic to compare
proportions of dichotomous variables **216**

APPENDIX 13.C. Total sample size required
when using the correlation coefficient (*r*) **218**

APPENDIX 13.D. Sample size for a descriptive
study of a continuous variable **219**

APPENDIX 13.E. Sample size for a descriptive
study of a dichotomous variable **220**

INTRODUCTION

Chapter 12 introduced the basic principles underlying sample size calculations; this chapter presents several cookbook techniques for using those principles to estimate the sample size needed for a research project. The first section deals with sample size estimates for an analytic study or experiment, and the second section considers studies that are primarily descriptive. The remaining sections present strategies for dealing with a fixed sample size, for maximizing the power of a study, and for estimating the sample size when there is insufficient information from which to work.

SAMPLE SIZE TECHNIQUES FOR ANALYTIC STUDIES AND EXPERIMENTS

There are several variations on the recipe for estimating sample size in an analytic study or experiment, but they all have certain steps in common:

1. State the **null hypothesis** and either a **one-** or **two-tailed alternative hypothesis**.
2. Select the appropriate **statistical test** from Table 13.1 based on the type of predictor variable and outcome variable in those hypotheses.
3. Choose a reasonable **effect size** (and **variability**, if necessary).
4. Set α and β. (If the alternative hypothesis is one-tailed, use a one-tailed α; otherwise, use a two-tailed α.)
5. Use the appropriate **table** or **formula** in the appendices of the chapter to estimate the sample size.

Table 13.1.
Simple statistical tests for use in estimating sample size[a]

| Predictor | Outcome variable | |
variable	Dichotomous	Continuous
Dichotomous	z statistic[b]	t test
Continuous	t test	Correlation coefficient

[a]See text for what to do about categorical variables, or if planning to analyze the data with another type of statistical test.
[b]A two-tailed z statistic for contingency table analysis is the same as the familiar Chi square statistic.

Even if the exact value for one or more of the ingredients is uncertain, it is important to *estimate the sample size early in the design phase*. Waiting until the last minute to prepare the sample size can be disastrous. It is often necessary to start over with new ingredients, which may mean redesigning the entire study.

Not all analytic studies fit neatly into one of the three main categories below; a few of the more common exceptions are discussed in the section called "special situations."

The *t* test

The *t test* is commonly used to determine whether the mean value of a continuous outcome variable in one group differs significantly from that in another group. The t test assumes that the distribution (spread) of the variable in the two groups approximates a normal (bell-shaped) curve.

To estimate the sample size for a study that will be analyzed with a t test, the investigator must:

1. State the null hypothesis, and decide whether the alternative hypothesis is one- or two-tailed.
2. Estimate the effect size as the difference in the mean value of the outcome variable between the study groups.
3. Estimate the variability of the outcome variable (as its standard deviation).
4. Set α and β.

The effect size and the variability can often be estimated from previous studies in the literature and consultation with experts;

occasionally, a pilot study will be necessary. In Table 13.A, the effect size is specified in standard deviation units, i.e., as the effect size divided by the standard deviation (a common measure of variability). This process, known as standardization, simplifies comparisons between the effect sizes of different variables. The larger the standardized effect size, the smaller the required sample size.

Appendix 13.A gives the sample size requirements for several combinations of α and β for a given standardized effect size. The table is easy to use, even by those who are unsure of the underlying concepts. Look down the leftmost column of Table 13.A for the standardized effect size. Next, read across the table to the chosen values for α and β for the sample size required *per group*. (The numbers in Table 13.A assume that the two groups being compared are of the same size; see the text below the table if that assumption is not true.)

Example 13.1.
Calculating sample size when using the t test in an experiment.

Problem: The research question is to compare the efficacy of metaproterenol and theophylline in the treatment of asthma. The outcome variable is FEV1 (forced expiratory volume in 1 second) 1 hour after treatment. A previous study has reported that the mean FEV1 in persons with treated asthma was 2.0 liters, with a standard deviation of 1.0 liter. The investigator would like to be able to detect a difference of 10% or more in mean FEV1 between the two treatment groups. How many patients are required in each group (metaproterenol and theophylline) at α (two-tailed) = 0.05 and power = 0.80?

Solution: The ingredients for the sample size calculation are as follows:

1. Null hypothesis: Mean FEV1 at 1 hour after treatment is the same in asthmatics treated with theophylline as in those treated with metaproterenol.
2. Alternative hypothesis: Mean FEV1 at 1 hour after treatment is different in asthmatics treated with theophylline than in those treated with metaproterenol.
3. Effect size = 0.2 liters (10% × 2.0 liters).
4. Standardized effect size = effect size ÷ standard deviation = 0.2 liters ÷ 1.0 liter = 0.2.
5. α (two-tailed) = 0.05; β = 1 − 0.80 = 0.20. (Recall that β = 1 − power).

Looking across from a standardized effect size of 0.20 in the leftmost column of Table 13.A, and down from α (two-tailed) = 0.05 and β = 0.20, 393 patients are required per group. This sample size calculation indicates that the investigator may need to reconsider the study design! See the section on the *t* test for paired samples (example 13.12) for a helpful suggestion.

The *t* test can also be used to estimate the sample size for a case-control study if the study has a continuous predictor variable. In this situation, the *t* test compares the mean value of the predictor variable in the cases with that in the controls.

Example 13.2.
Calculating sample size when using the *t* test in a case-control study.

Problem: The research question is whether serum cholesterol level is associated with stroke. The mean value for cholesterol in controls without stroke is about 200 mg/dl, with a standard deviation of about 20 mg/dl. A few previous studies have detected a difference of about +10 mg/dl between stroke patients and controls, and other studies have found no difference or even a tendency for serum cholesterol to be lower in stroke patients. How many cases and controls will be needed, at α (two-tailed) = 0.05 and β = 0.10, to detect a difference of 10 mg/dl between the two groups? Why was a two-tailed α used?

Solution: The ingredients for the sample size calculation are as follows:

1. Null hypothesis: There is no difference in mean serum cholesterol level in stroke cases and controls.
2. Alternative hypothesis: There is a difference in mean serum cholesterol level in stroke cases and controls.
3. Effect size = 10 mg/dl.
4. Standardized effect size = effect size ÷ standard deviation = 10 mg/dl ÷ 20 mg/dl = 0.5. (This assumes that the standard deviation of serum cholesterol level is the same in patients with and without stroke).
5. α (two-tailed) = 0.05; β = 0.10.

Reading across from a standardized effect size of 0.5 in the leftmost column of Table 13.A, and down from α (two-tailed) = 0.05 and β = 0.10, 84 cases and 84 controls will be required. A two-tailed α was chosen because the investigator was interested in both tails of the alternative hypothesis, namely that stroke is associated with either an increased or decreased serum cholesterol level.

The z statistic

The z statistic can be used to compare the proportion of subjects in each of two groups who have a dichotomous outcome. For example, the proportion of men who develop coronary heart disease (CHD) while treated with aspirin can be compared with the proportion who develop CHD while taking a placebo. The z statistic resembles the familiar X^2 (Chi square) test, with one important difference: the z statistic can be one- or two-tailed, whereas the X^2 test is always two-tailed.

In an experiment or cohort study, effect size is specified by the difference between P1, the proportion of subjects expected to have the outcome in one group, and P2, the proportion expected in the other group. In a case control study, P1 represents the proportion of cases expected to have a particular risk factor, and P2 represents the proportion of controls expected to have the risk factor. Variability is a function of P1 and P2, so it need not be specified directly.

To estimate the sample size for a study that will be analyzed with the z statistic, the investigator must:

1. State the null hypothesis, and decide whether the alternative hypothesis should be one or two-tailed.
2. Estimate the effect size and variability in terms of P1, the proportion with the outcome in one group, and P2, the proportion with the outcome in the other group.
3. Set α and β.

Appendix 13.B gives the sample size requirements for several combinations of α and β, and a range of values of P1 and P2. To estimate the sample size, look down the leftmost column of Table 13.B for the *smaller* of P1 and P2 (rounded to the nearest 0.05). Next, read across for the *difference* between P1 and P2. Based on the chosen values for α and β, the table gives the sample size required *per group*. Note that Table 13.B assumes that the two groups being compared are of the same size; see the text below the table if that assumption is not true.

Example 13.3.
Calculating sample size when using the z statistic in a cohort study.

Problem: The research question is whether elderly smokers have a greater incidence of skin cancer than nonsmokers. A review of previous literature suggests that the 5 year incidence of skin cancer is about 0.20 in elderly nonsmokers. At α (one-tailed) = 0.05 and power = 80%, how many smokers and nonsmokers will need to be studied to determine whether the 5 year skin cancer incidence is at least 0.30 in smokers? Why was a one-tailed alternative hypothesis chosen?

Solution: The ingredients for the sample size calculation are as follows:

1. Null hypothesis: The incidence of skin cancer is the same is elderly smokers and nonsmokers.
2. Alternative hypothesis: The incidence of skin cancer is higher in elderly smokers than nonsmokers.
3. P2 (incidence in nonsmokers) = 0.20; P1 (incidence in smokers) = 0.30. The smaller of these values is 0.20, and the difference between them (P1 − P2) is 0.10.
4. α (one-tailed) = 0.05; β = 1 - 0.80 = 0.20.

Looking across from 0.20 in the leftmost column in Table 13.B, and down from an expected difference of 0.10, the upper number (for α (one-tailed) = 0.05 and β = 0.20) is the required sample size of 231 smokers and 231 nonsmokers. A one-tailed alternative hypothesis was used because there is a great deal of evidence suggesting that smoking is a carcinogen, and none suggesting that it prevents cancer.

Often, the investigator will have specifed the effect size in terms of the **relative risk** (risk ratio) of the outcome in two groups of subjects, for example, whether women who use oral contraceptives are at least twice as likely as nonusers to have a myocardial infarction. In a cohort study (or experiment), it is straightforward to convert back and forth between relative risk and the two pro-

portions (P1 and P2), since the relative risk is just P1 divided by P2.

For a case-control study, however, the situation is a little more complex (see Chapter 8), because the relative risk must be approximated by the odds ratio (OR), which equals P1 x (1 − P2) ÷ P2 × (1 − P1). The investigator must specify P2 (the proportion of controls exposed to the predictor variable). Then P1 (the proportion of cases exposed to the predictor variable) equals

$$OR \times P2 \div (1 - P2 + OR \times P2).$$

For example, if the investigator expects that 10% of controls will be exposed (P2 = 0.1) and wishes to detect an odds ratio of 3 associated with the exposure, then

$$P1 = (3 \times 0.1) \div (1 - 0.1 + 3 \times 0.1)$$
$$= 0.3 \div 1.2 = 0.25.$$

Example 13.4.
Calculating sample size when using the z statistic in a case-control study.

Problem: The investigator plans a case-control study of whether a history of herpes simplex is associated with lip cancer. A brief pilot study finds that about 30% of persons without lip cancer have had herpes simplex. The investigator is interested in detecting, with α (one-tailed) = 0.025 and power = 90%, whether the odds ratio for lip cancer associated with herpes simplex infection is 2.5 or more. How many subjects will be required?

Solution: The ingredients for the sample size calculation are as follows:

1. Null hypothesis: The proportion of cases of lip cancer with a history of herpes simplex is the same as the proportion of controls with a herpes simplex history.
2. Alternative hypothesis: The proportion of cases of lip cancer with a history of herpes simplex is greater than the proportion of controls with a herpes simplex history.
3. P2 (proportion of controls expected to have the risk factor) = 0.30; P1 (proportion of cases expected to have the risk factor) = OR × P2 ÷ (1 − P2 + OR × P2) = (2.5 × 0.3) ÷ (1 − 0.3 + 2.5 × 0.3) = 0.75 ÷ 1.45 = 0.52. The smaller of P1 and P2 is 0.30; the difference between them is about 0.20.
4. α (one-tailed) = 0.025; β = 1 − 0.90 = 0.10.

Looking across from 0.30 in the leftmost column in Table 13.B, and down from an expected difference of 0.20, the lower number (for α (one-tailed) = 0.025 and β = 0.10) is the required sample size of 124 cases and 124 controls.

The correlation coefficient

Although the correlation coefficient (r) is not commonly used in sample size calculations, it can be useful when the predictor and outcome variables are both continuous. The correlation coefficient is a measure of the strength of the linear association between the two variables. It varies between -1 and $+1$. Negative values indicate that as one variable increases, the other decreases (like serum lead level and IQ in children). The closer the absolute value of r is to 1, the stronger the association; the closer to 0, the weaker the association. Height and weight in adults, for example, are highly correlated in some populations with an r of about 0.9. Such high values, however, are uncommon; many biologically important associations have correlation coefficients between 0.1 and 0.3.

To estimate sample size for a study that will be analyzed with a correlation coefficient, the investigator must:

1. State the null hypothesis, and decide whether the alternative hypothesis is one- or two-tailed.
2. Estimate the effect size as the absolute value of the smallest correlation coefficient (r) that you would like to be able to detect. (Variability is a function of r, and is already included in the table.)
3. Set α and β.

In Appendix 13.C, look down the leftmost column of Table 13.C for the *effect size (r)*. Next, read across the table to the chosen values for α and β, yielding the total sample size required. Note that Table 13.C yields the appropriate sample size when the investigator wishes to reject the null hypothesis that there is no association between the predictor and outcome variables (e.g., $r = 0$). If the investigator wishes to determine whether the correlation coefficient in the study differs from a value other than zero (e.g., $r = 0.2$), she should see the text below Table 13.C for the appropriate methodology.

Example 13.5.

Calculating sample size when using the correlation coefficient in a cross-sectional study.

Problem: The research question is whether urinary cotinine levels (a measure of the intensity of current cigarette smoking) and bone density in smokers are inversely correlated. The investigator believes that smokers with higher cotinine levels will have lower bone densities. A previous study found a modest correlation ($r = -0.2$) between serum carbon monoxide levels (another measure of cigarette consumption) and bone density; the investigator anticipates that urinary cotinines will be at least as well-correlated. How many smokers will need to be enrolled, at α (one-tailed) $= 0.05$ and $\beta = 0.10$?

Solution: The ingredients for the sample size calculation are as follows:

1. Null hypothesis: There is no correlation between urinary cotinine level and bone density in smokers.
2. Alternative hypothesis: There is an inverse correlation between urinary cotinine level and bone density in smokers.
3. Effect size $(r) = |-0.2| = 0.2$.
4. α (one-tailed) $= 0.05$; $\beta = 0.10$.

Using Table 13.C, reading across from $r = 0.20$ in the leftmost column, and down from α (one-tailed) $= 0.05$ and $\beta = 0.10$, 211 smokers will be required.

Special situations

Sample size techniques are unavailable or difficult to use for certain analytic techniques, such as logistic regression (1) and nonparametric tests (those that do not assume that a variable fits a particular statistical distribution, such as the normal curve). In these instances, the investigator can estimate the sample size as if a simpler analysis were planned; the actual study will then have a somewhat different power. Suppose, for example, that an investigator is studying whether dietary calcium (a continuous variable) predicts the occurrence of hip fracture (a dichotomous variable). Even if the eventual plan is to analyze the data with the logistic regression technique, a ballpark sample size can be estimated with the t test.

Categorical variables present a similar problem. Ordinal variables can be treated as continuous variables, especially if the number of categories is relatively large (6 or more) and the distribution of subjects within those categories is approximately normal (bellshaped). In other situations, the best strategy is to slightly change the research hypothesis by dichotomizing the categorical variable. As an example, suppose a researcher is studying whether sex predicts the number of times that someone visits a dentist in a year. The number of visits is unevenly distributed: many persons will have no visits, some will make 1 visit, and only a few will make 2 or more visits. In this situation, the investigator could estimate the sample size as if the outcome were dichotomous (0 visits versus 1 or more visits).

Occasionally, an investigator wishes to compare which of two treatments is more effective in prolonging life, or in reducing the symptomatic phase of a disease. Although the outcome variable, say weeks of survival, is continuous, the *t* test for equality of means is not as appropriate as survival analysis (or life table) techniques (2). Alternatively, the outcome variable can be dichotomized (such as survival for 6 months or more versus survival for less than 6 months), and sample size can be estimated with the z statistic.

For a variety of reasons (see Chapter 10), an investigator may choose to use a matched design. This usually has a minor effect on the sample size, and the techniques in this chapter provide reasonable (slightly high) estimates. More precise estimates can be made using approaches described by Schlesselman (3).

SAMPLE SIZE TECHNIQUES FOR DESCRIPTIVE STUDIES

Estimating the sample size for descriptive studies is based on somewhat different principles. Such studies do not have predictor and outcome variables, nor do they compare different groups. Thus the concepts of power and the null and alternative hypotheses do not apply. Instead, the investigator calculates descriptive statistics, such as means and proportions, and uses statistical techniques to make inferences about the population. Often, however, descriptive studies (*What is the prevalence of depression among elderly patients in a medical clinic?*) eventually ask analytic questions (*What are the predictors of depression among such patients?*). In this situation, sample size should be estimated

for the analytic study as well, to avoid the common problem of having inadequate power for what turns out to be the question of greater interest.

Descriptive studies commonly report **confidence intervals,** a range of values about the sample mean or proportion. Confidence intervals are discussed in Appendix 18 (see also 4-6). In simple terms, they can be thought of as measures of the precision of sample estimates. The **confidence level,** such as 95% or 99%, is set by the investigator. For example, an investigator might wish to estimate the mean diastolic blood pressure in a population. From a sample of 200 subjects, she might estimate that the mean diastolic blood pressure in the population is 80 mm Hg, with a 95% confidence interval from 78 to 82 mm Hg. A narrower confidence interval (say 79.5 to 80.5 mm Hg) is more precise than a wider one (78 to 82 mm Hg), and an interval with a higher confidence level (say 99%) is more likely to include the true population value than an interval with a lower one (90%).

When estimating sample size for descriptive studies, the investigator specifies the desired level and width of the confidence interval. The sample size can then be determined from the tables or formulas in the appendices to the chapter.

Continuous variables

When the variable of interest is continuous, a confidence interval around the mean value of that variable is often reported. To estimate the sample size for that confidence interval, the investigator must:

1. Estimate the standard deviation of the variable of interest.
2. Specify the desired precision (total width) of the interval.
3. Select the confidence level for the interval (e.g., 95%, 99%).

To use Appendix 13.D, standardize the total width of the interval (divide it by the standard deviation of the variable). Then look down the leftmost column of Table 13.D for the expected standardized width. Next, read across the table to the chosen confidence level for the required sample size.

Example 13.6.

Calculating sample size for a descriptive study of a continuous variable.

Problem: The investigator seeks to determine the mean birth weight in an urban area with a 99% confidence interval of ± 60 g. A previous study found the standard deviation of birth weight in a similar city was 600 g.

Solution: The ingredients for the sample size calculation are as follows:

1. Standard deviation of variable (SD) = 600g.
2. Total width of interval = 120 g (60 g above and 60 g below). Thus the standardized width of interval = total width ÷ SD = 120 g ÷ 600 g = 0.2.
3. Confidence level = 99%.

Reading across from a standardized width of 0.2 in the leftmost column of Table 13.D, and down from the 99% confidence level, the required sample size is 664 births.

Dichotomous variables

In a descriptive study of a dichotomous variable, results can be expressed as a confidence interval around the estimated proportion of subjects with one of the values. To estimate the sample size for that confidence interval, the investigator must:

1. Estimate the expected proportion with the variable of interest in the population. (If more than half of the population is expected to have the characteristic, then plan sample size based on the proportion expected not to have the characteristic.)
2. Specify the desired precision (total width) of the confidence interval.
3. Select the confidence level for the interval (e.g., 95%).

In Appendix 13.E, look down the leftmost column of Table 13.E for the expected proportion with the variable of interest. Next, read across the table to the chosen width and confidence level, yielding the required sample size.

Example 13.7.

Calculating sample size for a descriptive study of a dichotomous variable.

Problem: The investigator wishes to determine the sensitivity of a new diagnostic test for colon cancer. Based on a pilot study, she expects that 80% of patients with colon cancer will have positive tests. How many such patients will be required to estimate a 95% confidence interval for the test's sensitivity of 0.80 ± 0.05?

Solution: The ingredients for the sample size calculation are as follows:

1. Expected proportion = 0.20. (Because 0.80 is more than half, sample size is estimated from the proportion expected to have negative results, i.e., 0.20).
2. Total width = 0.10 (0.05 below and 0.05 above).
3. Confidence level = 95%.

Reading across from 0.20 in the leftmost column of Table 13.E, and down from a total width of 0.10, the middle number (representing a 95% confidence level) yields the required sample size of 246 patients with colon cancer.

Problem: Suppose the investigator also wishes to determine the specificity of the test for ruling out colon cancer. She expects that 90% of subjects without colon cancer will have negative tests. How many such patients will be required to estimate a 95% confidence interval for the test's specificity of 0.90 ± 0.05?

Solution: The ingredients for this part of the sample size calculation are as follows:

1. Expected proportion = 0.10 (1 − 0.90).
2. Total width = 0.10 (0.05 below and 0.05 above).
3. Confidence level = 95%.

Reading across from 0.10 in the leftmost column of Table 13.E, and down from a total width of 0.10, the middle number (representing a 95% confidence level) yields the required sample size of 139 subjects without colon cancer.

WHAT TO DO WHEN SAMPLE SIZE IS FIXED

Especially when doing secondary data analysis, the sample size may have been determined before the study was planned. In this situation, or if the number of patients who are available or affordable for study is limited, the investigator must work backwards from the sample size. She can estimate either the study's power to detect a given effect, or the effect size that can be detected at a given power. The investigator can use the sample size tables in the chapter appendices, interpolating when necessary, or solve the sample size formulas in the appendices for power or effect size.

A good general rule is that a study should have a power of 80% or greater to detect a reasonable effect size. It is often tempting to pursue research hypotheses that have lower levels of power if the additional cost of doing so is small. The investigator should keep in mind, however, that she may face the dilemma of deciding whether to report negative results that may simply have resulted from insufficient power.

Example 13.8.
Calculating power when sample size is fixed.
Problem: An investigator is interested in determining the correlation between family income and systolic blood pressure. She has access to a data set that includes the income and systolic blood pressure of 1000 individuals. What power does she have to detect a correlation coefficient of 0.10 or greater, at α (two-tailed) = 0.05?
Solution: In Table 13.C, reading across from $r = 0.10$ in the leftmost column and down from α (two-tailed) = 0.05, 1047 subjects would give the investigator a power of 90% ($\beta = 0.10$). Thus a sample size of 1000 would have slightly less than 90% power.

Example 13.9.
Calculating the detectable effect size when sample size is fixed.
Problem: There are 100 subjects willing to participate in a study of the effect of a lipid-lowering agent on serum cholesterol. If the standard deviation of the change in serum cholesterol is expected to be 10 mg/dl in both the placebo and the active drug groups, what size difference will the investigator be able to detect between the two groups, at α (one-tailed) = 0.05 and $\beta = 0.20$?
Solution: In Table 13.A, reading down from α (one-tailed) = 0.05 and $\beta = 0.20$ (the rightmost column), 49 subjects per group are required to detect a standardized effect size of 0.5, which is equal to 5 mg/dl (0.5 $\times$ 10 mg/dl). Thus the investigator (who will have 50 subjects per group) will be able to detect a difference of slightly less than 5 mg/dl between the two groups.

STRATEGIES FOR MINIMIZING SAMPLE SIZE

When the estimated sample size is greater than the number of subjects that can be realistically studied, the investigator should proceed through several steps. First, the calculations should be repeated: it is easy to make mistakes. Next, the "ingredients" should be reviewed. Is the effect size unreasonably small, or the variability unreasonably large? Could α and/or β be increased without

harm? Would a one-tailed alternative hypothesis be adequate? Is the confidence level too high, or the interval unnecessarily narrow?

These technical adjustments can be useful, but it is important to realize that statistical tests ultimately depend on the information contained in the data. Minor changes in the ingredients, such as switching from a two-tailed to a one-tailed alternative hypothesis, do not change the quantity or quality of the data that will be collected. There are, on the other hand, several strategies for reducing the required sample size (or increasing power for a given sample size) that actually increase the information content of the collected data. Many of these strategies involve modifications of the research hypothesis; the investigator should carefully consider whether the new hypothesis still answers the research question.

Use continuous variables

When continuous variables are an option, they permit smaller sample sizes than dichotomous variables. Blood pressure, for example, can be expressed either as millimeters of mercury (continuous), or as the presence or absence of hypertension (dichotomous). The former permits a smaller sample size for a given power, or a greater power for a given sample size.

Example 13.10.
Use of continuous versus dichotomous variables.
Problem: Consider a placebo-controlled experiment to determine the effect of prenatal vitamin supplements on birthweight in a population at risk for low birth weight (LBW) infants (<2500 grams). Suppose that a pilot study establishes that birth weight in the study population is normally distributed, with a mean of 3500 g and a standard deviation of 770 g. About 10% of infants are LBW. The placebo is anticipated to have no effect; vitamin supplements are anticipated to increase the mean birthweight by 300 g. This change in mean birth weight corresponds to a reduction in the proportion of LBW infants to 5%.
One design might treat birth weight as a dichotomous variable: LBW versus non-LBW. Another might use all of the information contained in the measurement, and treat birth weight as a continuous variable. How many live births would each design require, at α (one-tailed) = 0.05 and $\beta = 0.20$? How does the change in design affect the research question?

Solution: The ingredients for the sample size calculation using a dichotomous outcome variable (LBW or not LBW) are as follows:

1. Null hypothesis: The proportion of LBW babies born to mothers taking vitamin supplements is the same as that in mothers taking placebo.
2. Alternative hypothesis: The proportion of LBW babies born to mothers taking vitamin supplements is less than that in mothers taking placebo.
3. P1 (incidence of LBW in placebo group) = 0.10; P2 (incidence of LBW in vitamin group) = 0.05. The smaller of these values is 0.05, and the difference between them (P1 − P2) is 0.05.
4. α (one-tailed) = 0.05; β = 0.20.

Using Table 13.B, reading across from 0.05 in the leftmost column, and down from an expected difference of 0.05, the upper number (for α (one-tailed) = 0.05 and β = 0.20), this design would require 342 live births in each group.

The ingredients for the sample size calculation using a continuous outcome variable (birth weight) are as follows:

1. Null hypothesis: Mean birth weight among babies born to mothers taking prenatal vitamins is the same as among babies born to mothers taking placebo.
2. Alternative hypothesis: Mean birth weight among babies born to mothers taking vitamins is higher than among babies born to mothers taking placebo.
3. Effect size = 300 g.
4. Standardized effect size = effect size ÷ standard deviation = 300 g ÷ 770 g = 0.4.
5. α (one-tailed) = 0.05; β = 0.20.

Using Table 13.A, reading across from a standardized effect size of 0.40, with α (one-tailed) = 0.05 and β = 0.20, this design would require about 77 live births in each group, a substantially smaller sample.

The continuous outcome addresses the effect of vitamin supplements on the mean birth weight in the entire sample. The dichotomous outcome is concerned with its effects on the proportion of babies who have a categorically low birth weight, perhaps the more relevant question as a surrogate for neonatal morbidity and developmental abnormalities.

Use more precise variables

Because they reduce variability, more precise variables permit a smaller sample size in both analytic and descriptive studies. Techniques for increasing the precision of a vari-

able, such as making measurements in duplicate, are presented in Chapter 4. Increasing precision usually requires that more resources be put into measurement, thereby reducing the amount available for other aspects of the study, such as recruitment. This is particularly true in studies that make expensive measurements on a small number of subjects. At the conclusion of the study, the investigator may then be faced with the problem of having precise predictor variables, but too few subjects with outcomes to be able to draw any meaningful conclusions. A good general rule is that when balancing the expenses of measurement and recruitment, the investigator should lean toward making *fewer measurements* on *more subjects.*

Example 13.11.
Use of more precise measurements.

Problem: An investigator is describing the effects of sleep deprivation on serum norepinephrine levels. Two assays are available: the first, which costs $20, has a standard deviation of 25 ng/ml; the second, which costs $300, has a standard deviation of only 10 ng/ml. The investigator wishes to determine the 95% confidence interval for the mean serum norepinephrine level (± 2.5 ng/ml) in sleep-deprived persons. Which design will be more economic, assuming that there is no expense involved in recruiting sleep-deprived subjects? What if each subject must be paid $50? (Assume there are no other expenses involved).

Solution: The ingredients for the sample size calculation using the first assay are as follows:

1. Standard deviation of variable (SD) = 25 ng/ml.
2. Total width of interval = 5 ng/ml (2.5 ng/ml above and 2.5 ng/ml below). Standardized width of interval = total width ÷ SD = 25 ng/ml ÷ 5 ng/ml = 0.2.
3. Confidence level = 95%.

Using Table 13.D, a design using the first assay would require 385 subjects. If recruitment were free, the study would cost $7700 ($20 × 385). If subjects must be paid, a study using this assay would cost $26950 ($7700 + $50 × 385).

The ingredients for the sample size calculation using the second assay are as follows:

1. Standard deviation of variable (SD) = 10 ng/ml.
2. Total width of interval = 5 ng/ml (2.5 ng/ml above and 2.5 ng/ml below). Standardized

width of interval = total width ÷ SD = 5 ng/ml ÷10 ng/ml = 0.5.
3. Confidence level = 95%.

Using Table 13.D, the second assay would require 62 subjects. If recruitment were free, a study using this assay would cost $18600 ($300 × 62); thus the first design would be more economic. If subjects must be paid, a study using this assay would cost $21,700 ($18600 + $50 × 62), and this design would be more economic.

Use paired measurements

In certain experiments or cohort studies with continuous outcome variables, paired measurements—one at baseline, another at the conclusion of the study—can be made for each subject. The outcome variable is the *change* between these two measurements, and a *t* test on the paired measurements can be used to compare the mean value of this change in the two groups. This technique often permits a smaller sample size because it reduces the variation of the outcome variable. Sample size for this type of *t* test is estimated in the usual way, except that the standardized effect size (E/S in Table 13.2) is the anticipated change in the variable divided by the standard deviation of that change.

Example 13.12.
Use of the *t* test with paired measurements.
Problem: Recall Example 13.1, in which the investigator studying the treatment of asthma is interested in determining whether metaproterenol can improve FEV1 by 200 ml compared with theophylline. Sample size calculations indicated that 393 subjects per group are needed, more than are likely to be available. Fortunately, a colleague points out that asthmatic patients have great differences in their FEV1's before treatment. These differences account for much of the variability in FEV1 after treatment, thus obscuring the effect of treatment. She suggests using a *t* test to compare the *changes* in FEV1 in the two groups. A pilot study finds that the standard deviation of the change in FEV1 is only 250 ml. How many subjects would be required per group, at α (two-tailed) = 0.05 and β = 0.20?
Solution: The ingredients for the sample size calculation are as follows:

1. Null hypothesis: *Change* in mean FEV1 at 1 hour after treatment is the same in asthmatics treated with theophylline as in those treated with metaproterenol.

2. Alternative hypothesis: *Change* in mean FEV1 at 1 hour after treatment is different in asthmatics treated with theophylline than in those treated with metaproterenol.
3. Effect size = 200 ml.
4. Standardized effect size = effect size ÷ standard deviation = 200 ml ÷ 250 ml = 0.8.
5. α (two-tailed) = 0.05; β = 1 − 0.80 = 0.20.

Using Table 13.A, this design would require about 25 participants per group, a much more reasonable sample size than the 393 per group calculated previously.

Use unequal group sizes

Because an equal number of subjects in each of two groups usually gives the greatest power for a given total number of subjects, Tables 13.A and 13.B in the appendices assume equal sample sizes in the two groups. Sometimes, however, the distribution of subjects is not equal in the two groups, or it is easier or less expensive to recruit study subjects for one group than the other. It may turn out, for example, that an investigator wants to estimate sample size based on the 30% of the subjects in a cohort who are cigarette smokers (compared with 70% who are aren't). Or, in a case-control study, the number of persons with the disease may be small, but it may be possible to sample any number of controls. In general, the gain in power when the size of one group is increased to twice the size of the other is considerable; tripling and quadrupling one of the groups provide progressively smaller gains. Sample sizes for unequal groups can be computed from the formulas found in the text to Appendices 13.A and 13.B.

Here is a useful approximation (3) for estimating sample size for case-control studies of dichotomous risk factors and outcomes using *c* controls per case. If *n* represents the number of cases that would have been required for one control per case (at a given α, β, and effect size), then the approximate number of cases (n') with cn' controls that will be required is $[(c+1) \div 2c] \times n$. For example, with *c* = 2 controls per case, then $[(2+1) \div (2 \times 2)] \times n = 3/4 \times n$; thus only 75% as many cases are needed. As *c* gets larger, n' approaches 50% of *n* (when *c* = 10, for example, $n' = 11/20 \, n$).

Example 13.13.

Use of multiple controls per case in a case-control study.

Problem: An investigator is studying whether exposure to household insecticide is a risk factor for childhood leukemia. The original sample size calculation indicated that 25 cases would be required, using one control per case. Suppose that the investigator has access to only 18 cases. How should the investigator proceed?

Solution: The investigator should consider using multiple controls per case (after all, she can find lots of children who do not have leukemia). By using three controls per case, for example, the approximate number of cases that will be required is $[(3+1) \div (2 \times 3)] \times 25 = 17$.

Use a more common outcome

When the outcome is dichotomous, using a more frequent outcome is one of the best ways to increase power: if an outcome occurs more often (up to a frequency of about 0.5), there is more of a chance to detect its predictors. Power depends more on the number of outcomes that occur than it does on the number of subjects in the study. Studies with rare outcomes, like the occurrence of coronary heart disease in healthy men, usually require very large sample sizes in order to have adequate power (the MRFIT had to enroll more than 12,000 men in order to have about 250 CHD deaths during the 6-8 year study period).

One of the best ways to increase the number of outcomes is to extend the follow-up period (as the MRFIT investigators are doing). Another is to liberalize the definition of what constitutes an outcome. A third is to enroll subjects at higher risk of developing the outcome. All of these techniques, however, may change the research question, so they should be used with caution.

Example 13.14.

Use of a more common outcome.

Problem: Suppose an investigator is comparing the efficacy of an antiseptic gargle versus a placebo gargle in preventing upper respiratory infections (URI). Her initial calculations indicated that her sample of 200 volunteer college students was inadequate, perhaps because she expected that only about 20% of her subjects would have a URI during the 3-month follow-up period. Suggest a few changes in the study plan.

Solution. Here are two possible solutions: a) follow the sample for a longer period of time, say

6 or 12 months; and b) study a sample of pediatric residents, who are likely to experience a much higher incidence of URI's than college students. Both of these solutions involve modification of the research hypothesis, but neither change seems sufficiently large to affect the overall research question about the efficacy of antiseptic gargle.

HOW TO ESTIMATE SAMPLE SIZE WHEN THERE IS INSUFFICIENT INFORMATION

Often the investigator finds that she is missing one or more of the ingredients for the sample size calculation, and becomes frustrated in her attempts to plan the study. This is an especially frequent problem when the investigator is using an instrument of her design (such as a new questionnaire on quality of life), or enrolling a sample that has not previously been studied (such as Scandinavian sailors). How should she go about deciding what effect size or standard deviation to use?

The first strategy is an extensive search for previous findings on the topic, thoroughly reviewing the relevant literature, including nonmedical journals and texts. Roughly comparable situations and mediocre or dated findings may be good enough— the sample size calculation is just an estimate. If the literature review is unproductive, she should contact other investigators about their judgment on what to expect, and whether they are aware of any unpublished results that may be relevant. If there is still no information available, she may consider doing a small study (pretest) to obtain the missing ingredients before embarking on the main study.

Another strategy, when the mean and standard deviation of a continuous or categorical variable are in doubt, is to dichotomize that variable. Categories can be lumped into two groups, and continuous variables can be split at their mean or median. The z statistic can then be used to make a reasonable estimate of the sample size. Dividing the quality of life in Scandinavian sailors into "better than the median" or "the median or less" avoids having to estimate its standard deviation in the sample at the cost of slightly underestimating the actual power of the study.

If all of this fails, the investigator should just make an educated guess about the likely values of the missing ingredients. The process of thinking through the problem and imagining the findings will usually result in a reasonable estimate, and that is what sample size planning is about.

SUMMARY

1. When estimating sample size for an analytic study, the following steps need to be taken: a) *state the null and alternative hypotheses*, specifying the number of tails; b) *select a statistical test* that could be used to analyze the data, based on the types of predictor and outcome variables; c) *estimate the effect size and its variability* from the results of previous studies or pretests; and d) *specify appropriate values for α and β*, based on the importance of avoiding Type I and Type II errors.

2. The situation is slightly different for descriptive studies; the goal is to estimate the number of subjects required for a confidence interval of a given confidence level and precision. The steps are as follows: a) for a dichotomous variable, *estimate the proportion* of subjects with the variable of interest; for a continuous variable, *estimate its standard deviation*; b) *specify the desired precision* (width) of the confidence interval; and c) *specify the confidence level* (e.g., 95%).

3. *When sample size is predetermined*, the investigator can work backwards to esti-

mate the power or the detectable effect size.

4. Strategies are also available to *minimize the required sample size*. These include using continuous variables, more precise measurements, paired measurements, unequal group sizes, and more common outcomes.

REFERENCES

1. Whittemore AS: Sample size for logistic regression with small response probability. *J Am Stat Assoc* 76:27–32, 1981.
2. Friedman LM, Furberg CD, De Mets DL: *Fundamentals of Clinical Trials*. ed 2. Littleton, MA, PSG Publishing, 1985.
3. Schlesselman JJ: *Case-Control Studies*. New York, Oxford University Press, 1982.
4. Zar JH. *Biostatistical Analysis*. ed 2. Englewood Cliffs, NJ, Prentice-Hall, 1984.
5. Fleiss JL: *Statistical Methods for Rates and Proportions*. New York: John Wiley & Sons, 1981.
6. Browner WS, Newman TB: Confidence intervals. *Ann Intern Med* 105:973–974, 1986.

ADDITIONAL READINGS

(also see the references to Chapter 12)

Freiman JA, Chalmers TC, Smith H, Kuebler R: The importance of beta, the Type II error and sample size in the design and interpretation of the randomized controlled trial. *N Engl J Med* 299:690–4, 1978. (*Many clinical trials that have reported no difference between groups have been too small to discover important differences that might be revealed by a larger study.*)

Ingelfinger JA, Mosteller F, Thibodeau LA, Ware JH: *Biostatistics in Clinical Medicine*. New York, Macmillan Publishing Co, Inc., 1983. (*A well-written, accessible introduction to the area.*)

Kelsey JL, Thompson WD, Evans AS: *Methods in Observational Epidemiology*. New York, Oxford University Press, 1986. (*Chapter 10 discusses sample size calculations.*)

CHAPTER 14

Addressing Ethical Issues

Bernard Lo, David Feigal, Susan Cummins, and Stephen B. Hulley

INTRODUCTION 151

ETHICAL PRINCIPLES 151

FEDERAL GUIDELINES FOR RESEARCH ON
HUMAN SUBJECTS 151
Risks and benefits of research
Selection of subjects for research
Informed consent
Privacy and confidentiality

INSTITUTIONAL REVIEW BOARDS 154

SPECIAL TOPICS 155
Randomized blinded trials
Deception in research
The role of the investigator

SUMMARY 157

REFERENCES 157

ADDITIONAL READINGS 157

APPENDIX 14.A. Example of an informed
consent form 221

APPENDIX 14.B. Checklist for informed
consent 223

- - - - - - - - - - -

INTRODUCTION

Every study involving human subjects raises a unique set of ethical issues. A practical way to address these issues is to work from the regulations of federal agencies that fund research. Before coming to this, however, we will introduce the more important topic of the ethical standards the investigator should bring to her work.

ETHICAL PRINCIPLES

Three general ethical principles have evolved as guidelines for clinical research (2–4). The principle of **respect for persons** requires investigators to treat subjects as autonomous individuals and obtain their informed consent to participate in the research project. Research subjects must be regarded not as passive sources of data, but as individuals whose welfare and rights must be respected. Treating research subjects as partners and collaborators may also improve the scientific quality of the research by increasing enrollment and compliance.

The principle of **beneficence** requires investigators to design protocols that will provide valid and generalizable knowledge and to ensure that the benefits of the research are proportionate to the risks assumed by the subjects. Because subjects voluntarily agree to participate in research, often for the benefit of others, their well-being must be protected. The researcher must try to minimize the risks and maximize the benefits of participating in the study.

The principle of **justice** requires that the benefits and burdens of research be distributed fairly. Research participants assume some risk in order to benefit society as a whole. Therefore no single group, especially not disadvantaged, vulnerable, or minority groups, should be asked to bear a disproportionate share of the risk.

FEDERAL GUIDELINES FOR RESEARCH ON HUMAN SUBJECTS

The regulations of the Department of Health and Human Services (DHHS), summarized in Table 14.1, are intended to assure that clinical research is conducted in an ethically acceptable manner.

Table 14.1
Summary of DHHS guidelines for human research

- Risks to subjects are minimized and proportionate to the anticipated benefits and knowledge.
- Data are monitored to ensure safety of subjects.
- Selection of subjects is equitable.
- If subjects are vulnerable, additional safeguards are included.
- Informed consent is obtained if appropriate.
- Confidentiality is adequately protected.

Risks and benefits of research

Risks to subjects may include physical harm from complications of tests or treatments, psychosocial harm such as loss of privacy, and inconvenience from spending time and having blood or other clinical specimens collected. The DHHS regulations define minimal risk as that "ordinarily encountered in daily life or during the performance of routine physical or psychological tests" (1). For certain vulnerable populations, such as children, fetuses, and prisoners, research that involves more than minimal risk is either prohibited or subjected to more intensive scrutiny.

Much of the benefit of research accrues to society as a whole through the advancement of scientific knowledge. Often, however, individual research subjects also benefit directly if the research concerns their own illness and if they receive increased attention or improved care through participating in the research.

The principle of beneficence requires that the *risks of research be minimized and proportionate to the anticipated benefits*. Examples of strategies investigators can use to minimize risks include screening subjects to exclude those more likely to suffer adverse effects, using specimens that will be collected in any event for diagnosis or therapy, monitoring subjects for possible adverse effects, and establishing in advance criteria for intervening in the protocol or terminating the study if adverse effects are found. Examples of strategies investigators can use to maximize the benefits to subjects include screening them to select those who are most likely to benefit from treatments used in the study, informing subjects of potentially beneficial alternatives, and helping subjects to obtain continuing care after the study is completed.

Selection of subjects for research

Selection of subjects should be equitable. That is, the benefits and harms of research should be distributed fairly among different groups that could be studied. The principles of beneficence and justice require investigators to protect subjects who are disadvantaged, dependent, or vulnerable. Examples of subjects who lack the capacity to give informed consent include children and those who are mentally incapacitated. The DHHS regulations offer additional protection to children by requiring investigators to obtain both the permission of parents and the assent of the child (1). In addition, research involving more than minimal risk will not be acceptable if it does not benefit the child directly or provide generalizable knowledge about the child's particular illness or about a serious pediatric health problem. Other special DHHS regulations require extra protection when research is carried out on fetuses and embyros or on the pregnant women who bear them (1).

Mentally incapacitated patients, such as those with Alzheimer's disease, also may not be competent to consent to research. It seems reasonable to allow surrogates to consent for research that presents minimal risks and is directed toward understanding or improving their condition (5, 6). Another alternative is for an elderly patient to complete a durable power of attorney that allows a proxy to give permission for research studies if she should become incompetent (6).

Other subjects are vulnerable because their consent may be constrained. Since prisoners may not be truly free to refuse to participate in research and may be unduly influenced by cash payments or parole considerations, DHHS regulations limit the types of research that are permitted (1). Constraint may also occur when subjects depend on researchers for medical care, as in nursing homes, Veterans' Administration Hospitals, or municipal clinics. Similarly, students who depend on researchers for grades, or employees of researchers, may not be truly free to decline to participate. If the investigator is also the physician for a patient eligible for a research project, the patient may feel that her future care may be jeopardized if she declines to participate in research. In addition, subjects may not appreciate that the clinical investigator plays a different role than the personal physician. Such role conflicts should be anticipated and explained to subjects in advance. Whenever possible, the patient should be given the opportunity to receive care from a personal physician who is not associated with the study.

Justice requires that such vulnerable populations not be used as a source of research subjects when other populations would also be suitable subjects of study. Vulnerable populations are sometimes considered as sources of subjects merely because access and follow up are more convenient than with more autonomous individuals. The use of vulnerable subjects for research is more justifiable if the research will improve the understanding or treatment of the condition that makes the subjects vulnerable, if advocates for the vulnerable population approve of the research, and if the protocol takes steps to minimize the dependency and potential adverse effects.

Informed consent

The principle of respect for persons requires that subjects give informed consent to participate in the research project. The investigators must disclose information that will be relevant to the subject's decision on whether or not to participate. Such information should include:

The nature of the research project: The prospective subject should be told explicitly that the project involves research and how subjects are being recruited. The purposes

of the research and the names and affiliations of the investigators should be given.

The procedures of the study: What will being a research subject involve, and how long will the study last? From the patient's perspective, the fact that blood will be drawn means more than the names of the tests. In interview or questionnaire research, the subject will want to know the topics to be addressed and the length of time required. Procedures that are experimental rather than standard care should be identified. If treatment is involved, the subject will want to know how it differs from conventional care. Alternative procedures or treatments that may be available outside the study should be discussed. If the study involves blinding or randomization, these concepts should be explained.

The potential risks and benefits of the study: Medical, psychological, social and economic harms and benefits should be described in lay terms. The probability and magnitude of harms and benefits should be given.

Assurances that participation in the research is voluntary: The subject must be told that she can withdraw from the project at any time and that declining to participate or withdrawing from the study will not result in any penalty or loss of benefits.

Protection of confidentiality: The procedures that will be taken to assure privacy and protect confidentiality must be discussed.

Questions about the study: The investigator should offer to answer questions or provide further information. Furthermore, the subject should be told whom to ask about the rights of research subjects and about injuries resulting from the research.

Written consent forms are generally required to document that the process of informed consent—discussions between an investigator and the subject—has occurred. Researchers should appreciate, however, that the *process of consent* is more important that the subject's signature on a form. A signed consent form alone is not sufficient to establish that the process of informed consent occurred, nor does it provide protection from liability. Many consent forms contain technical jargon and complicated sentences that are incomprehensible to most lay-people. Informed decisions about participating in research are enhanced if the researchers take care to use clear, simple language during the disclosure process and to allow subjects sufficient time to make thoughtful decisions about participating. For instance, giving people written information about the project and suggesting that they take it home and discuss it with their family and friends may enhance the consent process.

When subjects are not capable of giving informed consent, surrogate consent should be obtained. More important, the protocol should be subjected to additional scrutiny, to ensure that the research question could not be studied in a population that is capable of giving consent.

Privacy and confidentiality

Maintaining confidentiality of medical information respects research subjects and their privacy. People generally wish to have control over what personal information is disclosed to others and feel violated when their privacy is not respected. Confidentiality protects subjects from adverse consequences that may occur if information about such issues as psychiatric illness, sexual preference, or substance abuse were disclosed to employers, insurers, or legal authorities. The AIDS epidemic has reminded researchers that concerns about confidentiality may deter potential subjects from participating in research (7). If confidentiality about HIV infection is broken, research subjects may be stigmatized and suffer discrimination in employment, housing, or insurance or even be subject to criminal charges in some situations.

Confidentiality may be threatened if sensitive information is inadvertently disclosed, if research records are subpoenaed in legal proceedings, if case studies or photographs are published, or if the research yields information about such problems as infectious diseases or child abuse that legally must be reported. Examples of *strategies for protecting* confidentiality include storing data in locked file cabinets, coding data to hide the identity of subjects, limiting access to the research data, destroying the data after the study is completed, and assuring that individual subjects cannot be identified when the findings are published. If the research data contain sensitive information that may create legal problems for the subjects if they are disclosed, researchers may wish to obtain confidentiality certificates from the DHHS and the Department of Justice (8). These certificates allow the identification of research subjects to be withheld if the research records are subpoenaed. If data are subpoenaed, the investigator has an ethical duty to seek legal counsel to have the subpoena quashed (9).

Potential threats to confidentiality, as well as measures that the investigators will take to maintain confidentiality, should be discussed explicitly with the study subjects before they decide to participate. Researchers must be careful not to make promises about confidentiality that may be impossible to uphold. Ultimately the integrity and sensitivity of the researcher may be the most effective guarantee to subjects that their privacy will be protected.

INSTITUTIONAL REVIEW BOARDS

Federal agencies that fund or regulate research on human subjects require that it be approved by an institutional review board (IRB). In addition, most institutions that are involved with research on human subjects require approval by an IRB, regardless of the source of funding. Such review is intended to ensure that the research is ethically acceptable and that the welfare and rights of the subjects are protected.

The IRB system is decentralized; each local IRB interprets and implements federal regulations using its own forms and guidelines. An IRB typically consists of faculty researchers, clinical staff, patient advocates, lay members, and persons knowledgeable about legal and ethical issues concerning research. Members or staff of the IRB are usually available to consult with investigators planning a research project. These individuals can provide information about the IRB's policies, suggest procedures for protecting subjects, and assist with designing consent forms.

The IRB may decide that certain types of research may be given expedited review, and that others may be exempted from IRB review or from requirements for informed consent. Examples of the latter are most types of survey and interview studies, observations of public behavior, educational evaluations, and reviews of existing data, records, and specimens (Table 14.2). Arguments for allowing such exemptions are that there is no risk and that most people would consent to such research. Furthermore, obtaining consent from each subject would make many such studies too expensive or difficult, and much important knowledge might be lost. Critics of such exemptions argue, however, that some subjects might object to the purposes of the research or resent the invasion of privacy. To resolve this problem, the investigator might ask a group of potential subjects or their representatives whether they object to the study.

The IRB system does not guarantee that research is ethically acceptable. Institutional review boards may place more emphasis on consent forms and on the risks and benefits of research than on other ethical issues. Review of the scientific design of the research and of the approach to selecting subjects is usually left to the funding agency and its extramural panels of experts (Chapter 17) . Institutional review boards are unable to monitor whether research was actually carried out in accordance with the protocols that were approved. For these reasons, DHHS regulations and IRB approval should be regarded only as a minimal ethical standard for research. The most important factors for assuring that research is ethically acceptable are the judgment and character of the investigator.

SPECIAL TOPICS

Randomized blinded trials

Randomized blinded trials are often the best design for studying treatment efficacy, thus satisfying the ethical principle of beneficence. They also lead, however, to special ethical concerns (10–12). In an experiment the investigator is actively doing something to the subject, and this creates more opportunity for both harm and benefit than is present in an observational study. In addition, there are some specific problems that result from randomization and blinding.

The ethical basis for assigning therapy by randomization is the judgment that the null hypothesis cannot be rejected on the basis of prior evidence. Reasonable people may disagree over this judgment. Physicians who believe that prior evidence indicates that one alternative offers better treatment cannot justify entering patients in the trial if this treatment is readily available outside the research project. Similarly, a patient's values and preferences may make one alternative preferable for that individual, such as when a medical and surgical intervention are compared. In this situation, random assignment of treatment may not be in the patient's best interests.

The use of placebo controls also raises ethical concerns. In some clinical situations, withholding active treatment from the control group may lead to serious medical com-

Table 14.2.
Exemptions from DHHS regulations

- Surveys or interviews, unless
  1. Subjects can be identified and
  2. Responses might lead to legal liability, financial loss, or reduced employability and
  3. Research deals with sensitive topics, such as sexual behavior or substance abuse.[a]
- Observations of public behavior, except if the above three conditions apply.
- Research on normal educational practices.
- Studies of existing records, data, or diagnostic or pathologic specimens, provided that the research data cannot be linked to individual subjects.

[a]Although DHHS exempts survey or interview research unless all three conditions hold, we believe IRB review is desirable if the first and *either* the second *or* the third conditions apply.

plications, although this possibility is often balanced by the potential hazards of active treatment. The blinding of the interventions may create problems in clinical management if, for example, the patient has emergency surgery, and it may be necessary to design a system (accessible 24 hours a day) for unblinding the intervention. Subjects need to be informed during the consent process if the control group will receive blinded placebos and what the risks might be.

Randomized trials sometimes have difficulty enrolling a high percentage of eligible patients. Requiring consent to randomization may be a major reason that patients decline to participate, but proposals to randomize subjects before obtaining informed consent have not been widely adopted because of ethical, practical, and biostatistical objections (10). Problems with enrollment of subjects may be successfully overcome by meeting potential subjects or their representatives. If potential subjects understand the reasons for the research, the problems facing the study, and the ways such problems might be handled, they may feel like partners in the research effort and be more willing to participate.

The analysis of preliminary data raises additional ethical issues. The principle of beneficence implies that it would be unethical to continue a study after it has been demonstrated that one therapy is safer or more effective. However, repeated analyses during the study (to see if the results are statistically significant) can undermine the power or validity of the study. Procedures for examining preliminary data and judging whether a significant difference is present (Appendix 11.B) should be established before the study begins. An independent panel of reviewers often is given the power to monitor preliminary data and to determine whether to terminate the study prematurely. Such procedures should be explained to subjects during the consent process.

Deception in research

In some projects, particularly in the realm of social psychology, investigators may not wish to fully inform subjects of the purpose of research. If covert observation is proposed, researchers may not even want to inform subjects that research is being done. Although withholding information or deceiving subjects may make it easier to conduct studies, several objections can be raised. Subjects are deprived of the opportunity to decide if they want to participate. Their self-esteem, privacy, and trust in others may be violated. Those who are deceived may be more concerned about such violations than are those who do the deceiving. In the long run, the public may become cynical about researchers and be less willing to participate in research.

Deception is difficult to justify if the research question can be studied without using deception, if the purpose of deception is merely to make the study more feasible, or if the use of deception may produce harm or discomfort. The investigator would be prudent to consult with a group of eligible subjects. Do they consider the deception unreasonable or unacceptable? If research is carried out using deception, the investigator should debrief subjects afterwards, explaining the true nature of the study and taking responsibility for any harmful consequences to the subjects (13).

The role of the investigator

Investigators should assure that research is ethically sound in several ways that are beyond the scope of regulations and IRB review. First, researchers must be scientifically competent, and protocols must be rigorously designed. If the research question is trivial or if the design of the study is so weak that valid conclusions are unlikely, then it is difficult to justify even minimal risk or inconvenience to human subjects. Second, researchers should promote appropriate attention to ethical issues in professional meetings and publications, in their institutions, and in their specific projects. Only if investigators are conscientious and sensitive to ethical issues can the safety and welfare of research volunteers be safeguarded.

Third, investigators must realize that the different roles they play may create conflicts of interest. An investigator who is also the personal physician for her study subjects must appreciate that what is best for the patient's medical care may conflict with what is best for the research project (such as whether to enroll or to remain on a standardized protocol rather than individualizing care when problems arise) (14). Other problems may arise when investigators have a financial interest in the therapy or procedure being studied (15), especially if those financial ties are not revealed when patients consent to participate or when manuscripts are submitted for publication. Even the appearance of a conflict of interest may undermine public and professional acceptance of the research.

Recent cases of fraud in biomedical research, with wholesale fabrication of data, have dramatized how difficult it may be to detect even blatantly unethical research practices (16). Ultimately the most important guarantee that research is conducted in an ethical manner is the professional and personal integrity of the investigator.

SUMMARY

1. In research involving human subjects, DHHS guidelines as well as an ethical and legal consensus require that the following conditions be met:
   a). The risks to subjects should be *minimized* and be *proportionate* to the anticipated *benefits* and knowledge.
   b). The *selection* of subjects should be *equitable*.
   c). If subjects are *vulnerable*, additional *safeguards* should be provided.
   d). *Confidentiality* should be adequately protected.
   e). *Informed consent* should be obtained from the subjects.
2. The *process* of obtaining informed consent is more important than the subject's signature on a form; there is a need to disclose the nature and procedures of the study and the potential risks and benefits, to assure the subjects that participation is voluntary and the results confidential, and to provide a continuing opportunity for answering questions.
3. For most research, an *institutional review board* must review the protocol to ensure that it complies with the above criteria.
4. To ensure that research meets the spirit as

well as the letter of federal regulations, *investigators must develop their own high standards* for the task of assuring that their research is ethical.

REFERENCES

1. Department of Health and Human Services Rule and Regulations. Title 45; Code of Federal Regulations; Part 46: Revised as of March 8, 1983. Washington, DC, U.S. Department of Health and Human Services, 1983
2. Levine RJ: *Ethics and Regulation of Clinical Research.* Baltimore, Urban & Schwarzenberg, 1986.
3. The National Commission for the Protection of Human Subjects of Biomedical and Behavioral Research: *The Belmont Report: Ethical Principles and Guidelines for the Protection of Human Subjects of Research.* (DHEW Publication No. (OS) 78–0012.) Washington, DC, U.S. Government Printing Office, 1978.
4. Veatch RM: *The Patient as Partner: A Theory of Human-Experimentation Ethics.* Bloomington, Indiana University Press, 1987.
5. Melnick VL, Dubler NM, Weisbard A, Butler RN: Clinical research in senile dementia of the Alzheimer type: suggested guidelines in addressing the ethical and legal issues. *J Am Geriat Soc* 32:531–536, 1984.
6. Annas GJ, Glantz LH: Rules for research in nursing homes. *N Engl J Med* 315:1157–1158, 1986.
7. Bayer R, Levine C, Murray TH: Guidelines for confidentiality in research on AIDS. *IRB* 6:1–7, 1984.
8. Levine RJ: *Ethics and Regulation of Clinical Research.* Baltimore, Urban & Schwarzenberg, 1986, pp 170–172.
9. Holder AR: When researchers are served subpoenas. *IRB* 7:5–7; 1985.
10. Ellenberg SS: Randomization Designs in Comparative Clinical Trials. *N Engl J Med* 310: 1404–1408, 1984.
11. Angell M: Patient preferences in randomized clinical trials. *N Engl J Med* 310:1385–1387, 1984.
12. Kopelman L: Randomized clinical trials, consent, and the therapeutic relationship. *Clin Res* 1983; 31:1–11.
13. American Psychological Association: *Ethical Principles in the Conduct of Research with Human Participants.* Washington, DC, American Psychological Association, 1982.
14. Holder AR: Do researchers and subjects have a fiduciary relationship? *IRB* 4:6–7, 1982.
15. Lind SE: Fee for service research. *N Engl J Med* 314:312–315, 1986.
16. Shapiro MF, Charrow RP: Scientific misconduct in investigational drug trials. *N Engl J Med* 312:731–736, 1985.

ADDITIONAL READINGS

Levine RJ: *Ethics and Regulation of Clinical Research.* Baltimore, Urban & Schwarzenberg, 1986. (*Highly recommended for further reading. Comprehensive, practical, and thoughtful, with detailed references.*)

Veatch RM: *The Patient as Partner: A Theory of Human-Experimentation Ethics.* Bloomington, Indiana University Press, 1987. (*Argues for increased participation of subjects in planning and conducting research.*)

Meinert C. *Clinical Trials.* New York, Oxford University Press, 1986, pp 153–158, 374–378. (*A good description of how to develop consent forms for clinical trials.*)

CHAPTER 15

Planning for Data Management and Analysis

David Feigal, Dennis Black, Deborah Grady, Norman Hearst, Cary Fox, Thomas B. Newman, and Stephen B. Hulley

INTRODUCTION **159**

THE DATA MANAGEMENT SYSTEM **159**

Setting up the rules for data entry
Choosing the computer
Choosing and using the data entry program
Designing the system for data management

THE STATISTICAL ANALYSIS SYSTEM **166**

Choosing the program

ANALYZING THE DATA **166**

Descriptive statistics: examining variables one at a time
Analytic statistics: examining variables two or more at a time

SUMMARY **170**

REFERENCES **170**

ADDITIONAL READINGS **170**

APPENDIX 15.A. Illustration of the use of a statistical analyses package to analyze the smoking questionnaire data **224**

APPENDIX 15.B. Classification of statistical analyses (and tests) by types of variables **226**

INTRODUCTION

A sometimes overlooked part of research planning is the preparation for the data entry, editing, and analysis. This is illustrated by an analogy to income tax preparation. Some taxpayers (*investigators*) take a shoe box (*file cabinet*) and keep their receipts (*data*) until the end of the year (*study*) when they take them to an accountant (*statistician*) who usually can't help very much until the receipts are organized (*data entered*) and veri-fied (*cleaned*). If the tax instructions (*methods sections*) are simple, without too many deductions (*variables*), then there is usually no problem unless receipts have been lost (*missing data*) or whole classes of documents have been neglected (*unmeasured variables*). Some receipts may not meet IRS guidelines (*invalid measurement techniques*) and are difficult to document at the end of the year (*study*). The taxpayers (*investigators*) could do their own taxes (*data analysis*) but would lose the advantage (*neglect some findings*) that the expertise of the accountant (*statistician*) could have provided. The taxpayers might also get too creative (*use inappropriate analyses*) and not discover until audit (*journal rejection*) that they paid the wrong amount (*got the wrong answer*).

The solution to problems of this sort is to have a good plan for data management and analysis, and to implement it well. The goal of this chapter is to introduce the investigator to the skills needed for dealing with her data, first for getting it edited and entered into the computer, and then for designing analyses that will answer the research questions. We will describe the types of **computers** (hardware) and **programs** (software) that are useful for these processes, illustrate how to go about using them, and indicate when and how to seek help from experts in **data processing** and **statistical analysis**.

THE DATA MANAGEMENT SYSTEM

The advent of the modern **microcomputer** has changed the way that data are collected, edited, stored, and analyzed. Most data entry and analyses can be done on moderately priced microcomputers with programs that are relatively easy to use. The technology in this field is changing so quickly that the specific hardware and software we describe here will be replaced by improved versions during the lifetime of this edition of this book. But the general approach will probably be more lasting. We use the questionnaire on smoking from Appendix 5 to demonstrate how to take data from the data collection instruments (described in Chapters 5 and 16) through various editing and organizing procedures to the stage of statistical analysis.

Setting up the rules for data entry

Planning for data management begins with developing rules for **coding the variables** for computer entry. Every variable is given a name that identifies its "field" (place) in the data set. For each variable, every possible value is then "coded" with a number so that it can be entered into the computer. This coding scheme is spelled out in a code book that is part of the operations manual.

Table 15.1 illustrates coding rules that might be set up for the questionnaire on smoking. Each variable has an abbreviated name that is self-explanatory; for example "StartSmo" is more informative than "1", the number of the question on the form, and this makes it easier to read the output from the computer. Each permitted response for every variable has a number. Missing data (coded 9 or 99 throughout the data set) have different codes from the response "don't know" (coded 8 or 98) because there may be different implications for editing and analyzing the data. Some questions do not include "don't know" as a permitted response in order to force the subject to respond.

In general, all coding decisions should be made before beginning to collect the data, and the coding instructions should be printed on the forms (the small numbers in the "yes" and "no" response boxes in Appendix 5). **Precoding** in this fashion makes data entry faster and more accurate. It also reminds the investigator that it is usually best to avoid open-ended questions and other measurements that require coding judgments

or interpretations to be made after the data have been collected (see Chapter 5).

Table 15.1 also establishes the basis for **editing ("cleaning") the data**. The column labeled "permitted responses" specifies the permissible values that will be used for **range checks**. For example, StartSmo can only have values between 7, the earliest age the investigator believes plausible for the onset of smoking, and 59, the upper age limit specified by the inclusion criteria for subjects in her study of middle-aged women. The column labeled **logic checks** specifies the rules for a different kind of editing. Here, the internal consistency of responses in several fields can be checked. For example, the answer to question 2 (StartSmo) should not be blank if the subject has indicated in question 1 that she smokes.

Choosing the computer

Having set up the rules for coding and editing the data, the next step is to choose a computer and program for entering it into a data base—a computerized file of the study observations. Some projects with large data sets or complicated analytic plans will need to rent time on one of the large **mainframe computers** that can be accessed by telephone in any major research institution. These offer enormous storage capacity, speed, analytic power, and graphic printing capacity. However, the current generation of **microcomputers** includes machines that can perform all the data processing and analysis functions that are needed for the average clinical research project, and that can be purchased for under $3000. Microcomputers are especially useful for data entry and may serve this function even when the data will eventually be analyzed on a mainframe computer. In this book, we will focus on the microcomputer approach to data management and analysis.[a]

Two microcomputers that are widely

---

[a] A third approach is to use a minicomputer, one that is intermediary between the mainframe and microcomputer in its performance. Minicomputers are actually quite large and powerful (despite their name) and, while expensive to purchase, may be cost-effective for large research projects or for shared use in a research organization.

Table 15.1.
Naming and coding the variables for the questionnaire in Appendix 5, and setting up the guidelines for editing

Question #	Variable name	Permitted responses		Logic checks
1.	EverSmo	Yes	= 1	
		No	= 2	
		Missing	= 9	
2.	StartSmo	7 to 59	= 7–59	Blank if, and only if,
		Don't know	= 98	response to #1 is 2.
		Missing	= 99	
		Does not apply	= blank	
3.	AvgCigs	0 to 96	= 0–96	Blank if, and only if,
		≥ 97	= 97	response to #1 is 2.
		Missing	= 99	
		Does not apply	= blank	
4.	NowSmo	Yes	= 1	Blank if, and only if,
		No	= 2	response to #1 is 2.
		Missing	= 9	
		Does not apply	= blank	
5.	StopSmo	7 to 59	= 7–59	Blank if, and only if,
		Don't know	= 98	response to #4 is 2;
		Missing	= 99	must be ≥
		Does not apply	= blank	response to #2 if that
				response is 7–59
6.	CigsNow	0 to 96	= 0–96	Blank if, and only if,
		≥ 97	= 97	response to #4 is 1
		Missing	= 99	
		Does not apply	= blank	

used by clinical investigators are the IBM personal computer (or any of the IBM-compatible computers produced by other vendors) and the Apple Macintosh. Both are excellent choices. A current (1988) advantage of the IBM is that better statistical analysis software packages are available; an advantage of the Macintosh is its user-friendliness (good for new staff and rotating fellows!). With either machine, the investigator should get advice in choosing a model that will be suitable for the programs she will be using and the data set she will create.

Choosing and using the data entry program

Having selected the hardware (computer) for the project, the investigator must next choose among a number of software options (the programs that give the computer its instructions). The main classes of software that are useful in clinical research are presented in Table 15.2. The first three classes—spreadsheet programs, data base managers, and statistical/graphics programs—can each be used for data entry and management. They differ chiefly in the ease of data entry, in the mechanisms for editing and accessing the data, and in the statistical analysis and reporting capabilities.

Spreadsheet software: Perhaps the most common and easily accessible approach to entering a modest number of observations and variables into a microcomputer is to use a spreadsheet program. This type of program arranges the data into a matrix of columns (for the variables) and rows (for the study subjects), as illustrated with hypothetical data for the smoking questionnaire in Table 15.3A. Spreadsheet programs make the entry of raw data easy. They can also be programmed to create a column of derived values, for example computing pack-years from the recorded age of onset of smoking, the current age, and the number of cigarettes smoked per day.

Spreadsheet programs can provide summary descriptive statistics and frequency distributions, and they can sort the data in

Table 15.2.
Research applications of microcomputer software[a]

Software	Research uses	Examples
Data entry software		
Spreadsheet	Data entry into a matrix of columns and rows; simple transformations, descriptions, sorting, and reporting	Excel Lotus 123 Multiplan
Data base management	Data entry with interactive editing and greater ability to manipulate, access, and report the data	dBase 3+ Helix Omnis RBase Reflex
Statistical/graphics	In addition to some of the above features: statistical analysis and graphics	BMDP Cricket SAS-PC SPSS-PC Statview Systat
Other microcomputer software commonly used in research		
Word processing	Text entry and revision: •protocols and reports •forms •correspondence •appointment reminders •bibliographies	MacWrite Word Wordperfect Wordstar
Drawing	Form design and printing Custom illustrations	MacDraw MacDraft PC-Paint
Telecommunication	Transfer data or messages Remote computing on the mainframe Literature search	Crosstalk MacTerm Procom Red Ryder

[a]This is a list of examples, and is not comprehensive. Investigators should seek advice from local experts in choosing microcomputers and programs.

ways that are helpful to the process of detecting and correcting errors in the data. In table 15.3B, the data have been sorted on the variables EverSmo, NowSmo, and AvgCigs. This makes it easier to carry out a *range check*, which reveals that the last line (ID #13) has an invalid value for column 1; the coding scheme in Table 15.1 did not permit 7 as a response. The investigator can correct this error by examining which box was checked on the original form.

Sorting is also helpful for carrying out *logic checks*; it becomes obvious, for example, that subject #10 has an illegal value for CigsNow (blank) since the value for NowSmo (1) indicates that she smokes. This error might either reflect a data entry error

(which the investigator can correct by examining what was written on the original form) or an incorrect response recorded on the form (which the investigator may be able to correct by making a telephone call to the subject). Spreadsheet programs can also facilitate logic checks by creating a calculated column of numbers; for example the quantity (StopSmo–StartSmo) cannot be a negative number.

The major drawbacks to spreadsheets are the fact that missing value codes (e.g., 99) cannot be ignored when calculating descriptive statistics, the slow speed when there are many observations, and the absence of many functions for editing, accessing, and analyzing the data. Nevertheless,

Table 15.3.
A set of data from 14 subjects

A. Before sorting

ID	1. EverSmo	2. StartSmo	3. AvgCigs	4. NowSmo	5. StopSmo	6. CigsNow
1	1	13	40	1		20
2	1	9	15	2	23	
3	2					
4	2					
5	1	22	10	1		10
6	2					
7	2					
8	1	14	20	2	28	
9	1	12	20	1		35
10	1	12	10	1		
11	2					
12	1	16	10	2	17	
13	7					
14	1	18	99	2	58	

B. Sorted by EverSmo, NowSmo, and AvgCigs

ID	1. EverSmo	2. StartSmo	3. AvgCigs	4. NowSmo	5. StopSmo	6. CigsNow
10	1	12	10	1		
5	1	22	10	1		10
9	1	12	20	1		35
1	1	13	40	1		20
12	1	16	15	2	17	
8	1	14	20	2	28	
2	1	9	95	2	23	
14	1	18	99	2	58	
3	2					
4	2					
6	2					
7	2					
11	2					
13	7					

C. Descriptive statistics for the eight smokers

	1. EverSmo	2. StartSmo	3. AvgCigs	4. NowSmo	5. StopSmo	6. CigsNow
count	8	8	8	8	4	3
mean		14.5	38.6[a]		31.5	21.7
s.d.		4.1	30.4[a]		18.2	11.8
min	1	9	10	1	17	10
max	1	22	99[a]	2	58	35

[a]The 99 response for AvgCigs is included in the descriptive statistics even though it is a code for missing data rather than an actual value, altering the values for these descriptive statistics (the mean of the seven actual values is 30). Spreadsheet software cannot ordinarily be programmed to ignore such code values but more sophisticated programs can (see Appendix 15A).

for small studies spreadsheets offer a simple tool for entering and cleaning the data, and for computing simple descriptive statistics.

Data base management software: Data base management programs are more suitable than spreadsheet programs for studies with large numbers of variables and observations. They also permit the investigator to carry out some editing functions *interactively*—to clean the data while they are being entered. The computer is programmed to expect responses to each specific variable on the data entry form; the screen shows the items on the form (or labels that represent them), and a "cursor" (marker) indicates the field for entering the value of the variable. The program can be made to require an entry before the cursor moves on to the next field, reducing the problem of missing data—the operator can still enter 9's, consciously indicating that the value is missing, but she cannot simply pass the item by, neglecting it altogether. The program can also check each value as it is entered to be sure that it is in the permissible range, reducing the problem of wildly aberrant values. For example, a data base management program could easily have prevented the erroneous entry for subject #13 in Table 15.3.

Most data base management software also offer a number of more sophisticated editing features, although in general these are considerably more difficult to program. Automatic logic checks can be included in the data entry procedure to make sure that questions are skipped when appropriate, and that the entries on the form are consistent with each other. This approach could have been used, for example, to prevent the erroneous entry for subject #10 in Table 15.3. Database management software can also be programmed for **duplicate data entry**. The fields are automatically blanked out after the subject's responses have been entered the first time, and values entered a second time must match the first set before they are accepted in the data base.

These approaches to customizing the data entry for a study can be an excellent strategy for minimizing errors in the data base, but they have some major disadvantages. Even an experienced programmer will find it time-consuming to program an interactive data entry system. Also, the complexity of the editing and checking parameters make modifications difficult, should there be changes in the data collection forms. Duplicate data entry doubles the time needed to enter the data. For these reasons, most investigators use data base management software without a great deal of custom programming.

Statistical software: It is possible to bypass the spreadsheet and data base management software described above by entering the data directly into a statistical analysis program, often in a format that resembles a spreadsheet program. This allows the investigator to skip the step (that would otherwise be necessary) of creating a mechanism for transferring data that have been entered into a spreadsheet or a data base management program over to the computer and program that will carry out the statistical analysis. A current (1988) disadvantage of entering data into some statistical packages is the limitations in the editing and data management functions.

Designing the system for data management

We have discussed coding and editing rules, and the computers and the programs for operating them. It is now necessary to bring together these components into a *system* for managing the study data. Collecting, editing, and storing the data requires attention to detail, and the investigator should develop for the operations manual a written systematic approach along the lines illustrated in Figure 15.1.

The data are recorded on forms that have been designed using the guidelines set forth in Chapters 5 and 16. It is important to record the data directly on the forms at the time the measurements are made (rather than keeping notes on scraps of paper as an intermediary step) to minimize the possibility of losses or transcription errors. The forms are then hand edited while the study subject is still available, looking for omissions, illegible entries, and gross errors that can be corrected on the spot. The next step, entering the data in the computer, should usually be done within the next several days. Entering the data promptly prevents backlogs from accumulating, allows early identification of data collection problems, minimizes the possibility of losses, and permits the investigator to examine periodic reports that keep track of her study. It also takes advantage of the computer's ability to edit the data at a time when it may still be

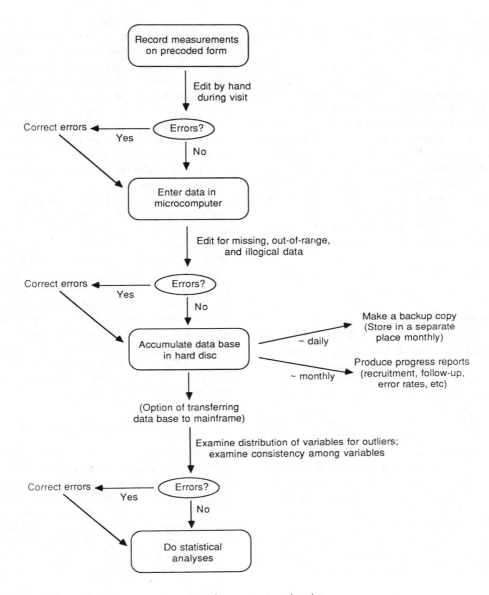

Figure 15.1. Schematic diagram of a system for managing the data.

possible to return to the source of the data and correct any errors.

If the study data base is relatively small it can be stored on a floppy disc, but in general it is best to store it on a hard disc that is attached to the microcomputer. A 20 megabyte hard disc will be large enough for most clinical research efforts (check with an expert to be sure), offers good speed of access and manipulation, and is suitable for sophis-

ticated data base management and statistical analysis programs. As the data base begins to accumulate, it is important to make a copy at regular intervals (in addition to filing the paper forms). "Backing up" the data set onto another set of floppies (or into the mainframe computer) is easy and cheap to do, and guards against losses due to such things as a failure of the hard disc. Storing the backup copy in a different building (for example the investigator's home) will provide a safeguard against rare but calamitous events like a fire or flood.

At periodic intervals during the study, typically once a month, the investigator should produce interim reports that monitor the technical progress of the study and tabulate such things as the rate of recruitment or missing data and the occurrence of tardy follow-up visits or data entry. She should keep these reports in a **study log**, which should also contain an ongoing record of relevant study events such as the date of each backup, the accomplishment of quality control procedures, any changes in protocol, and the occurrence of untoward events.

THE STATISTICAL ANALYSIS SYSTEM

Choosing the program

Three major packages of statistical programs (SAS, SPSS, and BMDP) have become standards for analyzing the data in clinical research. Each has a sophisticated set of programs that permit the investigator to carry out a broad range of statistical analyses. **SAS** offers the most flexibility for customizing the approach to data management and analyses, but is difficult to learn to use. **SPSS** is perhaps the easiest for a beginning investigator to learn, and comes with a manual that explains the philosophy as well as the mechanics of statistical techniques (1). **BMDP** (which is illustrated in Appendix 15A) has less data management capability but has many programs tailored to sophisticated biomedical data analysis.

In recent years SAS, SPSS, and BMDP have become available in microcomputer versions for the IBM AT and compatible machines. Running these statistical packages on microcomputers is less expensive in the long run than computing on the mainframe (after bearing the one-time cost of the microcomputer, hard disc, and program). These programs are much slower on the microcomputer than on the mainframe, but this is not a serious disadvantages unless the data set is extremely large.

Statistical program packages like Statview or SysStat are designed specifically for microcomputers (Macintosh- as well as IBM-compatible machines) and are easy to learn and operate. These programs offer a range of basic descriptive and analytic statistics (including t-test, chi-square, and multiple regression), and they permit immediate graphic display of the results. The chief disadvantage of these microcomputer statistical programs is their unsuitability for manipulating large data sets and for performing complex statistical tasks like survival analysis and logistic regression.

ANALYZING THE DATA

We recommend a deliberate approach to looking at data, using the same sequence for analyzing the study that was used for planning it: *first descriptive, then analytic* (Table 15.4). The investigator should always begin with **descriptive statistics**, examining the distribution of each study variable individually to complete the editing process and to reveal the basic structure of the findings. Next she

Table 15.4.
Steps in data analysis

Step		Examples	Purpose
Step 1.	Descriptive statistics (looking at distributions of variables, one at a time)	Mean, median Proportion Standard deviation Confidence interval Frequency distribution	Final step of editing Characterize study subjects Inform choice of analytic statisic
Step 2.	Analytic statistics (looking at associations among two or more variables)	Cross-tabulation Correlation Analysis of variance Regression	Estimate pattern and strength of associations among variables Test null hypotheses

can **analyze associations** between pairs of variables using simple scatterplots and correlation coefficients, and she can begin examining various predictor and confounding variables by stratification or multivariate analyses. Finally, she can carry out formal statistical tests of the study hypotheses and draw conclusions about the answers to the research questions.

The *details* of these steps are beyond the scope of this book, and we advise the reader to consult one of the excellent statistical analysis texts noted at the end of this chapter. We will, however, provide a brief overview to introduce the reader to the nature and rationale of the process.

Descriptive statistics: examining variables one at a time

The first step is to examine the **frequency distributions** of values for each variable collected. One reason for doing this is to *complete the editing* process, looking for outlying values that may represent errors that have survived previous efforts to edit the data set. The investigator can examine frequency distributions and consider whether the values at the ends of the distribution are implausible (e.g., in Figure 15.2, it would be a good idea to recheck a value of 95). The investigator can examine the internal consistency of the data, noting, for example, whether the distribution of change in weight from one visit to another contains any unlikely values. She can also use frequency distributions to reveal the number of missing values for each variable, distinguishing those that are due to problems in data

collection from those that are expected (e.g., number of cigarettes per day for a nonsmoker).

In general, the longer the investigator continues to examine her data, the longer potential errors will continue to emerge. At some point, however, these become infrequent enough to have no substantial effect on the overall conclusions. When the investigator judges that this point has been reached, we recommend "freezing" the data set—deciding not to make any more changes, even if further errors are discovered. This will free her from the burden of worrying about additional problems in the data set, and it means that all publications will have findings that are precisely consistent with each other.

In addition to their role in editing the data, frequency distributions are useful for *revealing the basic descriptive findings*. For categorical variables these graphs reveal the proportion of each response, and for continuous variables they reveal the shape of the distribution. If the data fit a **normal distribution** (roughly bell-shaped as in Fig. 15.2) then the investigator can use the mean to express the point estimate of the **central tendency** and the standard deviation (or confidence intervals) to express the **spread**. If the distribution is very *asymmetric* it may be better to use the median to express the central tendency and the range or 25th and 75th percentiles to express the spread.

Once the investigator has examined the frequency distribution of each variable and computed a statistic to estimate the central tendency and spread of the data, the next step is to stand back and think about these results. Is the distribution of values compatible with what was expected for the population sampled? If not, a more intensive search for possible errors is in order.

In a lengthy study, the investigator should carry out these steps at periodic intervals during the study as well as at the end. The earlier she knows about missing data and unexpected distributions, the sooner she can take corrective actions such as refining the study measurement techniques, taking steps to prevent missing data, and adjusting the sample size.

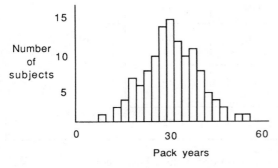

Figure 15.2. Illustration of a frequency distribution, or histogram.

Analytic statistics: examining variables two or more at a time

Once the distributions of individual variables have been described, the investigator can turn to analyzing associations among predictor and outcome variables. There are three steps: (1) inspection of the *pattern* of the association in the *sample*, (2) computation of the *magnitude* (measure) of the association in the *sample*, and (3) estimation of the *likelihood* that the association observed in the sample also exists in the *population* from which the sample was drawn (statistical significance). The choice of the specific technique for each step depends on the type of variables being examined (e.g., categorical or continuous).

Two dichotomous variables: For example, if both variables are dichotomous, then the pattern of a possible association is revealed by **cross-tabulation** in a simple **two-by-two table**. Suppose the investigator wants to examine whether the level of education of her subjects is a predictor of their ever having smoked cigarettes. In Table 15.5, an expanded hypothetical set of values for the variable "EverSmo" on the smoking questionnaire is cross-tabulated with the variable "years of education" (obtained from another form and merged in the data set using the subjects' ID number to assure correct linkage). Years of education has been dichotomized to produce two groups of subjects,

those with 12 or fewer years of education, and those with more than 12.

Now the investigator asks the question: Is there an association between education level and smoking? The first step in answering this question is to *inspect* the findings. The investigator notes that a higher proportion of the less educated group has smoked cigarettes at some time in their lives (51/81 = 63%) than of the more educated group (31/73 = 42%). The next step is to find a statistic that expresses the *magnitude* of this association. In this case the relative prevalence is 1.5 (63% / 42%), which means that less educated people in this sample are 50% more likely to have smoked cigarettes at some point in their lives than more educated people.

The final step is to draw an *inference* about whether the association observed in this sample exists in the population from which the sample was drawn (see Chapter 12). Here the investigator computes the statistical significance of the observed relative prevalence—the probability, given that the null hypothesis is true (i.e., that the relative prevalence in the population is actually 1.0), that a value of 1.5 or greater would be observed in the sample by chance. In this instance, the likelihood of this possibility can be computed using the chi-square test, and is $P = .02$. The investigator rejects the null hypothesis and draws the conclusion that there

Table 15.5.
Association between two dichotomous variables[a]

		Outcome variable: ever smoked?		
		yes	no	
Predictor variable: education	≤ 12 years	51	30	81
	> 12 years	31	42	73
		82	72	154

[a]By convention in a two-by-two table:
- the rows are for the predictor variable, with the condition under study (lower education) on top.
- the columns are for the outcome variable, with the presence of the outcome to the left, absence to the right.

is a real association between education and smoking in the population.

In addition to hypothesis testing in this way, another and sometimes more informative approach (2, 3) is to compute the 95% confidence interval of the observed relative prevalence (in this case 1.1 to 2.0). The confidence interval indicates that if a series of samples numbering 154 subjects each were drawn from this population, then 95% of these samples would give a relative prevalence between 1.1 and 2.0.

It should be noted that these two approaches to indicating statistical significance (hypothesis testing and confidence intervals) are concerned only with random error as a threat to drawing inferences from the sample to the population. The investigator must use judgment to assess the issue of bias— whether there may be *systematic* errors in sampling and measurement that threaten this inference.

Two continuous variables: When both variables are continuous, then a **scatterplot** of the two variables is the most informative way to inspect the pattern of an association. There are some types of associations (e.g., exponential and U-shaped relationships) that will be missed if the investigator goes directly to the task of analyzing the magnitude and statistical significance of the association without first inspecting the data in a scatterplot. Both of the common analytic approaches, correlation and linear regres-

sion, are designed to detect only straight line relationships; special statistical approaches will be needed if inspection suggests that a nonlinear association is present.

Figure 15.3 illustrates a hypothetical scatterplot of the association between education level and current number of cigarettes smoked per day among smokers. For regression analysis the investigator must specify one of the variables as the predictor, conventionally put on the abcissa, and she has decided that education is more likely to be a cause of current smoking habits than viceversa. Inspection of Figure 15.3 reveals an association that appears linear, so the magnitude of the association in the sample can be expressed as the regression coefficient. The inference that there is also an association in the population can be examined by testing the statistical significance of the difference between the observed value for the regression coefficient and zero.

Various other types of predictor and outcome variables: Using the general method described above (inspecting the data, calculating a measure of association and analyzing statistical significance), it is possible to examine the relationship between any two variables. There are many techniques for the evaluation of associations and the appropriate choice depends on the type of variable (dichotomous, categorical, continuous) and the probability distributions of the variables. We have summarized some of

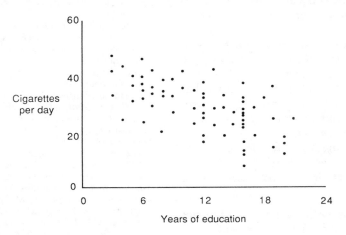

Figure 15.3. Illustration of a scatterplot.

these techniques in Appendix 15B. Readers who are already somewhat familiar with statistical analysis may find that the table in this appendix helps to organize their thinking and contributes to the choice of types of variables in the studies they are designing.

Examining multiple variables: In many epidemiologic studies it is important to carry the analysis beyond an examination of the association between a single predictor and outcome variable. The multivariate analytic techniques necessary to analyze multiple predictors, sequential outcomes, confounding variables and interaction are beyond the scope of this book. We refer the reader to the statistical texts referenced at the end of this chapter, and to an experienced statistician.

SUMMARY

1. In designing the *data management* system, the investigator begins with *coding rules* for the data collection instruments, and with a system for *editing the data* (including range checks and logic checks) that will minimize the occurrence of missing and erroneous data.
2. The investigator should then plan for *data entry*, choosing from a rapidly evolving assortment of *hardware* (microcomputers are an inexpensive and satisfactory option) and *software* (spreadsheet programs, data base management programs, and statistical software programs are all satisfactory options).
3. There is a need to develop a written *system* for managing the data, specifying the data collection, editing, and backup storage procedures, and setting out a mechanism for recording quality control activities, protocol changes, and other notable study events.
4. *Statistical analysis* also requires decisions about the choice of hardware and software. The investigator then examines the data:

   a. She begins with *descriptive statistics* that examine *distributions* of variables, one at a time, using means, medians, proportions, standard deviations, confidence intervals, and frequency distributions.

   b. She then turns to *analytic statistics* that examine (i) the *pattern*, (ii) the *magnitude*, and (iii) the *statistical significance* of *associations* among variables using cross-tabulation, scatterplots, correlation, regression, analysis of variance, and various multivariate approaches.

REFERENCES

1. SPSS Inc: *SPSS-X User's Guide.* New York, McGraw-Hill, 1983.
2. Rothman K: A show of confidence. *N Engl J Med* 299:1362–1363, 1978.
3. Poole C: Beyond the confidence interval. *AJPH* 7:195–199, 1987.

ADDITIONAL READING

Afifi AA, Clark V: *Computer-Aided Multivariate Analysis.* Belmont, CA; Lifetime Learning Publications, 1984. *(Multivariate methods, including multiple regression, logistic regression, and discriminant analysis are presented with discussion of the computer output from statistical packages such as BMDP, SAS, and SPSS.)*

Anderson S, Auquier A, Hauck W, et al: *Statistical Methods for Comparative Studies.* New York, John Wiley and Sons, 1980. *(A readable book on how to adjust for confounding.)*

Bailar JC, III, Mostiller F: *Medical Uses of Statistics.* Waltham MA, 1986. *(An excellent compilation of recent N Engl J Med articles.)*

Brown BW, Hollander M: *Statistics. A Biomedical Introduction.*, New York, John Wiley & Sons, 1977. *(An introductory level statistics text that presents commonly used nonparametric techniques and examples of survival analysis; assumes no prior knowledge of statistics.)*

Fleiss JL: *Statistical Methods for Rates and Proportions,* ed 2. New York, John Wiley & Sons, 1981. *(The standard reference text for dichotomous and categorical data; describes methods for confidence intervals for proportions, odds ratios, and matched designs and stratified analyses.)*

Friedman LM, Furberg CD, DeMets DL: *Fundamentals of Clinical Trials,* ed. 2, Boston, John Wright PSG, Inc., 1985. *(Introduction to statistical methods for clinical trials.)*

Ingelfinger JA, Mosteller F, Thibodeau L, et al: *Biostatistics in Clinical Medicine.* New York, Macmillan, 1983. *(An introductory level statistics text that illustrates quantitative methods in clinical contexts; a suitable first text, or a refresher course.)*

Kleinbaum DG, Kupper LL, Morgenstern H: *Epidemiologic Research: Principles and Quantitative Methods.* Belmont, CA, Lifetime Learning Publications, 1982. *(An advanced epidemiology text that emphasizes quantitative methodology.)*

Meinert CL: *Clinical Trials, Design, Conduct, and Analysis.* Monographs in Epidemiology and Biostatistics, Volume 8. New York, Oxford University Press, 1983. *(A good presentation of statistical methods for clinical trials.)*

Rothman KJ: *Modern Epidemiology.* Boston, Little, Brown and Company, 1986. *(An advanced text on epidemiologic approach to analyzing studies.)*

Snedecor GW, Cochran WC: *Statistical Methods,* ed 7. Ames, Iowa State University Press, 1980. *(A text of statistical methods for categorical and continuous data, with discussion of how sampling and special experimental designs are analyzed.)*

Tukey JW: *Exploratory Data Analysis,* Reading MA, Addison Wesley, 1977. *(Methods for graphical and tabular presentation and exploration of data, including nonparametric approaches such as box and whisker plots.)*

Zar JH: *Biostatistical Analysis,* ed 2. Englewood Cliffs, NJ, Prentice Hall, 1984. *(Good exposition of simple biostatistical methods, including sample size calculation methods.)*

CHAPTER 16

Implementing the Study: Pretesting, Quality Control, and Protocol Revisions

Stephen B. Hulley, David Siegel, and Steven R. Cummings

INTRODUCTION   172

PRETESTING   172
  Designing the study protocol
  Rehearsing the research team

QUALITY CONTROL   174
  The need for quality control
  Quality control of clinical procedures
  Quality control of laboratory procedures
  Quality control of the data
  Collaborative studies

PROTOCOL REVISIONS ONCE DATA
  COLLECTION HAS BEGUN   180
  Making minor revisions
  Making substantive revisions

SUMMARY   182

REFERENCES   182

ADDITIONAL READINGS   183

APPENDIX 16.A.   Example of an operations
  manual table of contents   227

APPENDIX 16.B.   Quality control check lists   228

INTRODUCTION

Most of this book has dealt with the left-hand side of the clinical research model (Fig. 16.1), addressing matters of design. In this chapter we turn to the right-hand, **implementation side**.

First, there is the issue of **pretesting**. Even the best of plans thoughtfully assembled in the armchair can work out very differently in practice. The response rates for acquiring or following subjects may be far lower than anticipated, and the measurements may turn out to be impractical. It is best to discover these problems in a series of pilot studies that can guide appropriate changes in the protocol before the study begins.

Second, there is the issue of **quality control**. Many investigators give insufficient attention to the task of implementing the study because they find it tedious and less intellectually stimulating than the design and the analysis phases. As a result, the conclusions of a well-designed study are often marred by carelessness and other errors in implementation. The solution is to develop systems for maximizing the completeness and quality of the data once the study is in progress.

These two aspects of implementation also lead to a topic that is usually swept under the rug: the inclination to **change the study protocol** after the study has begun. No matter how good the pretests, the investigator will inevitably discover, once the study is under way, a better way to apply the intervention or measure the outcome. This chapter provides some thoughts on the painful issue of when to tinker with the study protocol and when to leave it alone.

PRETESTING

The nature and timing of pilot studies that pretest the study methods depend on the needs of the study. The purpose is to guide the development of a study protocol that

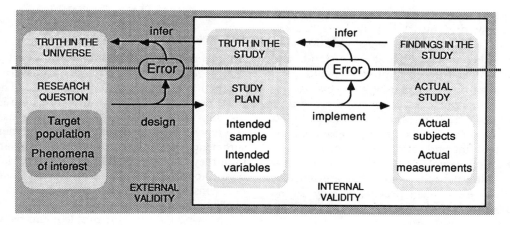

Figure 16.1.   Implementing a research project.

will produce better answers to the research questions at lower cost in time and money. Large collaborative studies can have large pilot studies; the feasibility trial for the Systolic Hypertension in the Elderly Program (SHEP), for example, studied 551 subjects for three years and produced its own set of publications (1). For most studies, however, small pilot studies that take only a few days or weeks serve very well, and a series of small pilot studies is generally more useful than one very large one.

Designing the study protocol

The main reason for pretesting is to guide decisions about how to design the recruitment and measurement approaches (Table 16.1). Pilot studies of the methods for **recruiting the study subjects** can provide estimates of the number of subjects who are available and willing to enroll, and test the efficiency of different recruitment approaches. They can also give the investigator an idea of the nature of the populations she will be sampling—of the distributions of age, sex, and other characteristics that may be important to the study.

Pilot studies are even more important in developing the **approaches to measuring variables.** Small exploratory pretests are used to examine alternatives at an early stage. The investigator can spend a few hours looking through clinic charts to see if the information she is seeking has been systematically recorded in previous years. She can select a small convenience sample of patients to test a new questionnaire, using open-ended responses to form the basis for constructing appropriate categorical responses in the final instrument. She can ask

Table 16.1.
Pretesting as a guide for developing recruitment and measurement approaches

Type	Purpose	Typical sample
Exploration	Examine major issues of content and feasibility	A convenience sample of 2–5 subjects
Refinement	Test recruitment approaches; improve clarity and efficiency of instruments and test distributions of responses	5–10 subjects who roughly represent the accessible population
Validation	Assess accuracy, validity, and reliability of instruments	Enough subjects sufficiently representative of the accessible population to produce the desired statistics

about subjective reactions to each procedure and any discomfort it may have caused, about whether there were questionnaire items the subject did not understand, and about other ways to improve the study.

Later on in the planning process, the investigator can use larger numbers drawn from the actual accessible population to test the logistics of making the measurements, and to refine and validate the instruments. If the study sample will include diverse ages and cultural backgrounds that are sensitive to the measurement process, it may be important to include representatives from each major subgroup in the pretest.

Pilot studies also play an important role in testing the **systems for data management.** Entering and editing some real data will help the investigator to know whether the data management system works, and tabulating the findings will reveal information on the quality and spread of responses for each questionnaire item.

Rehearsing the research team

Before the study begins, it is a good idea to test all the recruitment and measurement procedures in a full-scale **dress rehearsal.** This should involve subjects who would qualify for the study, including some with characteristics that may create difficulties during the study such as old age, cultural barriers, or illness. The purpose is to iron out problems with the final set of instruments and procedures using subjects who need not be counted in the study findings. Also, if several people will be involved in collecting the data, the principal investigator can take this opportunity to check on the research team and study plan. What appears to be a smooth, problem-free protocol on paper usually reveals both logistic and substantive problems in practice, and the dress rehearsal is sure to generate improvements in the approach. The investigator herself may decide to serve as a subject at this stage in order to experience the study and the research team from that viewpoint, and she may involve outside experts as mock subjects to solicit professional reactions to the study plan and its implementation.

QUALITY CONTROL

The need for quality control

An unheralded but very important aspect of clinical research is the approach to assuring the quality and consistency of the data. This topic receives insufficient attention because the data collection phase of a study is usually repetitive and tedious, and because measurements often seem more straighforward than they are. In the absence of appropriate quality control procedures to prevent them, problems with missing or erroneous data are likely to occur.

Missing data: This problem can be disastrous if it affects a large proportion of the measurements, and even a few missing values can sometimes bias the conclusions. A study of the long term sequellae of an operation that has a delayed mortality rate of 5%, for example, could seriously underestimate this complication if 10% of the patients were lost to follow-up and if death were a common reason for losing them. Erroneous conclusions due to missing data can sometimes be corrected after the fact—in this case by an intense effort to track down the missing patients—but often the measurement cannot be replaced.

The statistical techniques for dealing with the problem of missing data are **interpolation** (estimating a missing value that is in between two existing values), **extrapolation** (estimating a missing value that is outside the existing set of values based on the trends in those values), and **elision** (deleting the value—and often the subject—from the data set). Although these techniques are useful, they do not protect the conclusions from nonresponse bias if the number of missing observations is substantial. The only good solution is to *design and carry out the study in a way that avoids missing data.*

Inaccurate and imprecise data: This is an insidious problem that often remains undiscovered, particularly when more than one person is involved in making the measurements. In the worst case the investigator designs the study, then leaves the collection of the data to her research assistants. When she returns to analyze the data, some of the measurements may be seriously biased by the consistent use of an inappropriate technique. After the baseline examinations in the MRFIT had been completed, for example, a central review of the lung function tests showed that the water levels in the spirometry machines in some clinics had not been kept at an adequate level; the baseline vital capacity results had to be discarded for many subjects (2).

A worse problem arises when there are errors in the data that cannot be detected after the fact. If the interviews are carried out with leading questions in the place of neutral ones, or if blood pressure is measured differently in subjects known to be receiving placebo, the data base will have serious errors in it that are undetectable. The investigator will assume that the variables mean what she intended them to mean, and, blissfully ignorant of the problem, draw conclusions from her study that are wrong.

These problems are not restricted to studies that have a large research team of people collecting the data. Even when the investigator is working all alone on a small study, missing data and avoidable errors are common problems. The solution is to develop a systematic quality control program that will prevent them from occurring.

Quality control of clinical procedures

The quality control of clinical procedures begins during the planning phase and continues throughout the study (Table 16.2).

The operations manual: The operations manual is an expanded version of the methods section of the study protocol. It *operationally defines*—specifies exactly how to do—the approaches to recruiting study subjects, measuring variables, and all the other methods used in the study. An operations manual is essential for research that is carried out by several individuals, particularly when there is collaboration among investigators in more than one location. Even when a single investigator does the work all by herself, written specifications help to reduce random variation and changes in measurement technique over time (see Chapter 4).

The contents of an operations manual are illustrated in Appendix 16.A. They include all the instruments and forms used in the study, with instructions on such things as contacting the study subjects; carrying out interviews; filling in, coding, and editing forms; collecting and processing specimens; and managing and analyzing the data. There should also be a specific section that addresses the approach to assuring quality control.

Training and certification: Studies carried out by a research team will benefit from a formal system for training those who will carry out measurements of particular importance, and for testing and certifying their competence to do so. In the SHEP study of blood pressure treatment, for example (1), technical staff were trained in a standardized approach to preparing the pa-

Table 16.2.
Quality Control of Clinical Procedures
(e.g., blood pressure measurement, structured interview, chart review)

Steps that precede the study	Develop a manual of operations
	Operational definitions of recruitment and measurement procedures
	Standardized instruments and forms
	Approach to managing and analyzing the data
	Quality control systems
	Train the research team
	Certify the research team
Steps during the study	Provide steady and caring leadership
	Hold regular staff meetings
	Recertify the research team
	Periodically review performance
	Periodically tabulate measurements, categorized by technician

tient, applying the blood pressure cuff, locating the brachial artery, inflating and deflating the cuff, and recognizing which sounds represent the diastolic blood pressure. The technicians were then required to pass a written test on the relevant section of the operations manual, and to obtain satisfactory readings on pretest subjects who were assessed simultaneously by the instructor using a double stethoscope. This certification procedure was supplemented during the study by a scheduled program of recertification, periodically repeating aspects of the training and testing that took place before the study began.

Sometimes **role-playing** is a useful strategy in the process of training interviewers (3); one member of the research team can pretend to be a subject, coming up with some difficult responses. Afterward, the investigator can lead a discussion of how the interviewer handled the situation and what the alternatives were. The training experience should also include real subjects, however. It is often efficient to use the pretests and dress rehearsal in the training and certification, including subjects with characteristics that pose problems for data collection such as old age, cultural barriers, and illness.

Leadership and supervision: Quality control in a study that involves more than one person on the research team begins with the integrity and leadership of the principal investigator. She cannot watch every measurement her colleagues and staff make, but if she creates a sense that she is aware of all study activities and feels strongly about the accuracy of the data, most people will respond in kind. It is helpful to visit each member of the team from time to time, expressing a few pleasantries and a sense of appreciation. In addition to these intangibles, a good leader is adept in conventional management skills. This includes delegating authority appropriately (team members thrive on responsibility and independence) and at the same time setting up a hierarchical system of supervision that assures sufficient oversight of every aspect of the study.

Staff meetings: From the outset of the planning phase, the investigator should lead a series of meetings with all members of the research team. Each meeting should have an agenda that is distributed in advance and that is made up of progress reports from individuals who have been given responsibility for specific areas of the study. These meetings provide an opportunity to discover and solve problems, and to involve everyone in the process of developing the project and its timetable. Regular staff meetings are a great source of morale and interest in the goals of the study.

Performance review: It is important to set up a system for reviewing the techniques used by each member of the research team. The best systems for accomplishing this go beyond devices commonly used in clinical settings; we recommend that each supervisor directly review the way clinical procedures are carried out by periodically sitting in on representative clinic visits or telephone calls. After obtaining the study subject's permission, she can be quietly present for at least one complete example of every kind of interview or technical procedure each member of her research team performs. This may seem awkward at first (clinicians are used to being alone in a room with a patient and closing the door), but it soon becomes comfortable. Afterward, communication between the supervisor and the research team member can be facilitated with a standard checklist that covers the major topics; these notes can then be filed to record the fact of the visit and the resolution of any quality control issues that were noted. The discussion is most effective if it is carried out in a positive and nonpejorative fashion.

Involving *peers* in this system for reviewing clinical procedures is useful for building morale and teamwork, as well as for assuring the consistent application of standardized approaches among several members of the team who do the same thing. One advantage of using peers as observers in this system is that all members of the research team acquire a healthy sense of ownership of the quality control process. Another advantage is that the observer often learns as much from seeing how someone else handles things as she does when she is on the receiving end of the review procedure.

Periodic tabulations and reports: It is important to tabulate data on the technical quality of the clinical procedures or measurements at regular intervals. This can often give clues to the presence of missing, inaccurate, or imprecise measurements. Differences among the members of a blood pressure screening team in the mean levels each has observed over the past 2 months, for example, can lead to the discovery of differences in their measurement techniques. Similarly, a gradual change over a period of months in the standard deviation of large sets of readings can indicate a change in the technique for making the measurement.

Special procedures for drug interventions: Experiments that use drugs, particularly those that are blinded, require special attention to the quality control of this procedure. There are two main concerns: whether the correct drug and dosage has been provided, and whether the code number on each container is the proper one for the subject who receives it. The former is controlled by carefully planning with the manufacturer and pharmacy the nature of the drug and the approach to assuring its quality; the latter by developing a rigorous system for choosing and cross-checking the correct drug for a given individual (4).

Quality control of laboratory procedures

The quality of laboratory procedures can be controlled using many of the approaches described above for clinical procedures (Table 16.3). In addition, the fact that specimens are being removed from the subjects (creating the possibility of mislabeling) and the objective nature of laboratory tests lead to some special strategies. We summarize the major ones here, and refer the reader to other sources for more information on the topic (5-7).

Attention to labeling: When a subject's blood specimen or electrocardiogram is mistakenly labeled with another individual's name, it is usually impossible to correct or even discover the error later on. The only solution is to *avoid* such **transposition errors** by carefully checking the subject's name and number when labeling each specimen. The

microcomputer can print sets of gummed labels for blood tubes and records; these speed the process of labeling and also avoid the digit transpositions that can occur when numbers are handwritten. A good procedure to follow when transferring serum from one tube to another is to label the new tube in advance and hold the two tubes next to each other, reading one out loud while checking the other.

Blinding: The task of blinding the observer is a relatively easy one when it comes to measurements on specimens that have been taken from the patient, and it is always a good idea to label each specimen so that the technician has no knowledge of the study group or the value of other key variables. Even for apparently objective procedures like an automated blood glucose determination, this precaution will eliminate any small opportunities for bias, and provide a stronger methods section when it comes to reporting the results.

Use blinded duplicates or standard pools: When specimens are taken from the subjects for analysis or interpretation in a laboratory it is usually relatively easy to send blinded duplicates—a second specimen from a random subset of subjects that is given a separate and fictitious ID number— through the same system. This strategy gives the investigator a measure of the precision of the laboratory techniques, and can be designed in a way that tests either the consistency of a single observer or the consistency among observers. Another approach for serum specimens that can be stored frozen is to prepare a large pool of serum at the outset and periodically send aliquots through the system that are blindly labelled with a fictitious subject's ID numbers. A set of measurements carried out on the serum pool at the outset, using the best available technique, can establish the concentration of its constituents; the pool can then be used as a gold standard during the study, providing estimates of accuracy as well as precision.

Quality control of the data

One of the most common errors in research is the tendency to collect too many data. The fact that the baseline period is the only

Table 16.3.
Quality Control of Laboratory Procedures
(e.g., blood tests, X-rays, electrocardiograms)

Steps that precede the study	Use strategies in Table 16.2
	Establish good labelling procedures
	Blind the study group and other key variables
Steps during the study	Use strategies in Table 16.2
	Check equipment periodically
	Blind laboratory personnel
	Use blinded duplicates or standard pools

chance to measure baseline variables leads to an almost irresistable impulse to include everything that might conceivably be of interest, recording routine components of the physical examination that have no relation to the research question, for example, and expanding questionnaires to cover peripheral issues in excessive detail. Investigators tend to collect far more data than they ever analyze or publish.

One problem with this approach is the time consumed by measuring less important things; the subjects can become tired and annoyed, with the result that the quality of more important measurements deteriorates. Another problem is the added size and complexity of the database, which makes quality control and data analysis more difficult. It is wise to question the need for every variable that will be collected, eliminating most of those that are optional. Including a few intentional redundancies can serve the purpose of improving the reliability and validity of important variables, but the general rule is to *be parsimonious*.

The investigator should set up and pretest the data management system before the study begins. This includes designing the forms for recording measurements; choosing a computer; developing programs for data entry, management and analysis; and planning dummy tabulations to assure that the appropriate variables are collected (Table 16.4; see also Chapters 5 and 15).

Designing the forms: The design of the data collection forms will have an important influence on the quality of the data (8, 9). One vital step is **precoding**—specifying the data entry instructions in advance. This forces the investigator to standardize the responses during the planning steps, and reduces error in entering the data. It also reminds her to avoid open-ended responses, since these cannot be precoded.

Entries that involve judgment require explicit **operational definitions**; these should be summarized briefly on the form itself, and set out in more detail in the operations manual. The items should be **coherent** and the sequence of the items should be **clearly format-**

Table 16.4.
Quality Control of Data Management:
Steps that precede the study

Be parsimonious: collect only needed variables
Select appropriate computer hardware and software
Plan analyses with dummy tabulations
Design forms that are
    Precoded
    Self-explanatory
    Coherent (e.g., multiple-choice options are exhaustive and mutually exclusive)
    Clearly formatted with boxes for data entry and arrows directing skip patterns
    Printed in lower case using capitals, underlining, and bold font for emphasis
    Esthetic and easy to read
    Pretested and validated
    Labeled on every page with date, name and ID number

ted, with arrows indicating when questions should be skipped (see Appendix 5.A). Making the forms **readable and esthetic** will encourage careful attention among those who will use them. **Pretesting** will assure clarity of meaning and ease of use. **Labeling** every page with the date and ID number of the subject will safeguard the integrity of the data should the pages get separated.

Collecting and entering the data in the computer: The strategies for enhancing the completeness and accuracy of the data that were summarized in Chapter 15 are an important aspect of quality control.

The first area of concern, the accuracy of **collecting and recording the data**, should be addressed while the subject is still in the clinic (when it is relatively easy to correct errors that are discovered). The strategy is straightforward: a member of the research team edits what is written on the forms, checking the completeness and appropriateness of the entries (Table 16.5). If the editor can be someone who was not involved in collecting the data, this will increase the likelihood of detecting missing values and other errors.

A modern supplement to this hand editing process is to enter the data into a microcomputer that has been programmed to flag missing and out-of-range values. This strategy addresses the accuracy of **entering the data** into the computer as well as that of collecting and recording them. The classic antidote to data entry errors is more laborious— entering everything a second time, having

programmed the computer to accept only those values that are concordant with the first entries. This duplication doubles the time involved in entering the data and is generally not necessary (except perhaps on a subset of key variables) because the error rate is usually too low to influence the conclusions (10). For many small studies, the best approach is simply to take a random sample of the original forms and a printout of what is in the computer and compare the two by hand.

An important overall quality control strategy is to look at frequency distributions and cross-tabulations of important variables at regular intervals beginning early in the study. This allows the investigator to assess the completeness and quality of the data at a time when correction of past errors may still be possible (for example by calling the participant back in) and when further errors in the remainder of the study can be prevented. A useful list of topics for quality control reports compiled by Meinert is provided in Appendix 16.B.

A final aspect of quality control is the use of formal efforts to test the validity and reliability of the study measures. Such efforts include collecting particular sets of data twice to examine the concordance between the two sets of measurements, checking the internal consistency among related responses on a single occasion, using a gold standard to validate the measure on a sample of the study subjects, and other strategies described in Chapter 4.

Table 16.5.
Quality Control of Data Management:
Steps during the study

Check for omissions and major errors while subject is still in the clinic
    No errors or transpositions in ID number, name code, date on each page
    All the correct forms for the specified visit have been filled out
    No missing entries or faulty skip patterns (i.e., skip to question _____)
    Entries are legible
    Values of key variables are within permissible range (e.g., resting heart rate > 50 and < 130;
        values outside these levels would merit rechecking)
    Values of key variables are consistent with each other (e.g., age and birthdate)
Consider programming the computer to flag missing and out-of-range values
Enter data in duplicate or check accuracy of entries by hand on a random sample
Carry out periodic frequency distributions to discover aberrant values
Create other periodic tabulations to discover errors (see Appendix 16.B)

Managing quality control: In large studies it is a good idea to assign the duties of quality control coordinator to one member of the research team. That person is responsible for developing appropriate quality control techniques for all aspects of the study and overseeing their use by all members of the team. In small (one-person) studies the investigator should systematically oversee her own work in the same way.

Collaborative studies

Many research questions require larger samples than are available or feasible to study in a single center, and these are often addressed in collaborative studies that are carried out by research teams that will work in different locations. Sometimes these are all in the same city or state, and a single investigator can oversee all the research teams. Often, however, collaborative studies are carried out by investigators located in cities that are thousands of miles apart with separate grants and administrative structures.

Studies of this sort, of which the MRFIT is a good example, require special steps to assure that all centers are doing the same study and producing comparable data that can safely be combined in the analysis of the results. A coordinating center establishes a communication network, oversees data entry and analysis, and coordinates the development of the operations manual and other quality control aspects of the trial. A popular option these days is to locate a microcomputer at each data collection site. Such **distributed data processing** systems (10) put the responsibility for entering data in the hands of those who collect it, enhancing their involvement in the quality of the study.

There is also a need for establishing a governance system with a steering committee made up of the principal investigators and NIH representatives, and with various subcommittees (11) (Fig 16.2). One of the subcommittees can deal with quality control issues, drawing a member from each clinical center and working with the coordinating center to set up the standardization procedures and the systems for training, certification, and performance review. These tend to be complicated and expensive, providing centralized training for relevant staff from each center, for example, and coordinating site visits and data audits by peers from collaborating institutions (see Appendix 16.B).

PROTOCOL REVISIONS ONCE DATA COLLECTION HAS BEGUN

No matter how extensive the pretesting has been, further problems in design or in recruitment or measurement techniques inevitably appear once the study has begun. For those problems that will not have a major impact on the interpretation of the study, it is best to resist the inclination to change the protocol. The general rule is to *make as few changes as possible after the study has begun.* Sometimes, however, certain protocol modifications can strengthen the study.

Making minor revision

The decision on whether a minor change will improve the integrity of the study is often a trade-off between the benefit that results from the improved methodology and the cost of reducing the uniformity of the study. Decisions that simply involve making an operational definition more specific are relatively easy. For example, in a study that excludes alcoholics, can a reformed alcoholic be included? This decision should simply be made, one way or the other.

Other decisions are more difficult. A questionnaire to elicit symptoms of angina pectoris asks if the pain goes away within 10 minutes. Two months into the study the investigator realizes that this does not distinguish the brief sharp pains of a few seconds duration that probably originate in the rib cage from the pain of some minutes duration that is likely to represent an ischemic myocardium. The investigator could change the wording of a question to exclude instances of sharp pain lasting less than 10 seconds. Doing so might produce a variable that is more appropriate for the research question, but it would create a discontinuity in the data set—a change half way through the study in the nature of what is measured.

This is difficult to deal with in the analysis phase, and it may be best not to make the change. Sometimes it is possible to continue measuring the variable the old way, and to add the new approach in addition. The new version of the question should be asked last, so that it will not alter the responses to the original standard set of questions.

Changes in study methods should be noted in writing, making sure that everyone involved in the study is aware of them. These notes should be retained in the operations manual. It is important to recognize, however, that in the real world of research it is difficult to deal with protocol changes during the analysis phase. The investigator should undertake minor changes without any illusions, realizing that the data collected before and after the change will often end up being combined and interpreted as if the whole study had been carried out with the revised approach.

Making substantive revisions

Larger changes in the study protocol, such as including different kinds of subjects or substantially changing one of the major variables, can be a more serious problem. Although there may be good reasons for making these changes, they must be undertaken with a view to analyzing and reporting

the data separately if this will lead to a more appropriate interpretation of the findings. The judgments involved are illustrated by the different resolutions of these two examples from the MRFIT.

The initial inclusion criteria required each participant to have a risk of CHD in the top 10% of the population, based on the Framingham risk factor data. In fact, experience with recruitment soon showed that only 6% of the men who were screened met these criteria (because risk factor levels in the population had declined since the Framingham study began). The MRFIT investigators decided one third of the way through recruitment that changing the entry criterion from the top 10% to the top 15% would enhance the feasibility of recruiting enough subjects, and would not compromise the conclusions. This change was noted in reporting the findings (12), but the investigators did not consider it necessary to analyze the data separately for the two parts of the study cohort.

The second example concerns the approach for measuring one of the main endpoints in the MRFIT, nonfatal myocardial infarction. The approach specified in the protocol was a blinded reading of yearly

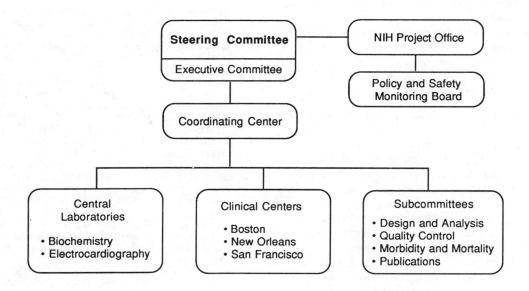

Figure 16.2 Organization and governance of a hypothetical collaborative study.

electrocardiograms. Near the end of the study, the investigators realized that it would also be desirable to use data from hospitalizations for assessing this important outcome. In order not to change the previously established hypothesis, however, the findings for nonfatal heart attack were reported separately for the two ascertainment approaches (13).

These are examples of substantive revisions that have not compromised the overall integrity of the study. Tinkering with protocol is not always so successful, however. Substantive revisions should only be undertaken after thoughtfully weighing the pros and cons with members of the research team and with appropriate advisors. The investigator must then deal with the potential impact on the findings when she draws and reports the conclusions.

SUMMARY

1. The process of designing the study should include a series of *pilot studies* to improve the nature and efficiency of the methods for recruiting subjects and making measurements. These begin as small and informal explorations, and they end with larger and more systematic pilot studies to refine and validate the methods and to rehearse the research team.

2. Even well-designed studies can yield erroneous conclusions because of *missing, inaccurate or imprecise data*. Quality control strategies to minimize these problems include:

   a. Efforts to enhance the *quality of the clinical procedures*—developing an operations manual, training and certifying the research team in the standard techniques, providing high-quality leadership, meeting regularly with the research team, creating performance review systems, and looking at periodic tabulations on the recruitment and measurement procedures.

   b. Efforts to enhance the *quality of the laboratory procedures*—in addition to the procedures noted above, developing systems for blinding and systemat-

ically labeling the specimens taken from the study subjects, and for using standard pools and blinded duplicates.

   c. Efforts to enhance the *quality of the data management*—in addition to the procedures noted above, improving the design of the forms and developing systems to oversee the accuracy of collecting, editing, entering, and analyzing the data.

3. After the study has started, it is inevitable that new ideas for improving the study will tempt the investigator to make changes in the study plan. However, *protocol revisions* after the data collection has begun should be undertaken cautiously, and only when it is clear that they will not compromise the overall integrity of the study and its conclusions.

REFERENCES

1. Siegel D, Kuller L, Lazarus NB, et al: Predictors of cardiovascular events and mortality in the Systolic Hypertension in the Elderly Pilot Project (SHEP). *Am J Epidemiol* 126:385–399, 1987.
2. Townsend MC, Morgan J, Durkin D, et al: Quality control aspects of pulmonary function testing in the MRFIT. *Contr Clin Trials* 7:179S–192S, 1986.
3. Russell ML, Ghee KL, Probstfield JL, et al: Development of standardized simulated patients for quality control of the clinical interview. *Contr Clin Trials* 4:429–440, 1983.
4. Friedman LM, Furberg CD, DeMets DL: *Fundamentals of Clinical Trials*, ed 2. Littleton, MA, PSG Publishing Co, Inc, 1985, p 143.
5. Canner PL, Krol WF, Forman SA: External quality control programs. *Contr Clin Trials* 4:441–466, 1983.
6. Habig RL, Thomas P, Lippel K, et al: Central laboratory quality control in the National Cooperative Gallstone Study. *Contr Clin Trials* 4:101–123, 1983.
7. Widdowson BM, Kuehneman M, DuChene AG, et al: Quality control of biochemical data in the MRFIT. *Contr Clin Trials* 7:17S–33S, 1986.
8. Knatterud GL, Forman SA, Canner PL: Design of data forms. *Contr Clin Trials* 4:429–440, 1983.
9. Wright P, Haybittle J: Design of forms for clinical trials. *Br Med J* 2:529–530, 590–592, 650–651, 1979.
10. Bagniewska A, Black D, Molvig K, et al: Data quality in a distributed data processing system: The SHEP Pilot Study. *Contr Clin Trials* 7:27–37, 1986.
11. Sherwin R, Kaelber CT, Kezdi P, et al: The MRFIT: II The development of the protocol. *Prev Med* 10:402–425, 1981.
12. The MRFIT Research Group: MRFIT: Risk factor

changes and mortality results. *JAMA* 248:1465–1477, 1982.

13. The MRFIT Research Group: CHD death, nonfatal acute MI and other clinical outcomes in the MRFIT. *Am J Cardiol* 58:1–13, 1986.

ADDITIONAL READINGS

Friedman LM, Furberg CD, DeMets DL: *Fundamentals of Clinical Trials*, ed 2. Littleton, MA, PSG Publishing Co, Inc, 1985, pp 135–146. (*An excellent chapter on quality control with many specific illustrations of useful procedures.*)

Meinert C: *Clinical Trials: Design, Conduct, and Analysis*, New York, Oxford University Press, 1986, pp 166–176. (*Another excellent chapter on quality assurance with detailed specific check-lists, some of which are provided in Appendix 16.B*)

MRFIT Research Group: The MRFIT: quality control of technical procedures and data acquisition. *Contr Clin Trials* 7:1S–202S, 1986. (*A supplement containing 12 quality control chapters addressing data management, blood chemistries and electrocardiograms, and clinical procedures such as measuring blood pressure, assessing pulmonary function, and providing nutrition intervention.*)

CHAPTER 17

Writing and Funding a Research Proposal

Steven R. Cummings, A. Eugene Washington, Christine Ireland, and Stephen B. Hulley

INTRODUCTION 184

WRITING PROPOSALS 184
  Organize a team and designate a leader
  Follow the guidelines of the funding agency
  Establish a timetable and meet periodically
  Find a model proposal
  Work from an outline on a word processor
  Review, pretest, and revise repeatedly

ELEMENTS OF A PROPOSAL 186
  The beginning
  The administrative parts
  The goals and rationale
  The scientific methods
  Ethics and miscellaneous parts

CHARACTERISTICS OF GOOD PROPOSALS 190

FINDING SUPPORT FOR RESEARCH 192
  NIH grants and contracts
  Foundation grants
  Corporate support
  Intramural research support

SUMMARY 195

REFERENCES 196

ADDITIONAL READINGS 196

APPENDIX 17. NIH institutes and DRG study
  sections 230

INTRODUCTION

The **protocol** is the detailed written plan of the study. Writing the protocol forces the investigator to organize, clarify, and refine all of the elements of the study, and this enhances the scientific rigor and the efficiency of the project. Thus, even if the investigator does not require funding for a study, a protocol is necessary for guiding the work.

A **proposal** is a document written for the purpose of obtaining funds from granting agencies or approval from institutional review boards. It contains the study protocol and other administrative and supporting information that is required by the specific agency or board. This chapter will focus on the structure of a proposal and on how to write one that will be successful.

WRITING PROPOSALS

The task of preparing a proposal generally requires several months of organizing, writing, and revising. The following steps can help the project to get off to a good start.

Organize a team and designate a leader

Most proposals are written by a team of several people who will eventually carry out the study. This team may be small (just the investigator and her mentor) or large (including a nurse coordinator, a biostatistician, a data manager, a psychologist, a fiscal administrator, several medical specialists, and a support staff). It is important that this team include or have access to the main expertise needed for designing and implementing the study.

One member of the team must assume the responsibility for leading the effort. Often this is the **principal investigator** (PI), the individual who will have ultimate authority and accountability for the study. The PI should be an experienced scientist whose knowledge and wisdom are useful for design decisions and whose track record with previous studies will increase the likelihood of funding (reviewers give considerable weight to the value of experience). Some studies also have a project director, a younger scientist who will serve as the day-to-day manager of the study, and who can coordinate the proposal-writing effort. Either the PI or the project director must exert steady leadership, delegating responsibilities for writing and other tasks, setting deadlines, conducting periodic meetings of the team, and assuring that all of the necessary tasks are completed on time.

Follow the guidelines of the funding agency

All funding sources provide written guidelines that the investigator must study before starting to write the proposal. However, these guidelines do not contain all the important information that the investigator needs to know about the operations and the preferences of the funding agencies. The National Institutes of Health (NIH) and private foundations have scientific administrators whose job is to help investigators tailor their proposals to be more responsive to the agency's funding policies. Early in the development of the proposal, it is a good idea to discuss the plan with the individual at the agency who will coordinate the review of the applications. This will clarify what the agency prefers (such as budgetary limits and the scope and detail required in the proposal) and confirm that the research plan is within the bounds of the agency's interests. The initial contact can be made by letter, but a telephone call or visit is often a better way to get information that will lead to a more fundable proposal.

Establish a timetable and meet periodically

A schedule for completing the writing tasks keeps gentle pressure on team members to meet their obligations on time. In addition to addressing the scientific components specified by the funding agency, the timetable should take into account the administrative requirements of the institution that will sponsor the research. Universities often require a time-consuming review of the budget and submission to the local Institutional Review Board before a proposal can be submitted to the funding agency. Leaving these details to the end can precipitate a last-minute crisis that damages an otherwise well done proposal.

A timetable generally works best if it specifies deadlines for written products, and if each individual participates in setting her own assignments. The timetable should be reviewed at periodic meetings of the writing team to check that the tasks are on schedule and the deadlines still realistic.

Find a model proposal

It is helpful to borrow from a colleague a copy of a successful recent proposal to the agency from which funding is being sought. Successful applications illustrate in a concrete way the format and content of a good proposal. The investigator can adapt the best ideas from the model and then design and write a proposal that is even clearer, more logical, and more persuasive. It is also a good idea to borrow examples of written criticisms that have been provided by the agency for either successful or unsuccessful proposals. This will illustrate the kinds of issues that are important to the scientists who will be reviewing the proposal.

Work from an outline on a word processor

Begin by setting out the proposal in outline form (Table 17.1). This provides a starting point for writing and is useful for organizing the tasks that need to be done. If several people will be working on the grant, the outline helps in assigning responsibilities for writing parts of the proposal. Writing a proposal entails frequent revisions that are much more easily and quickly made on a word processor. Word processing also makes it easy to produce a final document that is perfect in appearance.

One of the most common road blocks to creating an outline is the feeling that an entire plan must be worked out before starting to write the first sentence. The investigator should put this notion aside and let her thoughts flow onto paper, creating the raw material for editing, refining, and getting specific advice from colleagues.

Review, pretest, and revise repeatedly

Writing a proposal is an iterative process; there are usually many versions, each reflecting new ideas, advice, and pretest experiences. Before the final draft is written, the proposal should be reviewed by colleagues who are familiar with the funding agency. Particular attention should go to the quality of the research question, the validity of the design and methods, and the clarity of the writing. It is better to have sharp and detailed criticism before the proposal is submitted than to have the project rejected because of failure to anticipate and address potential problems. When the proposal is nearly ready for submission, the final step is to review it carefully for internal consistency, format, and typographical errors.

ELEMENTS OF A PROPOSAL

The elements of a proposal are set out in Table 17.1 in the sequence required by the NIH and ADAMHA[a] (1). Some funding institutions may require less information or a different format, and the investigator should organize the proposal according to the guidelines of the agency that will receive the proposal. The scientific elements of the study plan are emphasized in boldface type in Table 17.1; these should be written out for all studies, including those that do not need funding.

The beginning

The Title should be descriptive and concise. It provides the first impression and a lasting reminder of the content and design of the study. A good title manages to summarize these elements, achieving brevity by avoiding unnecessary phrases like "A study to determine the . . . ." In an NIH grant appli-

---

[a] ADAMHA, the Alcohol, Drug Abuse, and Mental Health Administration, is the other major federal agency (besides NIH) that funds medical research.

Table 17.1.
Elements of a Proposal[a]

Title

Abstract

Table of contents

Budget

Biosketches of investigators (2-page curricula vitae)

Resources, equipment, and physical facilities

Specific objectives (the research questions)

Significance

Preliminary studies and competence of the investigators

Methods

- **Overview of design**
  time frame and nature of control

- **Study subjects**
  selection criteria that specify the target and accessible populations
  design for sampling and plans for recruiting subjects

- **Measurements**
  main predictor variables (intervention, if an experiment)
  potential confounding variables
  outcome variables

- **Pretest plans**

- **Statistical issues**
  approach to statistical analyses
  hypotheses and sample size estimates

- **Quality control and data management**

- **Timetable and organizational chart**

Ethical considerations

Consultants and arrangements between institutions

References

Appendices

---

cation, the choice of words in the title is particularly important because it influences the decision on which study section (review group) will receive the protocol (2).

The **Abstract** is a concise summary of the protocol that should begin with the research question, then set out the design and methods, and conclude with a statement of the importance of potential findings of the study (3). Most agencies require that the abstract be kept within a limited number of words, so it is best to use efficient and descriptive terms. The abstract should be written last, when the other protocol elements are settled, and it should go through enough revisions to assure that it is first rate. This will be the only page read by some reviewers, and a convenient reminder of the major features of the proposal for everyone else. It must therefore be able to stand on its own, incorporating all the features of the proposed study and persuasively revealing the strengths.

The **Table of Contents** is an essential aid to the reader. It may be useful to include a more detailed table of contents than the summary version suggested in the NIH instructions. This is especially true for proposals that are large or have complex or unusual sections. The items in the table of contents should correspond to prominently labeled headings or subheadings in the text.

The administrative parts

The **Budget** section is generally organized according to guidelines from the funding institution. The NIH has a prescribed format that requires a detailed budget for the first 12-month period and a summary budget for the entire proposed project period (usually 3–5 years). The detailed 12-month budget includes the following categories of expenses: personnel (including names and positions of all persons involved in the project, the percent of time each will devote to the project, and the dollar amounts of salary and fringe benefits listed separately for each individual); consultant costs; equipment (itemized); supplies (itemized); travel (itemized); patient care costs; alterations and renovations; consortium/contractual costs; and other expenses (e.g., the costs of telephones, mail, copying, illustration, publication, books, computer use, and fee-for-service contracts).

The amounts requested for each category of the budget must be justified with a clear and concise text. Salaries will generally comprise 80-90% of the overall cost of a typical clinical research project, so it is important to show the need for each person in the payroll. Brief job descriptions for the investigators and other members of the research team should leave no doubt in the reviewers' minds that each individual is essential to the success of the project.

Reviewers often look at the percentages of time committed by key members of the project. Occasionally, proposals may be criticized because key members of the research team have only a very small (5%) commitment of time listed in the budget (implying that they have too many other commitments to be able to devote the necessary energy to the proposed study). On the other hand, the reviewers may also balk at percentages that are inflated beyond the requirements of the job description.

The budget should not be left until the last minute. An administrator can begin working on it as soon as the outline of the proposal is formulated, recommending the amounts for budget items and anticipating institutional procedures, pitfalls, and delays. The administrator can also be very helpful in drafting the text of the sections on budget and resources, and in collecting the curricula vitae and other supporting materials.

Even the best planned budgets change as the needs of the study change or there are unexpected expenses and savings. In general, the investigator is free to spend money in different ways from those specified in the budget provided that the expenditures are all appropriate to the study and that money is not moved from one major category to another (e.g., from personnel to travel). When the investigator does want to move money across categories, or to spend it for a purpose that is restricted in the grant award, she will need to get approval from the funding agency. Agencies generally approve reasonable requests for rebudgeting so long as the investigator is not asking for an increase in total funds.

The **Biosketches of Investigators** are two-page resumes that include academic degrees, administrative and research positions, honors and national committee work, and publications. A senior investigator with a lengthy curriculum vitae should pick the most important positions and a recent set of publications that are relevant to the research project.

The **Resources** available to the project, including computer and technical equipment and office and laboratory space, should be fully described. Components of these sections are usually available in prior grant proposals written by colleagues in the investigator's institution.

The goals and rationale

The **Specific Objectives** are statements of the research question using a format that specifies the desired outcome. Each objective should be described in one or two sentences. Most research proposals have several objectives and these should be presented in a logical sequence. Sometimes this means putting them in order of importance, sometimes in chronological order (objectives served by baseline data first, then those related to follow-up). Sometimes, as in the following example, the most logical approach is to present the descriptive aims first, then the analytic aims:

1. To describe the prevalence of coffee consumption, and of fibrocystic breast disease, in middle-aged U.S. women.
2. To determine whether coffee drinking is a risk factor for fibrocystic breast disease.

The specific aims section can also serve as an outline for organizing later sections; the components of the significance and methods sections should follow a parallel sequence.

When a study has many facets, it is tempting to impress the reader with a long and detailed listing of specific aims. This strategy may backfire, creating a proposal that is overly ambitious or cluttered. When numerous specific aims are possible, it is best to propose only the most important and interesting ones. In general, this should not exceed one page.

The **Significance** section sets the proposal in context, describing the background in the field under study. It should be written, as much as possible, in a way that is comprehensible to someone who is not an expert in that field. Enough information should be given to make clear what this particular study will accomplish and why it is important. How, specifically, will the study benefit patients, advance understanding, or influence policy?

The purpose of this section is to demonstrate that the investigator understands what has been accomplished, what the problems are, and what needs to be done. The appropriate breadth or detail of the review depends on the scope of the specific aims, the complexity of the field, and the expectations of the review panel. Usually, a critical review of the best and most recent 20 or 30 references will suffice.

The **Preliminary Studies and Competence of the Investigators** section should describe relevant previous work by the investigator, making reference to detailed reports and preprints in the appendices. Emphasis should be placed on the importance of the previous work and on the reasons why it should be continued or extended. This is also a good place to put one or two paragraphs about each investigator, emphasizing background, previous research experience, and skills pertinent to the proposed research.

Pilot studies that support the research question and the feasibility of the study are important to many types of proposals, especially when the research team has little previous experience in the area to be studied, when the question is novel, and when there may be doubts about the feasibility of the proposed procedures or recruitment of subjects. Results of these studies should be highlighted here, with details provided in the appendices.

The scientific methods

The **Methods** section generally receives close scrutiny from reviewers and it will later serve as the basis for the operations manual for carrying out the study. Weakness in the technical methods is a common reason why proposals fail to be approved or funded by the NIH (4). For these reasons, this section deserves careful attention to detail.

The first concern is how to organize the section, a topic on which the NIH instructions offer surprisingly little guidance. We recommend the components and sequence listed in Table 17.1. A detailed table of the contents of the methods section can be very helpful at this point, and an **overview of the design,** accompanied by a schematic diagram of the sort illustrated in Figure 17.1, is essential for orienting the reader.

The other specific components of the methods section have been discussed in other parts of this book. The **subjects** and **measurements** (Chapters 3 and 4) and the **pretest plans, data management,** and **quality control** (Chapters 15 and 16), are the centerpiece of the proposal, and require sufficient detail so that sophisticated reviewers will understand exactly how the study will be performed, and why the design choices were made. Long descriptions of some techniques, such as the details of biochemical assays or of questionnaires, can be put into an appendix.

The **statistical issues** subsection should usually begin with the plans for analysis. This can be set out in the sequence noted in Chapter 15, first the descriptive tabulations and then the approach to analyzing associations among variables. This will lead logically to the topic of sample size (Chapters 12 and 13) which should begin with a statement of the null hypotheses and the choice of statistical test before giving the sample size and power estimates at the specified alpha, beta and effect size. Most NIH review panels attach considerable importance to the statistical issues, so it is a good idea to involve a statistician in writing, or at least in reviewing, this component of the proposal.

The protocol must provide a realistic work plan and **timetable,** including dates when each major phase of the study will be started and completed (Table 17.2). Similar timetables can be prepared for staffing patterns and other components of the project. An **organizational chart** describing the research team should indicate levels of authority and accountability, and show how the team will function (Figure 17.2).

Ethics and miscellaneous parts

The **Ethical Considerations** section is devoted to the ethical issues raised by the study, setting forth the issues of safety, privacy, and confidentiality. This section should indicate the specific plans to inform potential subjects of the risks and benefits, and to obtain their consent to participate (Chapter 14).

The proposed use and value of each **Consultant** should be described, accompanied by a letter of agreement from that individual and a copy of her curriculum vitae (in an appendix). An explanation of the programmatic and administrative arrangements between the applicant organization and collaborating institutions should be included, accompanied by letters of support from responsible officials addressed to the investigator.

References should be cited, preferably by

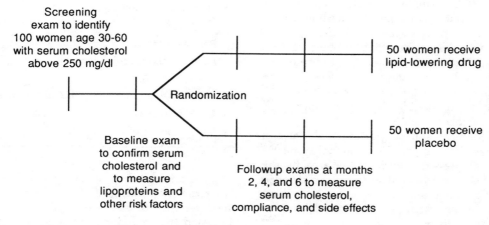

Figure 17.1.   Example of a schematic diagram of the study design.

Table 17.2.
Hypothetical Timetable

Date	Activity
Jan 1, 1989	Funding starts
	Final stages of recruiting research associate
	Begin designing interview
February	Hire and begin training research associate
	First draft of interview completed—review by consultants
March	Begin pretests of interview
	Begin planning data management system
April	Complete pretests
	Revise interview
May–June	Final pretest and revisions
	Write computer programs for data entry
	Complete operations manual
July	Begin recruiting and interviewing subjects
	Begin data entry
September	Recruitment and interviewing completed
	Begin to clean and prepare data for analysis
Oct–Dec	Analyze data and begin to prepare reports
Dec 31, 1989	Submit final report
	Submit paper for publication

author and date (e.g., Miller, 1984), with the complete citation listed alphabetically at the back. (It is permissible to cite references by number, but this means that adding a citation in the final stages of preparing a proposal will change the other numbers.) Errors in these citations or misinterpretation of the work can be irritating to reviewers who are familiar with that field of research, so it is important to double-check the accuracy of the references.

Technical and supporting material can be placed in Appendices. Examples are reports of previous work in the area by the investigators, letters of support, and detailed questionnaires and instruments for making measurements that are particularly important or challenging.

CHARACTERISTICS OF GOOD PROPOSALS

A good proposal has several attributes (Table 17.3). First is the scientific quality of the research plan: it must be based on a good research question, use a design and methods that are rigorous and feasible, and have a research team with sufficient experience, skill, and commitment to carry it out.

Table 17.3.
Characteristics of a Good Proposal

1. Overall quality of the study
   - Good research question
   - Appropriate and efficient design
   - Rigorous and feasible methods
   - Qualified research team
2. Specific sections
   - Informative title
   - Self-sufficient and convincing abstract
   - Specific aims that state the research question clearly
   - Scholarly and pertinent background and rationale
   - Relevant previous work, expertise, pilot studies
   - Appropriate population and sample
   - Appropriate measurement and intervention methods
   - Good pretest and quality control plans
   - Adequate sample size
   - Scientifically sound analysis plan
   - Ethical issues well addressed
   - Tight budget
   - Realistic timetable
3. Quality of the presentation
   - Clear, concise, well-organized
   - Helpful table of contents and subheadings
   - Good schematic diagrams and tables
   - Neat and free of errors

A second attribute is the technical quality of the proposal itself. One study of the characteristics of successful proposals has suggested that the clarity of presentation is the single most important determinant of the fate of NIH grant applications (5). Even if the research question is important and the study plan excellent, a poor presentation can leave the reviewer confused and uninterested. The proposal should be concise and engaging, and not lose the attention of the reviewer with writing that wanders vaguely through peripheral topics. A proposal that is well organized, thoughtfully written, and free of errors (including typographic errors) reassures the reader that the conduct of research is likely to be of similar quality.

When writing a proposal, it is essential to keep the reviewer in mind. Reviewers are often overwhelmed by a large stack of lengthy proposals, so the merits of the proj-

ect must stand out in a way that will not be missed even with a quick and cursory reading. Clear outlines, short sections with meaningful subheadings, brief point-by-point summaries, concise tables, and simple diagrams can guide the reviewers' understanding of the most important features of the proposal.

Most reviewers are sophisticated, and easily put off by overstatement and other heavy-handed forms of grantsmanship. Proposals that exaggerate the importance of the project or overestimate what it can accomplish will generate skepticism. Writing with enthusiasm is a good idea, but the investigator should be realistic about the limitations of the project. Most reviewers are adept at iden-

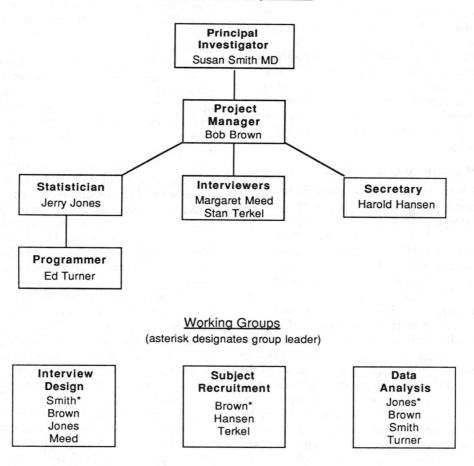

Figure 17.2. A hypothetical organizational chart.

tifying potential problems in the design or feasibility of a research project. Rather than ignore potential flaws, an investigator can address them explicity, discussing the advantages and disadvantages of the various trade-offs in reaching the chosen plan. It is not a good idea to overemphasize these problems, however, for this may lead a reviewer to focus disproportionately on the weaker aspects of the proposal and to overlook its strengths. The goal is to reassure the reviewer that the investigator has anticipated the potential problems and has a realistic and thoughtful approach to dealing with them.

FINDING SUPPORT FOR RESEARCH

There are four main sources of funds for medical research: (a) the government (notably the NIH), (b) private non-profit institutions (notably foundations), (c) private profit-making corporations (notably drug companies), and (d) intramural resources (e.g., from the investigator's university). Getting support from one of these sources is a complex and competitive process that favors investigators with experience and tenacity.

NIH grants and contracts

The NIH, which supports about $7 billion in research each year, typically requires 10 months to process lengthy and detailed applications through a **peer review** mechanism in which the NIH staff function as administrators and the funding decisions are largely made by scientists selected from universities not involved in the application. This process, although laborious, is reasonably fair and tends to enhance the quality of medical research in the same way that journal reviewers enhance the quality of the medical literature. A similar process is used by the ADAMHA and other federal and state agencies to determine research funding priorities.

The NIH funds two main types of research proposals: those conceived by the investigator on a topic of her choosing and those written in response to a publicized request by one of the institutes at NIH (Fig.

17.3). An investigator-initiated grant application is called an **RO-1** unless it is part of a program project grant (several proposals on a given topic, reviewed as a set) in which case it is called a **PO-1**. Institute-initiated proposals are designed to stimulate research in areas designated by NIH advisory committees, and respond either to Requests for Proposals (**RFPs**) or to Requests for Applications (**RFAs**). RFPs and RFAs differ from each other chiefly in the type of agreement: under an RFP, the investigator contracts to perform certain research activities determined by the NIH. Under an RFA, the investigator conducts research in a topic area defined by the NIH, but the specific research question and study plan are proposed by the investigator. RFPs use the contract mechanism to reimburse the contractor for the costs involved in achieving the prespecified objectives, and RFAs use the grant mechanism to support activities that are more open-ended.

RO-1s are usually reviewed by one of several dozen NIH **"study sections."** Each of these deals with projects on a particular topic, and is composed of experts in that area drawn from institutions around the country. A list of the study sections is given in Appendix 17; their membership is published by NIH (6), and many investigators use this information to make sure their applications will be responsive to the particular individuals who will provide their peer review. Proposals sent in response to an RFA or RFP are usually reviewed by ad hoc committees of peers that follow the same procedures as the study sections in passing on the merits of a proposal.

When an investigator submits an RO-1 grant proposal to the NIH it is assigned by the Division of Research Grants (DRG) to a particular study section (Figure 17.4). After review and discussion of the proposal, each member of the study section votes for approval or disapproval. (A few applications are deferred to the next cycle four months later, pending clarification by the investigator on points that were unclear.) If the majority approve, the members then vote a priority score from 100 (best) to 500 (worst); this is done by secret ballot, and the average is computed. The DRG also assigns each grant proposal to a particular institute at NIH (the institutes of the NIH are categorized, unlike the study sections, by disease, e.g., the National Cancer Institute—see appendix 17). Each institute then funds the grants assigned to it, in order of priority score, until the budget it has received from Congress is exhausted. Roughly two-thirds of all grant applications are approved at the present time, but only one-third of these are funded; the cutoff point needed for funding, which varies by year and by institute, is a score of about 150.

The investigator should decide in advance, with advice from senior colleagues, on the outcome she prefers for the two key assignments that are made by the DRG—to a study section and to an institute. It makes a big difference; study sections vary a great deal in the stringency and nature of their review, and there is a considerable difference among institutes in the extent and quality of the competition. Although the assignments are not fully controllable (2), the investigator can influence them by: (a) choosing words in the title that make it obvious what the best assignment would be; (b) stating her preference in the cover letter for the application; (c) asking the NIH scientist in charge of the study section of choice (the "executive secretary") or the NIH scientist who will handle the grant at the institute of choice (the "project officer") for advice on how to steer the application.

After a proposal has been reviewed by the appropriate committee, the investigator receives written notification of the committee's action. This notification, called the "pink sheets" because it is often printed on pink paper, includes detailed comments and criticisms from the committee members who reviewed the proposal.

Proposals that fail to win funding, as is

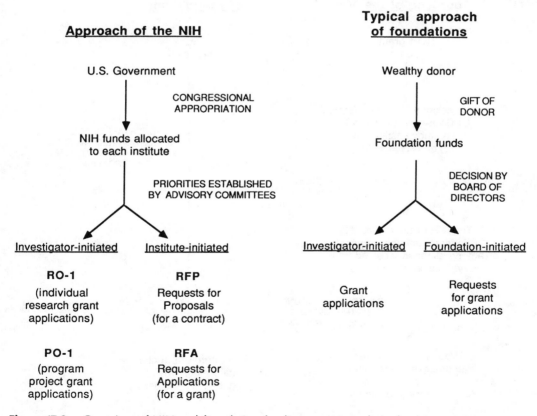

Figure 17.3. Overview of NIH and foundation funding sources and mechanisms.

often the case for the first submission, can be revised and submitted again. If the reviewers' criticisms suggest that the proposal can be made more acceptable to the committee, then a thoughtfully revised proposal may have an excellent chance of obtaining funding when it is resubmitted. An investigator need not automatically make all of the changes suggested by reviewers, but she should adopt revisions that will satisfy the reviewer's criticisms wherever possible and justify any decision not to do so. A good format for the resubmission is to begin with an introduction that quotes each major criticism from the pink sheets and summarizes the corresponding changes in the proposal.

Foundation grants

Foundations and other private sources generally restrict their funding to specific areas of interest. The total amount of research support is far smaller than that provided by NIH, and most foundations have the goal of using this money to fill the gaps, funding projects of merit that for one or another reason would not be funded by NIH. Decisions about funding follow procedures that vary from one institution to another, but that usually respond rapidly to relatively short proposals. The decisions are made by an executive process rather than by peer review—typically the staff of the foundation makes a recommendation that is ratified by a Board of Directors (Fig 17.4).

To determine whether a foundation might be interested in a particular proposal, an investigator should check with her senior advisors, or look in directories (7) that describe the goals and purposes of individual foundations and that list projects that have

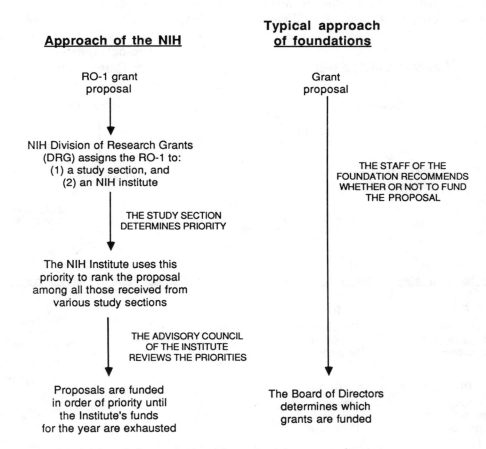

Figure 17.4   NIH and foundation procedures for reviewing grant applications.

recently been funded. Most foundations ask that investigators send a short (three to five page) letter describing the background and principal goals of the project, the qualifications of the investigators, and the approximate duration and costs of the research. If the proposal is of sufficient interest, the foundation may request a more detailed proposal.

Corporate support

Support for studies of how well a drug or a piece of equipment works can be sought by contacting the research director of the manufacturer. However, support from profit-making companies can be a mixed blessing. The chief **disadvantages** are the channeling of the research question to meet the corporate goals, and the financial motive that always underlies this source of funding. The latter infringes, at least in subtle ways, on the scientific integrity of the work, and the pursuit of a favorable effect of a drug can replace the pursuit of truth as the goal of the research. In fairness, however, all medical research (regardless of the source of support) is susceptible to pressure from the fact that society places a premium on a favorable result. Negative results are dull and hard to publish, even though we all recognize that a conclusive negative finding is often as important as a conclusive positive one.

One **advantage** of corporate support is that it is the only practical way to address some research questions; there would be no other source of funds, for example, for testing a new antibiotic that is not yet on the market. Another advantage is the relative ease with which this source of funding can be acquired; drug companies are often eager to sign up additional physicians and clinics to participate in their multicenter clinical trials. Third, most drug companies place a high premium on maintaining a reputation for integrity (which has the secondary gain for them of enhancing their dealings with an increasingly vigilant Food and Drug Administration), and the research expertise, measurement instruments, and statistical support they provide can favorably influence the quality of the research effort.

Intramural support

Universities often have local research funds for their own investigators which can be discovered through the Dean's Office. Grants from these intramural funds are generally limited to small amounts (a few thousand dollars) but they are usually available much more quickly (weeks to months) and to a higher proportion of applicants (71% at our university last year) than grants from the NIH or private foundations. Intramural funds may be restricted to special purposes, such as pilot studies that may lead to external funding, or the purchase of equipment that will permit a study to be done by scientists whose salary is supported by training funds. Such funds are often earmarked for junior faculty members or fellows, and provide a unique opportunity for a beginning investigator to acquire the experience of being principal investigator of a funded project.

SUMMARY

1. The *protocol* is the detailed written plan of the study. It is the scientific component of a *proposal for funding*, which also contains administrative and supporting information required by the funding agency.

2. An investigator who has developed a research question and a 1–3 page outline of the study plan should begin by getting *advice* from senior colleagues about the choice of funding agency. The next steps are to study that agency's written guidelines and to contact the appropriate officer in the agency for advice.

3. The process of *writing a proposal*, which often takes much longer than expected, includes organizing a team with the necessary expertise, designating a project leader, establishing a timetable for written products, finding a model proposal, outlining the proposal along agency guidelines, and reviewing progress at regular meetings. The proposal should be reviewed by knowledgeable colleagues, revised often, and polished at the end with attention to details.

4. A good proposal requires not only a

good research question, study plan, and research team, but also a *good presentation:* the proposal must communicate clearly and concisely, following a logical outline and indicating the advantages and disadvantages of the trade-offs in the study plan. The merits of the proposal should stand out so that they will not be missed by a busy reviewer.

5. There are four main sources of support for clinical research:

a. The *NIH* and other governmental sources are the largest providers of support, using a complex system of peer and administrative review that moves slowly but encourages good science.

b. *Foundations* are often interested in research questions that would not be funded at NIH, and have review procedures that are quicker and more partial than those of NIH.

c. Profit-making *corporations* are a readily accessible source of support that is usually channelled to tests of specific new drugs and medical devices.

d. *Intramural funds* can provide small amounts of money quickly, and are suitable for pilot studies and beginning investigators.

REFERENCES

1. Anonymous: *Instruction Sheet for Grant Application Form PHS 398.* U.S. Department of Health and Human Services, OMB No. 0925–0001.
2. Stallones RA: Research grants: advice to applicants. *Yale J Biol Med* 48:451–458, 1975.
3. Cremmins ET: *The Art of Abstracting.* Philadelphia, ISI Press, 1982.
4. Cuca JM: NIH grant applications for clinical research: reasons for poor ratings or disapproval of clinical research. *Clin Res* 31:453–463, 1983.
5. Norman KL: Importance of factors in the review of grant proposals. *J Appl Psychol* 71: 156–162, 1986.
6. Committee Management Staff: *NIH Public Advisory Groups: Authority, Structure, Function, Members.* U.S. Department of Health and Human Services, NIH Publication No. 86–10 October 1985.
7. Kurzig CM: *Foundation Fundamentals: A Guide for Grantseekers.* New York, The Foundation Center, 1980.

ADDITIONAL READINGS

Anonymous: *NIH Extramural Programs.* U.S. Department of Health and Human Services, NIH Publication No 83–33, 1983. (*Summary of the funding policies and procedures of the NIH.*)
Anonymous: *NIH Guide for Contracts and Grants.* U.S. Department of Health and Human Services. (*A biweekly periodical which announces RFPs and RFAs, and provides policy and administrative information.*) Available from The Distribution Center, NIH, Room B3BE07, Bldg. 31, Bethesda, MD 20892.
Anonymous: *National Heart, Lung, and Blood Institute: Fiscal Year 1985 Fact Book.* U.S. Department of Health and Human Services, October 1985. (*Detailed presentation of the current budget and the trends since 1950 of the second largest institute at NIH.*) Available from the NHLBI Information Office, 9000 Rockville Pike, Bethesda, MD 20205.
Lohr KN, Draper D: *Preparing a Demonstration Grant Proposal.* Santa Monica, CA, The Rand Corporation, 1986. (*A monograph about preparation of proposals for submission to the Health Care Financing Administration.*) Available from The Rand Corporation, PO Box 2138 Santa Monica, CA, 90406–2138.
Renz L, Read P: *The Foundation Directory,* ed 10. New York, The Foundation Center, 1985. (*900-page compilation of information on the finances, governance, and giving interests of U.S. foundations with assets of at least $1 million.*) Available from The Foundation Center, 79 Fifth Avenue, New York, NY 10003.

APPENDIX 1.
Outline of an AIDS study protocol

Element	Example
Title	AIDS Virus Infection in i.v. Drug Addicts
Research questions (objectives)	1. To determine the prevalence of AIDS virus infection in i.v. drug addicts in San Francisco.
	2. To discover the risk factors for infection in this population, and to test whether race is one of them.
Significance (background)	1. The AIDS epidemic is a serious public health problem.
	2. I.v. drug addicts are a likely mode of spread of the epidemic in San Francisco.
	3. Knowledge of the prevalence of infection in this population will contribute to the design of preventive programs.
	4. Knowledge of the risk factors for infection will provide information on the mode of spread, and will identify high-risk groups (e.g., blacks) who should be the target of screening and health education programs to prevent further spread.
Design	A cross-sectional study with descriptive and analytic components.
Subjects	
Selection criteria	I.v. drug addicts attending methadone clinic at San Francisco General Hospital.
Sampling design	A consecutive sample of those attending clinic.
Variables	
Predictor variables	Weight loss, needle-sharing habits, age, sex, race.
Outcome variable	ELISA test for AIDS virus antibodies.
Statistical issues	
Hypotheses and analytic approach	1. The prevalence objective (a descriptive finding that requires no hypothesis) will be analyzed as the proportion who have antibodies, with 95% confidence intervals in various age, sex, and race groups.
	2. The analytic objective has the hypothesis that black subjects will have a greater prevalence of AIDS antibodies than white subjects. Predictors of serological status will be analyzed by logistic regression.
Sample size and power	(to be covered in Chapters 12 and 13)

APPENDIX 2.
Developing the research question: A hypothetical example

While reading about the risks of passive smoking for heart and lung disease, and recalling that cigarette smoking by the mother during pregnancy reduces the birthweight of the infant, an investigator gets an idea. Perhaps the health of newborns would be adversely affected if a non-smoking mother was passive exposed during pregnancy to the cigarette smoking of others. He begins with the question: *Is passive smoking harmful to a fetus?* This is an important question, but the variables "passive smoking" and "harmful to a fetus" are ambiguous and broad. In its present form the question is not researchable.

To translate this research question into a study plan the investigator discusses his idea with his advisor and with colleagues who have done research in the area of smoking and health. They agree that the question is important and novel, and suggest several articles to review. In reviewing these the investigator finds that there is strong evidence that active maternal smoking reduces birth weight, but that the effects on the fetus of passive maternal exposure to cigarette smoke has not been studied.

From his literature review he learns that passive smoking can be estimated by measuring concentrations of cotinine (a metabolic product of nicotine in tobacco smoke) in the urine of nonsmokers. After telephone inquiries with scientists at another university who have reported studies using cotinine, he learns that the test would be available at a reasonable price by mailing samples to a reference laboratory. Although not an ideal measure of fetal health, birth weight is easily measured and has been used in many other studies. He decides to use birth weight as the primary outcome variable for the study and rewrites his question: *Among nonsmoking pregnant women, is*

there an association between higher concentrations of cotinine in urine and reduced birth weight of their newborn infants?

The investigator writes a 1-2 page outline of the study plan that specifies the approaches to selecting study subjects and making measurements. To be certain that there will be enough subjects, he estimates the sample size needed for the study, then surveys the records of the hospital's obstetrical unit to estimate the number of births each month to nonsmoking women. In a small pilot study he talks with 20 of these women to confirm that they do not smoke, and to determine their interest in participating in the study. He measures their urinary cotinine to test the feasibility of using the reference laboratory and to determine whether there will be enough women with elevated levels to allow meaningful data analysis. He estimates that it would require about 12 months to collect an adequate number of subjects and that the cost of measuring cotinines, and of collecting and analyzing the data, is small enough to be feasible with the $10-15,000 that may be available through an intramural research grant.

Having determined that the project is important and feasible, he writes out the research question in its final specific form: *Among nonsmoking pregnant women admitted to this hospital in the next year, is an elevated concentration of urinary cotinine associated with reduced birth weight in their newborn babies?* This question meets all the criteria for a good ("FINER") research question (Table 2.1). It provides a clear focus for the study, describes the variables in terms that can be measured, and specifies the population that will be studied.

The investigator rewrites the 1-2 page outline of the study for review by colleagues and advisors. This process leads to other helpful modifications of the study plan and eventually to the submission of a detailed proposal to attract funding by an intramural research grant.[a]

---

[a] After this hypothetical study was designed for the purposes of illustrating this chapter, a real study of similar design was reported (1). Smoking was assessed by questionnaire, however, rather than by cotinine. The findings were that nonsmoking mothers living with men who smoked at least one pack of cigarettes daily gave birth to babies that weighed 120 g less than the babies of nonsmoking mothers living with men who did not smoke.

REFERENCE

1. Rubin DH, Krasilnikoff PA, Leventhal JM, et al: Effect of passive smoking on birth-weight. *Lancet* 2:415–417, 1986.

APPENDIX 3.
Selecting a random sample from a table of random numbers

10480	15011	01536	81647	91646	02011
22368	46573	25595	85393	30995	89198
24130	48390	22527	97265	78393	64809
42167	93093	06243	61680	07856	16376
37570	33997	81837	16656	06121	91782
77921	06907	11008	42751	27756	53498
99562	72905	56420	69994	98872	31016
96301	91977	05463	07972	18876	20922
89572	14342	63661	10281	17453	18103
85475	36857	53342	53998	53060	59533
28918	79578	88231	33276	70997	79936
63553	40961	48235	03427	49626	69445
09429	93969	52636	92737	88974	33488
10365	61129	87529	85689	48237	52267
07119	97336	71048	08178	77233	13916
51085	12765	51821	51259	77452	16308
02368	21382	52404	60268	89368	19885
01011	54092	33362	94904	31273	04146
52162	53916	46369	58569	23216	14513
07056	97628	33787	09998	42698	06691
48663	91245	85828	14346	09172	30163
54164	58492	22421	74103	47070	25306
32639	32363	05597	24200	38005	13363
29334	27001	87637	87308	58731	00256
02488	33062	28834	07351	19731	92420
81525	72295	04839	96423	24878	82651
29676	20591	68086	26432	46901	20949
00742	57392	39064	66432	84673	40027
05366	04213	25669	26422	44407	44048
91921	26418	64117	94305	26766	25940

To select a 10% random sample, begin by enumerating (listing and numbering) every element of the population to be sampled. Then decide on a rule for obtaining an appropriate series of numbers; for example, if your list has 741 elements, your rule might be to go vertically down each column using the first three digits of each number (beginning at the upper left, the numbers are 104, 223, etc.) and to select the first 74 different numbers that fall in the range 1-741. Finally, pick a starting point by an arbitrary process—closing your eyes and putting your pencil on some number in the table is a good way to do it.

APPENDIX 4.
Operations manual: An example

The operations manual describes the method for conducting and recording the results of all of the measurements made in the study. This example is taken from the operations manual of our Study of Osteoporotic Fractures. It describes the use of a dynamometer to measure grip strength. Note that in order to standardize the instructions from examiner to examiner and from subject to subject, the protocol includes a script of instructions to be read to the participant verbatim.

Protocol for measuring grip strength with the dynamometer

Grip strength will be measured in both hands. The handle should be adjusted so that the individual holds the dynamometer comfortably. Place the dynamometer in the right hand with the dial facing the palm. The participant's arm should be flexed 90° at the elbow with the forearm parallel to the floor.

1. Demonstrate the test to the subject: As you demonstrate, instruct the individual to squeeze the hand as hard as he can while simultaneously lowering the arm on a three second count. His grip should be released when his arm is completely extended, hanging straight at his side. While demonstrating, use the following description: *"This device measures your arm and upper body strength. We will measure your grip strength in both arms. I will demonstrate how it is done. Bend your elbow at a 90° angle, with your forearm parallel to the floor. Don't let your arm touch the side of your body. Lower the device slowly as you squeeze as hard as you can. Once your arm is fully extended, you can loosen your grip."*
2. Allow one practice trial for each arm. On the second trial, record the kilograms of force from the dial to the nearest 0.5 kg.
3. Reset the dial. Repeat the procedure for the left arm.

Precautions

The arm should not contact the body. The gripping action should be a slow sustained squeeze rather than an explosive jerk.

APPENDIX 5.
An example of a questionnaire about smoking

The following items are taken from a self-administered questionnaire used in our Study of Osteoporotic Fractures. Note that the branching questions are followed by arrows that direct the subject to the next appropriate question, that the form is precoded with the data entry instructions (the small numbers in the boxes), and that the format is uncluttered with the responses consistently lined up on the left of each text area.

1. Have you smoked at least 100 cigarettes in your entire life?

Yes ☐₁ →

No ☐₂

2. About how old were you when you smoked your first cigarette?

☐☐ years old

3. On the average over the entire time since you started smoking, about how many cigarettes did you smoke per day?

☐☐ cigarettes per day

4. Have you smoked any cigarettes in the past week?

Yes ☐₁ →

No ☐₂

5. About how many cigarettes per day did you smoke in the past week?

☐☐ cigarettes per day

Please skip to next page, question #7

6. How old were you when you stopped smoking?

☐☐ years old

Please go to next page, question #7

202

7. Have you ever lived for at least a year in the same household with someone who smoked cigarettes regularly?

☐1
Yes

☐2
No

8. For about how many years, in total, have you lived with someone who smoked cigarettes regularly at the time?

☐☐ years

9. On the average over the entire time you lived with people who smoked, about how many cigarettes a day were smoked while you were at home?

☐☐ cigarettes per day

10. Do you now live in the same household with someone who smokes cigarettes regularly?

☐1
Yes

☐2
No

11. etc.

APPENDIX 8.A.
Calculating measures of association

Cross-sectional studies

The research questions for Example 8.1 were: What is the prevalence of *Chlamydia* in the population, and is it associated with the use of oral contraceptives (OCs)? The hypothetical findings are that 50 of the women report taking oral contraceptives, and that 10 of these women have positive cultures, compared with 5 of the 50 women not taking oral contraceptives. A two-by-two table of these findings is as follows:

Predictor variable: Contraceptive history	Outcome variable: Cervical culture results	
	Chlamydia present	Chlamydia absent
Users of Oral Contraceptive	10(a)	40(b)
Nonusers of Oral Contraceptive	5(c)	45(d)

Prevalence of Chlamydia infection in users $= a/(a+b) = 10/50 = 20\%$
Prevalence of Chlamydia infection in nonusers $= c/(c+d) = 5/50 = 10\%$
Prevalence of Chlamydia infection overall $= (a+c)/(a+b+c+d) = 15/100 = 15\%$

Relative prevalence[a] $= \dfrac{\text{prevalence of Chlamydia in OC users}}{\text{prevalence of Chlamydia in nonusers}} = \dfrac{a/(a+b)}{c/(c+d)} = \dfrac{10/50}{5/50} = 2.0$

Excess prevalence[a] $= a/(a+b) - c/(c+d) = 10/50 - 5/50 = 5/50 = 10\%$

Thus, the prevalence of Chlamydia infection in this population of venereal disease clinic patients (who may not represent the general population) is 20% among OC users, 10% among nonusers, and 15% overall. There is an association between OC use and Chlamydia infection that is characterized by a relative prevalence of 2.0 and by an excess prevalence of 10%.

---

[a] Relative prevalence and excess prevalence are the cross-sectional analogs of relative risk and excess risk.

Case-control studies

The research question for Example 8.2 was whether there is an association between use of aspirin by children with viral illnesses and the development of Reye's syndrome. The hypothetical findings were that 28 of the 30 cases reported taking aspirin during the viral illness that preceded the Reye's syndrome, whereas only 35 of the 60 controls took aspirin. A two-by-two table of these findings is as follows:

Predictor variable	Outcome variable	
Medication history	Diagnosis	
	Reye's	No Reye's
Aspirin	28(a)	35(b)
No aspirin	2(c)	25(d)

$$\text{Relative risk} \approx \text{Odds ratio} = \frac{ad}{bc} = \frac{28 \times 25}{35 \times 2} = 10.0$$

Thus, there is a strong association; patients who take aspirin are approximately 10 times more likely to develop Reye's syndrome than those who do not. Note that this relatively inexpensive study has revealed a risk factor for this rare disease that could not have been discovered with any other design. However, the study provides no information on the incidence of Reye's syndrome or the excess risk associated with aspirin.

APPENDIX 8.B.
Why the odds ratio can be used as an estimate for relative risk in a case-control study

The data in a case-control study represent two samples: the cases are drawn from a population of people who have the disease (in this instance children with Reye's syndrome), and the controls from a population of people who do not have the disease. The predictor variable is measured (in this instance history of aspirin use), and the following two-by-two table produced:

	Disease	No disease
Risk factor present	a	b
Risk factor absent	c	d

If this two-by-two table represented data from a cohort study, then the incidence of the disease in those with the risk factor would be $a/(a+b)$ and the relative risk would be simply $[a/(a+b)] \div [c/(c+d)]$. However, it is not appropriate to compute either incidence or relative risk in this way because the two samples are not drawn from the population in the same proportions—usually there are roughly equal numbers of cases and controls in the study samples, but many fewer cases than controls in the population. Instead, relative risk in a case-control study can be approximated by the **odds ratio**, computed as the cross-product of the two-by-two table, ad/cb.

The basis for this extremely useful fact cannot be understood intuitively, but is relatively easy to demonstrate algebraicly. Consider the situation for the full population, represented by a', b', c', and d'.

	Disease	No disease
Risk factor present	a'	b'
Risk factor absent	c'	d'

Here, it *is* appropriate to calculate the risk of

disease among people with the risk factor as $a'/(a'+b')$, the risk among those without the risk factor as $c'/(c'+d')$, and the relative risk as $[a'/(a'+b')] \div [c'/(c'+d')]$. We have already discussed the fact that $a'/(a'+b')$ is not equal to $a/(a+b)$. However, if the disease is relatively uncommon (as most are) then a' is much smaller than b', and c' is much smaller than d'. This means that $a'/(a'+b')$ is closely approximated by a'/b', and that $c'/(c'+d')$ is closely approximated by c'/d'. Thus, the relative risk *of the population* can be approximated as:

$$\frac{a'/(a'+b')}{c'/(c'+d')} \approx \frac{a'/b'}{c'/d'}$$

The latter term is the odds ratio of the population (literally, the ratio of the odds of disease in those with the risk factor, a'/b', to the odds of disease in those without the risk factor, c'/d'). This can be rearranged as the cross-product:

$$\frac{a'}{b'} \times \frac{d'}{c'} = \frac{a'}{c'} \times \frac{d'}{b'}$$

However, a'/c' in the population equals a/c in the sample if the cases are representative of the population (i.e., have the same prevalence of the risk factor). Similarly, b'/d' equals b/d if the controls are representative.

Thus, the population parameters in this last term can be replaced by the sample parameters, and we are left with the fact that the odds ratio observed in the sample, ad/bc, is a close approximation of the relative risk in the population, $[a'/(a'+b')] \div [c'/(c'+d')]$, provided that the disease is rare and sampling error (systematic as well as random) is small.

APPENDIX 10.A.
Hypothetical example of confounding

Confounding by cigarette smoking can be the cause of an apparent association between coffee drinking and MI. The entries in these tables are numbers of subjects. Thus, the top left entry of Panel 1 means that, among the smokers, 80 MI cases drank coffee (out of $80+20=100$ total MI cases).

1. Both in smokers and in nonsmokers, coffee drinking is *not* associated with MI.

	Smokers		Nonsmokers	
	MI	No MI	MI	No MI
Coffee	80	40	10	20
No Coffee	20	10	40	80

Odds ratio for MI associated with coffee:

$$\text{in smokers} = \frac{80 \times 10}{20 \times 40} = 1$$

$$\text{in nonsmokers} = \frac{10 \times 80}{40 \times 20} = 1$$

2. However, if we did not stratify on smoking, (i.e., if we did not consider smokers and nonsmokers separately), coffee drinking and MI would appear to be related. Combining the two tables above gives:

Smokers and nonsmokers combined		
	MI	No MI
Coffee	90	60
No Coffee	60	90

Odds ratio for MI associated with coffee:

$$\text{in smokers and non-smokers combined} = \frac{90 \times 90}{60 \times 60} = 2.25$$

3. Smoking is a confounder because it is strongly associated with coffee drinking (below, left) and with MI (below, right)[a]:

	MI and no MI combined		Coffee and no coffee combined	
	Coffee	No coffee	MI	No MI
Smokers	120	30	100	50
Nonsmokers	30	120	50	100

$$\text{Odds ratio for coffee drinking associated with smoking} = \frac{120 \times 120}{30 \times 30} = 16$$

$$\text{Odds ratio for MI associated with smoking} = \frac{100 \times 100}{50 \times 50} = 4$$

[a] These tables were obtained by rearranging numbers in Panel 1, then combining tables.

207

APPENDIX 10.B.
A simplified example of adjustment

Suppose that a study finds two major predictors of the IQ of children: the parental education level and the child's blood lead level. Consider the following hypothetical data on children with normal and high lead levels:

	Average years of parental education	Average IQ of child
High lead level	10.0	95
Normal lead level	12.0	110

Note that the parental education level is also associated with the child's blood lead level. The question is: is the difference in IQ more than can be accounted for on the basis of the difference in parental education? To answer this question we look at how much difference in IQ the difference in parental education levels would be expected to produce. We do this by plotting parental educational level versus IQ in the children with normal lead levels (Fig. 10.B).[b]

[b] This description of analysis of covariance (ANCOVA) is simplified. Actually, parental education is plotted against the child's IQ in both the normal and high lead groups, and the single slope that fits both plots the best is used. The model for this form of adjustment thus assumes linear relationships between education and IQ in both groups, and also that the slopes of the lines in the two groups are the same.

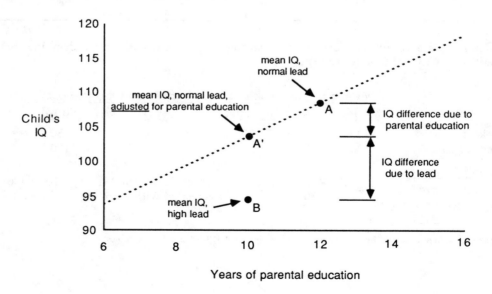

Figure 10.B. Hypothetical graph of child's IQ as a linear function (dotted line) of years of parental education.

The dotted line in Figure 10.B shows the relationship between the child's IQ and parental education in children with normal lead levels; there is an increase in the child's IQ of 5 points for each 2 years of parental education. Thus, we can **adjust** the IQ of the normal lead group to account for the difference in mean parental education by sliding down the line from point A to point A'. (Because the group with normal lead levels had 2 more years of parental education on the average, we adjust their IQs downward by 5 points to make them comparable in mean parental education to the high-lead group.) This still leaves a 10-point difference in IQ between points A' and B, suggesting that lead has an independent effect on IQ of this magnitude. Thus, of the 15-point difference in IQ of children with low and high lead levels, 5 points can be accounted for by their different education levels and the remaining 10 are attributable to the lead exposure.

APPENDIX 11.A.
Randomization procedures for studies of small or moderate sample size

Experiments of small to moderate size may have a small gain in power if special randomization procedures are used to balance the study groups in the numbers of subjects they contain, and in the distribution of baseline variables known to predict the outcome. These strategies are only suitable, of course, for variables that are known in advance to predict outcome. They are the design phase alternative to statistically adjusting (in the analysis phase) for maldistribution of baseline variables.

Blocked randomization is a commonly used technique to assure that the *number* of subjects is equally distributed among the study groups at periodic intervals during the process of randomization. The randomization is set up in "blocks" of predetermined size. For example, if the block size is six, randomization procedes normally within each block until the third person is randomized to one group, after which subjects are automatically assigned to the other group until the block of six is completed. This means that in a study of 30 subjects exactly 15 will be assigned to each group, and in a study of 33 subjects, the disproportion could be no greater than 18:15. If blocked randomization is to be used in nonblinded studies, the size of the blocks should be varied randomly (ranging, for example, from four to eight) according to a schedule set up in advance and not known to the investigator; otherwise, the treatment assignment of the subjects at the end of each block could be predicted and manipulated.

Stratified blocked randomization is a technique for assuring that an important baseline prognostic variable (one that predicts outcome) is more evenly distributed between the study groups than chance alone would dictate. In a study of the effect of an antihypertensive drug, baseline blood pressure is an important predictor of outcome, so it is best if the mean level is the same (or nearly so) in each group. This can be achieved by dividing the study cohort at baseline into patients with mild, moderate, and severe hypertension at the outset, and then carrying out a blocked randomization within each of these three "strata". Stratified blocked randomization increases the power of a study by reducing the variation in outcome that comes from chance disproportions in the way the baseline variable is allocated to the study groups. A limitation is the small number of baseline variables, not more than two or three, that can be balanced by this technique.

Adaptive randomization is a technique that uses a "biased coin" to alter the probability of assigning each subject in order to balance the distribution of baseline prognostic variables between study groups (1). Adaptive randomization has an advantage over stratified randomization in its suitability for simultaneously balancing a large number of baseline variables and for weighting them according to their strength as predictors. A disadvantage is the complexity of the system, which requires an interactive microcomputer and increases the possibility of technical error.

Both adaptive and stratified blocked randomization also have the disadvantage that special analytic techniques should be used for testing statistical significance. If the investigator ignores this and uses the *t* test, chi square, and other ordinary tests of significance she will lose the increased power that is the reason for using these special randomization techniques (1). In general, therefore, these techniques do not offer great advantages for most studies (2). They should be considered when the sample size is small (say less than 50 per group) and there are variables known to have a strong influence on outcome. In addition, multicenter experiments that are carried out in several discrete sites often stratify the randomization on the clinical site for reasons analogous to those discussed in the Chapter 10 section on matching.

REFERENCES

1. Friedman LM, Furberg CD, DeMets DL: *Fundamental of Clinical Trials.* ed 2. Littleton, MA, PSG Publishing Co, 1985.
2. Pocock SJ: Current issues in the design and interpretation of clinical trials. *Brit Med J* 1985; 296:39-42.

APPENDIX 11.B.
Three analysis issues pertinent to designing an experiment

Intention-to-treat analysis

This is an analytic approach that compares the outcomes with every subject analyzed according to her randomized group assignment. At issue here is what to do with **crossovers**, subjects who in effect change study groups. In a drug versus placebo study a crossover is either someone assigned to the active drug who does not take it, or someone assigned to the placebo who ends up taking the active drug (or a congener). **Intention-to-treat** means that an individual assigned to a particular intervention group is included in that group's outcome statistics even if she never receives the intervention.

An alternative to intention-to-treat is to analyze only those who comply with the intervention. This seems reasonable—subjects can only be affected by an intervention they actually receive—but the problem arises that compliant patients may be inherently different from those who drop out in ways that have an effect on the outcome. The Coronary Drug Project provides an empirical demonstration of the wrong conclusions that this type of confounding can produce (1). Subjects were randomly assigned to receive either the lipid-lowering agent clofibrate or a placebo, and the effects on CHD mortality are shown in Example 11.1.

Example 11.1
Here is the first half of the published abstract of the Coronary Drug Project study of the effect of clofibrate in preventing CHD mortality.

The Coronary Drug Project was carried out to evaluate the efficacy and safety of several lipid-influencing drugs in the long-term treatment of CHD. The five-year mortality in 1103 men treated with clofibrate was 20.0%, as compared with 20.9% in 2789 men given placebo (P = .55) Good adherers to clofibrate, i.,e., patients who took 80% or more of the protocol prescription during the five-year follow-up period, had a substantially lower five-year mortality than did poor adherers to clofibrate (15.0% versus 24.6%; P = .00011).

Before reading the second half of the abstract (below), stop and think about the implications of these findings. Is it sensible to conclude that clofibrate decreased the CHD death rate in those who complied well? Now read the second half of the Coronary Drug Project abstract:

. . . However, similar findings were noted in the placebo group, i.e., 15.1% mortality for good adherers and 28.3% for poor adherers (P = 4.7 x 10^{-16}) These findings and various other analyses of mortality in the clofibrate and placebo groups of the project show the serious difficulty, if not impossibility, of evaluating treatment efficacy in subgroups determined by patient responses (e.g., adherence or cholesterol change) to the treament protocol after randomization. (1)

The complete abstract of the clofibrate study clarifies the conclusions that should be drawn from this study. Looking only at the findings within the clofibrate group, those who faithfully took the drug had a CHD mortality rate half that observed in those who complied poorly with the drug. Exactly the same effect was observed in the placebo group, however—those who faithfully took the placebo had a CHD mortality rate half that of those who adhered poorly to the placebo. Therefore, the apparent benefit in those who adhered well to the clofibrate was confounded by undetected differences between compliers and noncompliers, and had nothing to do with the clofibrate. This problem did not affect the intention-to-treat comparison of the overall CHD rates, which correctly revealed no difference between the two study groups.

Example 11.1 is an excellent illustration of the fact that the *intention-to-treat analytic approach is the only one that preserves the full value of randomization*, and guarantees control over baseline confounders. The disadvantages of intention-to-treat are obvious: subjects who choose not to take the assigned intervention will nevertheless be included in the statistics that estimate of the effects of that intervention. These crossovers reduce the power of the study and attenuate the size of the estimated intervention effect. (The attenuation of the intervention effect can actually enhance generalizability, however, if the study's compliance problems match those that will occur in the population.)

In summary, the integrity of the main hypothesis test in an RBT depends on (a) the use of the intention-to-treat rule, and (b) the investigator's ability to achieve high rates of compliance. On the other hand, as we shall see in the next section, analyses which are not intention-to-treat can provide additional information when cautiously interpreted.

Subgroup analyses

Subgroup analyses examine the findings in subsets of the randomized study groups. These strategies have a mixed reputation because they are easy to misuse and can lead to wrong conclusions. With proper care, however, they can provide useful ancillary information and expand the inferences that can be drawn from a clinical trial. The likelihood of drawing erroneous inferences depends a great deal on whether the predictor variables that define the subgroups are measured before or after randomization.

Subgroup analyses based on **postrandomization factors** are the more dangerous. An example is the "explanatory analysis" proposed by Sackett and Gent (2), which analyzes only the subgroups of subjects who turned out to comply well with the intervention. Example 11.1 illustrates vividly the misleading conclusions that can result when the explanatory findings do not jibe with those of the overall intention-to-treat analysis.

Subgroup analyses based on postrandomization factors can produce useful secondary inferences in some circumstances. For example, the investigator may wish to estimate the magnitude of the treatment effect in compliant patients once an intention-to-treat analysis has revealed an overall benefit. The strategy can also be used to look for clues to help explain an unexpected negative result in the intention-to-treat analysis. In the MRFIT, regression analysis within the intervention group showed that men who decreased their cholesterol and smoking levels in the first year of the study subsequently had lower CHD rates than those who did not, but that men who decreased their blood pressure levels tended to have *higher* CHD rates (3). The implication—that the cholesterol and smoking interventions had had their expected beneficial effects and that antihypertensive treatment had produced an unexpected adverse response—is not conclusive enough to base health policy on, but it does indicate the need for future studies of this possibility.

Subgroup analyses that are based on **prerandomization factors** are further classified according to whether the comparison is within- or between-group. **Within-group** analyses are really just ordinary cohort study analyses that take advantage of the opportunity to examine risk factors within one of the study groups; when the analysis is carried out within an untreated group, the result is useful natural history information that is often quite independent of the goals of the experiment. A good example is the MRFIT study of whether Type A behavior pattern is a risk factor for CHD (4), discussed in Chapter 4. These within-group analyses do not take advantage of the randomization and therefore have the usual problem of analytic cohort studies: their findings are susceptible to confounding.

Between-group analyses in subgroups stratified by **prerandomization factors** do not have this problem. The BHAT (β-blocker Heart Attack Trial) produced the overall finding that β-blocking drugs reduced the death rate after a heart attack; subgroup analysis revealed that this benefit occurred mostly in the subgroup of patients who had poor myocardial function at the outset of the study (5). β-blockers do have some side effects, and many physicians have used this subgroup finding as a reason for restricting the routine use of β-blockers to this relatively small subgroup of the population of men who have had a heart attack. Between-group analyses preserve the control over confounding factors provided by randomization, but their *power* to detect effects that exist in the population is limited by the size of the subgroup. There may also be the problems that arise from having multiple hypotheses, particularly if the subgroups were not defined before the study began (see Chapter 12).

Early stopping rules

Sometimes it is useful to include an early stopping rule for ending the study when the outcome has become clear, one way or the other. This is best accomplished by testing the statistical significance at several preset points, and considering whether continuing the study is likely to produce more conclusive or comprehensive answers. There are ethical and fiscal advantages to being able to stop the study once benefit or harm has been established, but the trade-off is the disadvantage that taking "multiple peeks" is a form of multiple hypothesis testing, and can increase the sample size requirements (see Chapter 12). For many studies, however, particularly those of several years' duration, the advantages of considering whether the study can be stopped predominate. One of the best of the several approaches available (6) is that of O'Brien and Fleming (7), which minimizes the problem of multiple hypothesis testing by requiring very small P values in the early statistical tests.

The issue of looking at the outcome data during the study brings up the issue of who should do the looking. Some authors recommend that this should be done by an external group of experts, and that the investigators should be kept blind to their own outcome data until the very end (6). However, except in an unblinded study (when knowledge of outcome trends might influence how the subjects were cared for), this seems an unnecessary complexity and expense. Even worse, it removes the investigators from the control of one of the important scientific decisions of their own study. In our opinion, investigators in an RBT may look at their own outcome findings if they have previously specified the guidelines by which they will decide whether to stop the study.

REFERENCES

1. The CDP Research Group: Influence of adherence to treatment and response of cholesterol on mortality in the CDP. *N Engl J Med* 303:1038–1041, 1980.
2. Sackett DL, Gent M: Controversy in counting and attributing events in clinical trials. *N Engl J Med* 301:1410–2, 1979.
3. The MRFIT Group: The MRFIT: Coronary death, non-fatal MI and other clinical outcomes. *Am J Cardiol* 58;1–13, 1986.
4. Shekelle RB, Hulley SB, Neaton JD, et al: The MRFIT Behavior Pattern Study: II. Type A behavior and the inc:.dence of CHD. *Am J Epidemiol*, 122:550–570, 1985
5. Furberg CD, Hawkins CM, Lighstein E: Effect of propranolol in post infarction patients with mechanical or electrical complications. *Circulation* 69:761–765, 1984.
6. Friedman LM, Furberg CD, DeMets DL: *Fundamental of Clinical Trials.* ed 2. Littleton, MA, PSG Publishing Co, 1985.
7. O'Brien PC, Fleming TR: A multiple testing procedure for clinical trials. *Biometrics* 35:549–556, 1979.

APPENDIX 13.A.
Sample size required per group when using the t test to compare means of continuous variables

Table 13.A.
Sample size per group for comparing two means

E/S[a]	One-tailed $\alpha =$ 0.005 Two-tailed $\alpha =$ 0.01 $\beta =$ 0.05	0.10	0.20	One-tailed $\alpha =$ 0.025 Two-tailed $\alpha =$ 0.05 $\beta =$ 0.05	0.10	0.20	One-tailed $\alpha =$ 0.05 Two-tailed $\alpha =$ 0.10 $\beta =$ 0.05	0.10	0.20
.10	3563	2977	2337	2599	2102	1570	2165	1713	1237
.15	1584	1323	1038	1155	934	698	962	762	550
.20	891	744	584	650	526	393	541	428	309
.25	570	476	374	416	336	251	346	274	198
.30	396	331	260	289	234	174	241	190	137
.40	223	186	146	162	131	98	135	107	77
.50	143	119	93	104	84	63	87	69	49
.60	99	83	65	72	58	44	60	48	34
.70	73	61	48	53	43	32	44	35	25
.80	56	47	36	41	33	25	34	27	19
.90	44	37	29	32	26	19	27	21	15
1.00	36	30	23	26	21	16	22	17	12

[a]E/S is the standardized effect size, computed as E (expected effect size) divided by S (standard deviation of the outcome variable). To estimate the sample size, read across from the *standardized effect size*, and down from the specified values of α and β for the required sample size in each group.

Calculating Variability

Variability is usually reported as either the standard deviation (SD) or the standard error of the mean (SEM). For the purposes of sample size calculation, the standard deviation of the variable is most useful. Fortunately, it is easy to convert from one measure to another: the standard deviation is simply the standard error times the square root of N, where N is the number of subjects that make up the mean. Suppose a study reported that the weight loss in 25 persons on a low-fiber diet was 10±2 kg (mean ± SEM). The standard deviation would be 2 × $\sqrt{25}$ = 10 kg.

General Formula for Other Values

The general formula for other values of E, S, α and β, or for unequal group sizes, where E and S are defined above, follows. Let:

z_α = the standard normal deviate for α (For those unfamiliar with this concept, see ref 5. If the alternative hypothesis is two-tailed, z_α = 1.96 when α = 0.05, and z_α = 1.645 when α = 0.10. If the alternative hypothesis is one-tailed, z_α = 1.645 when α = 0.05).

z_β = the standard normal deviate for β. (z_β = 0.84 when β = 0.20, and z_β = 1.282 when β = 0.10).

q_1 = proportion of subjects in group 1
q_2 = proportion of subjects in group 2
N = **total** number of subjects required.

Then:

$$N = [(1/q_1 + 1/q_2)\ S^2\ (z_\alpha + z_\beta)^2] \div E^2.$$

(Because this formula and Table 13.A are based on approximating the *t* statistic with a *z* statistic, they slightly underestimate the sample size when *N* is less than about 30.)

APPENDIX 13.B.
Sample size required per group when using the z statistic to compare proportions of dichotomous variables.

Table 13.B.
Sample size per group for comparing two proportions

Smaller of P1 and P2[a]	Upper number: $\alpha = 0.05$ (one-tailed) or $\alpha = 0.10$ (two-tailed); $\beta = 0.20$ Middle number: $\alpha = 0.025$ (one-tailed) or $\alpha = 0.05$ (two-tailed); $\beta = 0.20$ Lower number: $\alpha = 0.025$ (one-tailed) or $\alpha = 0.05$ (two-tailed); $\beta = 0.10$									
	Expected difference between P1 and P2									
	0.05	**0.10**	**0.15**	**0.20**	**0.25**	**0.30**	**0.35**	**0.40**	**0.45**	**0.50**
.05	342	110	59	38	27	21	17	13	11	9
	434	140	75	49	35	27	21	17	14	12
	581	187	100	65	46	35	28	22	19	15
.10	539	156	78	48	33	25	19	15	12	10
	685	199	99	62	43	31	24	19	16	13
	916	266	133	82	56	42	32	25	21	17
.15	712	197	95	57	38	28	21	16	13	11
	904	250	120	72	49	35	27	21	17	14
	1210	334	161	96	65	47	35	28	22	18
.20	860	231	108	64	42	30	23	17	14	11
	1093	293	138	81	54	38	29	22	18	14
	1462	392	184	108	72	51	38	29	23	19
.25	984	258	119	69	45	32	24	18	14	11
	1249	328	152	88	58	41	30	23	18	14
	1672	439	203	117	77	54	40	30	24	19
.30	1083	280	128	73	47	33	24	18	14	11
	1375	356	162	93	60	42	31	23	18	14
	1840	476	217	124	80	56	41	31	24	19
.35	1157	295	133	75	48	33	24	18	14	11
	1469	375	169	96	61	42	31	23	18	14
	1966	502	226	128	82	56	41	30	23	18
.40	1206	305	136	76	48	33	24	17	13	10
	1532	387	173	97	61	42	30	22	17	13
	2050	518	231	129	82	56	40	29	22	17
.45	1231	308	136	75	47	32	23	16	12	9
	1563	391	173	96	60	41	29	21	16	12
	2092	523	231	128	80	54	38	28	21	15
.50	1231	305	133	73	45	30	21	15	11	—
	1563	387	169	93	58	38	27	19	14	—
	2092	518	226	124	77	51	35	25	19	—
.55	1206	295	128	69	42	28	19	13	—	—
	1532	375	162	88	54	35	24	17	—	—
	2050	502	217	117	72	47	32	22	—	—

216

Table 13.B. continued

Smaller of P1 and P2[a]	Expected difference between P1 and P2									
	0.05	0.10	0.15	0.20	0.25	0.30	0.35	0.40	0.45	0.50
.60	1157	280	119	64	38	25	17	—	—	—
	1469	356	152	81	49	31	21	—	—	—
	1966	476	203	108	65	42	28	—	—	—
.65	1083	258	108	57	33	21	—	—	—	—
	1375	328	138	72	43	27	—	—	—	—
	1840	439	184	96	56	35	—	—	—	—
.70	984	231	95	48	27	—	—	—	—	—
	1249	293	120	62	35	—	—	—	—	—
	1672	392	161	82	46	—	—	—	—	—
.75	860	197	78	38	—	—	—	—	—	—
	1093	250	99	49	—	—	—	—	—	—
	1462	334	133	65	—	—	—	—	—	—
.80	712	156	59	—	—	—	—	—	—	—
	904	199	75	—	—	—	—	—	—	—
	1210	266	100	—	—	—	—	—	—	—
.85	539	110	—	—	—	—	—	—	—	—
	685	140	—	—	—	—	—	—	—	—
	916	187	—	—	—	—	—	—	—	—
.90	342	—	—	—	—	—	—	—	—	—
	434	—	—	—	—	—	—	—	—	—
	581	—	—	—	—	—	—	—	—	—

[a]P1 represents the proportion of subjects expected to have the outcome in one group; P2 in the other group. (In a case-control study, P1 represents the proportion of cases with the predictor variable; P2 the proportion of controls with the predictor variable). To estimate the sample size, read across from the *smaller* of P1 and P2, and down the *expected difference* between P1 and P2. The three numbers represent the sample size required in each group for the specified values of α and β.

General Formula for Total Sample Size

The general formula for calculating the *total* sample size (N) required for a study using the z statistic, where P1 and P2 are defined above, is as follows (see Appendix 13.A for definitions of z_α and z_β). Let

q_1 = proportion of subjects in group 1
q_2 = proportion of subjects in group 2
N = *total* number of subjects
$P = q_1 P1 + q_2 P2$

Then:

$$N = \frac{[z_\alpha\sqrt{P(1-P)(1/q_1+1/q_2)}+z_\beta\sqrt{P1(1-P1)(1/q_1)+P2(1-P2)(1/q_2)}]^2}{(P1 - P2)^2}$$

(This formula and Table 13.B do not include the Fleiss-Tytun-Ury continuity correction (5), and thus slightly underestimate the required sample size.)

APPENDIX 13.C.
Total sample size required when using the correlation coefficient (r)

Table 13.C.
Sample size for revealing a correlation

r[a]	One-tailed $\alpha =$ 0.005 Two-tailed $\alpha =$ 0.01			One-tailed $\alpha =$ 0.025 Two-tailed $\alpha =$ 0.05			One-tailed $\alpha =$ 0.05 Two-tailed $\alpha =$ 0.010		
$\beta =$	0.05	0.10	0.20	0.05	0.10	0.20	0.05	0.10	0.20
0.05	7118	5947	4663	5193	4200	3134	4325	3424	2469
0.10	1773	1481	1162	1294	1047	782	1078	854	616
0.15	783	655	514	572	463	346	477	378	273
0.20	436	365	287	319	259	194	266	211	153
0.25	276	231	182	202	164	123	169	134	98
0.30	189	158	125	139	113	85	116	92	67
0.35	136	114	90	100	82	62	84	67	49
0.40	102	86	68	75	62	47	63	51	37
0.45	79	66	53	58	48	36	49	39	29
0.50	62	52	42	46	38	29	39	31	23
0.60	40	34	27	30	25	19	26	21	16
0.70	27	23	19	20	17	13	17	14	11
0.80	18	15	13	14	12	9	12	10	8

[a]To estimate the total sample size, read across from r (the expected correlation coefficient) and down from the specified values of α and β.

General Formula for Other Values

The general formula for other values of r, α, and β is as follows (see Appendix 13.A for definitions of z_α and z_β). Let

r = expected correlation coefficient
$C = 0.5 \times \ln [(1+r)/(1-r)]$
N = Total number of subjects required

Then:

$$N = [(z_\alpha + z_\beta) \div C]^2 + 3.$$

Estimating Sample Size for Difference between Two Correlations

If testing whether a correlation, $r1$, is different from $r2$ (i.e., the null hypothesis is that $r1 = r2$; the alternative hypothesis is that $r1 \neq r2$), let

$C1 = 0.5 \times \ln [(1+r1)/(1-r1)]$
$C2 = 0.5 \times \ln [(1+r2)/(1-r2)]$

Then:

$$N = [(z_\alpha + z_\beta) \div (C1 - C2)]^2 + 3.$$

APPENDIX 13.D.
Sample size for a descriptive study of a continuous variable

Table 13.D.
Sample size for common values of W/S[a]

W/S	Confidence Level		
	90%	**95%**	**99%**
0.10	1083	1537	2665
0.15	482	683	1180
0.20	271	385	664
0.25	174	246	425
0.30	121	171	295
0.35	89	126	217
0.40	68	97	166
0.50	44	62	107
0.60	31	43	74
0.70	23	32	55
0.80	17	25	42
0.90	14	19	33
1.00	11	16	27

[a]W/S is the standardized width of the confidence interval, computed as W (desired total width) divided by S (standard deviation of the variable). To estimate the total sample size, read across from the *standardized width,* and down from the specified confidence level.

General Formula for Other Values

For other values of W, S, and a confidence level of $(1 - \alpha)$, the total number of subjects required (N) is:

$$N = 4z_\alpha^2 \, S^2 \div W^2$$

(see Appendix 13.A for the definition of z_α).

APPENDIX 13.E.
Sample size for a descriptive study of a dichotomous variable

Table 13.E.
Sample size for common values of P[a]

	Upper number: 90% confidence level Middle number: 95% confidence level Lower number: 99% confidence level				
	Total width of confidence interval (W)				
Expected proportion (P)	**0.10**	**0.15**	**0.20**	**0.25**	**0.30**
0.10	98	—	—	—	—
	139	—	—	—	—
	239	—	—	—	—
0.15	138	62	—	—	—
	196	88	—	—	—
	339	151	—	—	—
0.20	174	77	43	—	—
	246	110	62	—	—
	425	189	107	—	—
0.25	203	91	51	33	—
	289	128	73	47	—
	498	221	125	80	—
0.30	228	101	57	37	26
	323	144	81	52	36
	558	248	139	90	62
0.40	260	116	65	42	29
	369	164	93	60	41
	638	283	160	102	71
0.50	271	121	68	44	31
	384	171	96	62	43
	664	294	166	107	74

[a]To estimate the sample size, read across from the *expected proportion* (P) who have the variable of interest and down from the desired *total width* (W) of the confidence interval. The three numbers represent the sample size required for 90%, 95%, and 99% confidence levels.

General Formula for Other Values

The general formula for other values of P, W, and a confidence level of $(1 - \alpha)$, where P and W are defined above, is as follows. Let

z_α = the standard normal deviate for a two-tailed α, where $(1 - \alpha)$ is the confidence level (for example, since $\alpha = 0.05$ for a 95% confidence level, $z_\alpha = 1.96$).

Then the total number of subjects required is:

$$N = 4 \, z_\alpha^2 \, P \, (1-P) \div W^2$$

(see Appendix 13.A for the definition of z_α).

APPENDIX 14.A.
Example of a Consent Form

CONSENT TO PARTICIPATE IN A RESEARCH STUDY

Title of Research Study

Hypertension Arrhythmia Reduction Trial (HART)

Investigator

Dr. Davida Siegel, Clinical Epidemiology program, University of California, San Francisco, Phone (415) 476-XXXX.

Purpose and Background

This is a study of the side effects of different medicines for high blood pressure (hypertension), particularly the risk of irregularities of the heartbeat (arrhythmias). The purpose of this study is to learn which of two commonly prescribed treatments for high blood pressure causes the fewest irregularities of the heartbeat.

Procedures:

If I agree to participate, the following things will happen:

1. I will answer some questions about my medical history. This will take about 15 minutes.
2. I will have an ordinary physical examination to confirm that I have mild hypertension. This will take about 20 minutes.
3. I will have blood drawn with a needle from my arm for potassium and other tests. The needle often causes discomfort lasting less than a minute; occasionally a bruise or minor infection may occur, but these are very unlikely.
4. I will have an electrocardiogram (ECG) and an echocardiogram. These are not painful, do not involve needles, and are not dangerous. The electrocardiogram, which traces my heart rhythm, takes about 2 or 3 minutes. The echocardi-ogram, which measures heart dimensions, takes about 10 or 15 minutes.
5. I will have continuous recording of my heart rhythm for 24 hours. For this, I will wear a portable recorder about the size of a book on a strap over my shoulder for 24 hours. This test is not painful, does not involve needles, and is not dangerous.
6. I will then be given some pills to take twice a day. The pills will either hydrochlorothiazide (a commonly prescribed medicines for high blood pressure), or hydrocholothiazide with potassium (a commonly prescribed combination), or a placebo (an inactive sugar pill). The choice of medicine will be determined by chance, not by the research doctor. Neither I nor the research doctor will know which drug I am taking, although in case of an emergency it can be revealed. I will take this medicine for 2 months.
7. While I am taking the medicine I will have my blood pressure checked each month. At the end of the two months I will have a second 24-hour recording of my heart rhythm. I will also have blood drawn again and answer some questions about side effects.

Benefits

There may be no direct benefit to me from participating in the study. However, I may find out the safest way to treat my high blood pressure. I will receive several heart tests free.

Risks

My blood pressure may rise during the 2 months I am taking a drug or placebo. The risk of developing medical complications, such as a heart attack or stroke, are very small. Steps have been taken to reduce any risk. My blood pressure will be checked periodically, and if it rises above a certain level, it will be measured a second time the next day. If my blood pressure remains above this level, I will be treated with known medicine.

The medicine that I am given may cause side effects that are bothersome but rarely serious. I may experience dizziness, tiredness, weakness, or impotence.

Reimbursement

I will be paid $25 for the first time, and $50 for the second time I complete the 24-hour continuous recording of my heart rhythm. If I am injured as a result of being in this study, treatment will be available. The costs of such treatment may be paid by the University of California, depending on a number of factors. The University does not normally provide any other form of compensation for injury. For further information about this, I may call the Committee on Human Research at (415) 476-XXXX.

Alternatives

The medicines used in this study are standard treatments for high blood pressure that can be obtained without participating in the study.

Confidentiality

The results of all the study tests will be discussed with me, and sent to my personal physician (unless I wish otherwise). Except for this disclosure, all information obtained in this study will be considered confidential and used only for research purposes. My identity will be kept confidential in so far as the law allows.

Questions

_____, the research assistant, has discussed this information with me and offered to answer my questions. If I have further questions, I can contact her at 476-XXXX or Dr. Siegel the director of the study, at 476-XXXX.

Right to Refuse or Withdraw

My participation in the study is entirely voluntary, and I am free to refuse to take part or withdraw at any time without affecting or jeopardizing my future medical care.

Consent

I agree to participate in this study. I have been given a copy of this form and had a chance to read it.

Signature: _____
Date: _____
Signature of
clinician: _____

APPENDIX 14.B.
Checklist for informed consent

- **The nature of the research project**
  Explicit statement that the project involves research.
  Identification of investigators.
  Purposes of the research.
  Procedure for selection of subjects.

- **Procedures** of the study
  Time required.
  Assignment of treatments.
  Explanation of randomization and blinding.
  Procedures that are experimental rather than standard care.

- **Benefits and harms** of procedures
  Probability and magnitude of benefits and harms.
  Procedures to maximize benefits and minimize harms.

  Alternative procedures or treatments available outside the study.
  Potential costs.
  Information about results that will or will not be disclosed to subjects.

- Procedures to maintain **confidentiality**

- Assurances that **participation in research is voluntary**
  Assurance that subject may decline to participate or withdraw at any time without penalty.

- An explicit offer to **answer questions** or provide further information.
  Directions on whom to contact with questions about the study and the rights of research subjects, or about injuries resulting from the research.

APPENDIX 15A.
Illustration of the use of a statistical analysis package to analyze the smoking questionnaire data

Statistical analysis programs vary in the amout of time needed to learn how to use them. They all begin, as illustrated in the table, with a description of the data and a specification the analysis. The program is not so formidable as it looks at first glance. Each line consists of a statement about the data which is almost self explanatory. The first line simply specifies a title to be printed on the report at the top of each page, to which the computer will also add a date and time. The second line says that there are 8 variables (we are going to add ID number and pack-years, to be calculated from our original 6) and that they are in a free format, such as a comma-delimited file (i.e., each field is separated from the next by a comma). The next section specifies the names of the variables and the missing values.

The next section tells the program how to calculate pack years. Even though calculating pack years is something we can all do quickly in our head during an interview, it is a bit more complicated to tell a computer how to do this. The instructions tell the computer that if the subject has never smoked, the pack years are zero. If she currently smokes, pack years are computed by subtracting her current age from the age when she started and multiplying by the number of cigarettes smoked on average, and dividing the whole by the number in a pack (20). If she has quit, the year she quit must be subtracted from the year she started before doing this. Letting the computer do the math prevents math errors and forces the investigator to think out the logic of the variables that are being measured.

The next two sections in the table below are a list of the values of the variables, and of the results. This illustration is for a program which was preset to produce the mean, standard deviation, and range, with the missing values coded with 9's omitted from the statistics.

```
/PROBLEM        TITLE IS 'SMOKING DATA SET'.
/INPUT          VARIABLES = 8
                FORMAT IS FREE.
/VARIABLES         ADD=1. NAMES ARE ID, EverSmo, StartSmo, AvgCigs,
                   NowSmo, StopSmo, CigsNow, Age
                MISSING = 9999, 9, 99,99,9,99,99,99
                BLANKS ARE MISSING.
/TRANSFORM      IF (EverSmo=2) THEN PACKYRS=0
                IF (EverSmo=1) AND NowSmo=1) THEN
                   PACKYRS=(Age-StartSmo) *AvgCigs/20.
                IF (EverSmo=1 AND NowSmo=2) THEN
                   PACKYRS=(StopSmo-StartSmo) *AvgCigs/20
/PRINT LEVEL=MIN. LINE=80.
/END
```

SMOKING DATA SET   8/8/88   8:08 am

```
1,    1,13,40,1,99,20,55
2,    1,9,15,2,23,99,52
3,    2,99,99,9,99,99,52
4,    2,99,99,9,99,99,52
5,    1,22,10,1,99,10,44
6,    2,99,99,9,99,99,53
7,    2,99,99,9,99,99,52
8,    1,14,20,2,28,99,44
9,    1,12,20,1,99,35,43
10,   1,12,10,1,99,10,48
11,   2,99,99,9,99,99,47
12,   1,16,10,2,17,99,43
13,   2,99,99,9,99,99,42
14,   1,18,99,2,58,99,57
```

NUMBER OF CASES READ 14

VARIABLE NO. NAME VALUE	TOTAL FREQ.	MEAN	STANDARD DEVIATION	SMALLEST VALUE	LARGEST
1 ID	14	7.500	4.183	1.000	14.000
2 EverSmo	14	1.429	0.514	1.000	2.000
3 StartSmo	8	14.500	4.071	9.000	22.000
4 AvgCigs	7	17.857	10.746	10.000	40.000
5 NowSmo	8	1.500	0.535	1.000	2.000
6 StopSmo	4	31.500	18.230	17.000	58.000
7 CigsNow	4	18.750	11.815	10.000	35.000
8 Age	14	48.857	5.021	42.000	57.000
9 PACKYRS	12	14.042	24.125	0.000	84.000

APPENDIX 15B.
Classification of statistical analyses (and tests) by types of variables

The table below presents many of the most common approaches to analyzing (and testing the significance of) associations between a predictor and an outcome variable. The table is intended as an organizing tool for the reader who already has some familiarity with the philosophy and meaning of statistical analysis. The main point is that the choice of analytic approach (or test of significance) chiefly determined by the type of predictor and outcome variable (see also Chapters 4 and 12).

Predictor variable	Outcome Variable			
	Continuous, normally distributed	Continuous, not normally distributed, *or* Ordinal with > 2 categories	Nominal with > 2 categories	Dichotomous
Continuous, normally distributed	Correlation, Linear regression (F test)	*Spearman rank correlation*	Analysis of variance (F test)	Logistic regression (likelihood ratio test)
Continuous, not normally distributed, *or* Ordinal with > 2 categories	*Spearman rank correlation*	*Spearman rank correlation*	*Kruskall-Wallis*	*Wilcoxon rank sum*
Nominal with > 2 categories	Analysis of variance (F test)	*Kruskall-Wallis*	Contingency table (Chi-square test)	Contigency table (Chi-square test)
Dichotomous	Comparison of means (t test)	*Wilcoxon rank sum*	Contingency table (Chi-square test)	Contingency table (Chi-square test or z statistic for one tail)

Nonparametric tests, shown in italics, are tests that do not require that the data follow a specific distribution (e.g., normal).

Categorical variables are classified ordinal if the categories are ordered (e.g., classifying a heart murmur as grades I through VI), and nominal if they are not (e.g., classifying a heart murmur as aortic stenosis, mitral regurgitation, or functional).

APPENDIX 16.A.
Example of an operations manual table of contents based on the Systolic Hypertension in the Elderly Project (SHEP)

Chapter 1. Introductory summary
Specific objectives of the study
Study design

Chapter 2. Background and rationale

Chapter 3. Organization and policies
Participating units (clinical centers,
laboratories, coordinating center,
etc.)
Administration and governance
(committees, funding agency, safety
and data monitoring, etc.)
Policy concerns (publications and
presentations, ancillary studies, etc.)

Chapter 4. Recruitment
Eligibility and exclusion criteria
Sampling design
Recruitment approaches (publicity,
referral contacts, screening, etc.)
Informed consent

Chapter 5. Clinic visits
Content of baseline visit
Randomization procedures
Content and timing of followup visits
Followup procedures for non-
responders

Chapter 6. Predictor variables
Measurement procedures
Intervention protocol
Drug handling procedures
Assessment of compliance

Chapter 7. Outcome variables
Assessment and management of side-
effects
Assessment of fatal and non-fatal
cardiovascular events

Chapter 8. Quality control
Overview and responsibilities
Training in procedures
Certification in procedures
Equipment maintenance
Peer review and site visits
Periodic reports

Chapter 9. Data management and analysis
Data collection and recording
Data entry
Editing, storage, and backup
Confidentiality
Analysis plans

Appendices
Letters to subjects, primary providers,
etc.
Questionnaires, forms
Details on procedures, criteria, etc.

N.B. This is a model for a large multi-center study. The manual of operations for a small study can be less elaborate.

APPENDIX 16.B.
Quality control checklists[a]

I. Tabulations for monitoring performance characteristics:

A. Clinic characteristics

1. Patient recruitment

- Number of patients screened for enrollment; proportion rejected and tabulation of reasons for rejection*

- Current rate of recruitment compared with that required to achieve a pre-stated recruitment goal

2. Patient follow-up

- Distribution of enrollment times and median length of follow-up

- Number of completed follow-up examinations*

- Number of missed examinations*

- Total number of dropouts and estimated dropout rate*

- Number of patients who cannot be located for follow-up

3. Data quantity and quality

- Number of forms completed since last report and number that generated edit messages*

- Current edit message rate per form*

- Number of forms received with missing parts or missing supporting records*

- Number of unanswered edit queries*

4. Protocol adherence

- Number of ineligible patients enrolled*

- Number of patients who did not accept the assigned treatment*

- Number of patients who received a treatment other than the one assigned*

- Summary of data on pill counts and other adherence tests by treatment group*

- Number of departures from the treatment protocol*

B. Data center characteristics

- Number of random allocations issued*

- Number of allocations returned unused

- Number of forms received*

- Total number of forms awaiting data entry*

- List of coding and protocol changes implemented since last report

- List of data processing and programming errors and likely impact on study results

- Summary of major events, such as computing malfunctions necessitating use of backup tapes to restore the data system

- Timetable for unfinished tasks

C. Central laboratory characteristics

- Number of samples received*

- Number of samples received improperly or inadequately identified*

- Number of samples lost or destroyed*

- Number of samples requiring reanalysis and tabulation of reasons for reanalysis*

- Backlog of samples remaining to be analyzed*

- Summary of major events affecting laboratory operations, such as power outages, particularly those resulting in possible degradation of frozen samples

- Mean and variance of inter-aliquot differences over time for specified tests

- Secular trend analyses based on repeat determinations of known standards

---

[a]Reproduced in slightly revised form and with permission, from Meinert C: *Clinical Trials: Design, Conduct, and Analysis*, New York, Oxford University Press, 1986 pp 166–176.

D. Reading center characteristics

- Number of records received and read*

- Number of records received that were improperly labelled or had other deficiencies (tabulate deficiencies)*

- Analyses of repeat readings as a check on reproducibility of readings and as a means of monitoring for time shifts in the reading process

E. Other performance characteristics

- Status of papers being written

- Progress in locating patients lost to follow-up

- Labelling errors made in drugs dispensed from the central pharmacy

*Report should contain results for the entire study period, and for the time period covered since production of the last report. Rates and comparisons among centers should be provided when appropriate.

II. Site visit components:

A. Site visit to Clinical Center

- Private meeting of the site visitors with the clinic director

- Meeting of the site visitors with members of the clinic staff

- Inspection of examining and record storage facilities

- Comparison of data contained on selected data forms with those contained in the computer data file

- Review of file of data forms and related records to assess completeness and security against loss or misuse

- Observation of clinic personnel carrying out specified procedures

- Check of handbooks, manuals, forms, and other documents on file at the clinic to assess whether they are up-to-date

- Observation or verbal walk-through of certain procedures (e.g., the series of examinations needed to determine patient eligibility, or the components of the follow-up visits)

- Conversations with actual study patients during or after enrollment as a check on the informed consent process

- Private conversations with key support personnel to assess their practices and philosophy with regard to data collection

- Private meeting with the clinic director's chief concerning special issues

B. Site visit to Data Center

- Review of methods for inventorying forms received from clinics

- Review of methods for data entry and verification

- Assessment of the adequacy of methods for filing and storing paper records received from clinics, including the security of the storage area and methods for protecting records against loss or unauthorized use

- Review of available computing resources

- Review of method of randomization and of safeguards to protect against breakdowns in the randomization process

- Review of data editing procedures

- Review of computer data file structure and methods for maintaining the analysis database

- Review of programming methods both for data management and analysis, including an assessment of program documentation

- Comparison of information contained on original study forms with that in the computer data file

- Review of methods for generating analysis data files and related data reports

- Review of analysis philosophy

- Review of methods for backing up the main data file

- Review of methods for restoring the main data file or original study records if lost or destroyed

- Review of master file of key study documents, such as handbooks, manuals, data forms, minutes of study committees, etc., for completeness

APPENDIX 17.
NIH institutes and DRG study sections

I. NIH institutes (projected fiscal year 1987 budget, in millions):*

National Cancer Institute	($1,158)
National Heart, Lung, and Blood Institute	(786)
National Institute of Diabetes, and Digestive and Kidney Diseases	(419)
National Institute of General Medical Sciences	(472)
National Institute of Neuro, and Communicative Disorders and Stroke	(399)
National Institute of Allergy and Infectious Diseases	(331)
National Institute of Child Health and Human Development	(309)
National Institute of Environmental Health Sciences	(188)
National Eye Institute	(179)
National Institute on Aging	(146)
National Institute on Arthritis	(107)
National Institute of Dental Research	(97)

* In addition to the Institutes at NIH, there are also three Institutes heavily involved in extramural medical research funding in another agency of the Public Health Service, the Alcohol, Drug Abuse, and Mental Health Administration (ADAMHA). These are the National Institute on Drug Abuse (NIDA, $83), the National Institute on Mental Health (NIMH, $242), and the National Institute on Alcohol Abuse and Addiction (NIAAA, $68). In addition, there are other parts of the federal government which fund health-related research, notably the National Science Foundation (oriented toward basic science), and to a lesser extent the Centers for Disease Control (CDC, oriented to research on the delivery of public health measures). Research funding is also available from state and local agencies, and in small amounts from voluntary organizations like the American Heart Association and the American Cancer Society.

*II. NIH Division of Research Grants (DRG) study sections** *

Allergy and Immunology	Endocrinology
Bacteriology and mycology	Epidemiology and Disease Control
Behavioral and Neurosciences	Experimental Cardiovascular Sciences
Behavioral Medicine	Experimental immunology
Bio-Organic and Natural Products	Experimental Therapeutics
Chemistry	Experimental Virology
Biochemical Endrocrinology	General Medicine A
Biochemistry	Genetics
Biomedical Sciences	Hearing Research
Biophysical Chemistry	Hematology
Biopsychology	Human Development and Aging
Cardiovascular and Pulmonary	Human Embryology and Development
Cardiovascular and Renal	Immunobiology
Cellular Biology and Physiology	Immunological Sciences
Chemical Pathology	Mammalian Genetics
Clinical Sciences	Medicinal Chemistry
Diagnostic Radiology	Metabolism

Metallobiochemistry
Microbial Physiology and Genetics
Molecular and Cellular Biophysics
Molecular Biology
Molecular Cytology
Neurological Sciences
Neurology A
Nutrition
Oral Biology and Medicine
Orthopedics and Musculoskeletal
Pathobiochemistry
Pathology A
Pharmacology
Physical Biochemistry

Physiological Chemistry
Physiology
Radiation
Reproductive Biology
Respiratory and Applied Physiology
Sensory Disorders and Language
Social Sciences and Population
Surgery and Bioenginereing
Surgery, Anesthesiology and Trauma
Toxicology
Tropical Medicine and Parasitology
Virology
Visual Sciences B

** In addition to the study sections that are administered through the Division of Research Grants, there are also review groups within each of the NIH institutes (see reference (1)), and review groups within ADAMHA for the NIMH, the NIDA, and the NIAAA.

REFERENCE

1. Committee Management Staff: *NIH Public Advisory Groups: Authority, Structure, Function, Members*. U.S. Department of Health and Human Services, NIH Publication No. 86–10 October 1985.

APPENDIX 18.*
Are All Significant *P* Values Created Equal?

The Analogy Between Diagnostic Tests and Clinical Research

Warren S. Browner, MD, MPH, Thomas B. Newman, MD, MPH

Just as diagnostic tests are most helpful in light of the clinical presentation, statistical tests are most useful in the context of scientific knowledge. Knowing the specificity and sensitivity of a diagnostic test is necessary, but insufficient: the clinician must also estimate the prior probability of the disease. In the same way, knowing the *P* value and power, or the confidence interval, for the results of a research study is necessary but insufficient: the reader must estimate the prior probability that the research hypothesis is true. Just as a positive diagnostic test does not mean that a patient has the disease, especially if the clinical picture suggests otherwise, a significant *P* value does not mean that a research hypothesis is correct, especially if it is inconsistent with current knowledge. Powerful studies are like sensitive tests in that they can be especially useful when the results are negative. Very low *P* values are like very specific tests; both result in few false-positive results due to chance. This Bayesian approach can clarify much of the confusion surrounding the use and interpretation of statistical tests.

(*JAMA* 1987;257:2459-2463)

IN THE four ORIGINAL CONTRIBUTIONS in this issue of THE JOURNAL, the authors report the results of statistical tests of 76 hypotheses.[1-4] Of these, 32 had significant *P* values (*P*<.05). But do these *P* values imply that the 32 hypotheses are true? Or that 95% of them are true? Are all significant *P* values created equal?

The answer to these questions is "No!" What then is a *P* value? It is the likelihood of observing the study results under the assumption that the null hypothesis of no difference is true. Probably because this definition is elusive and intimidating, understanding *P* values (and other statistical concepts like power, confidence intervals, and multiple hypothesis testing) is often left to experts in the field. It is easier just to check whether a *P* value is .05 or less, call the result "statistically significant," regard the tested hypothesis as probably true, and move on to the next paragraph.

Readers of medical literature need not give up quite so quickly, however. As Diamond and Forrester[5] pointed out, many statistical concepts have remarkably similar analogues in an area famil-

From the Departments of Medicine (Dr Browner), Pediatrics (Dr Newman), and Epidemiology and International Health (Drs Browner and Newman), School of Medicine, University of California at San Francisco, and the Clinical Epidemiology Program, Institute for Health Policy Studies, San Francisco (Drs Browner and Newman).

Reprint requests to the Division of General Internal Medicine 111A1, Veterans Administration Medical Center, San Francisco, CA 94121 (Dr Browner).

iar to clinicians—the interpretation of diagnostic tests. In the diagnosis of Cushing's syndrome, for example, most clinicians recognize that an elevated serum cortisol level is more useful than an elevated blood glucose level, and that an elevated cortisol level is more likely to be due to Cushing's syndrome in a moon-faced patient with a buffalo hump and abdominal striae than in an overweight patient with hypertension.[6,7] Why? Because the interpretation of a test result depends on the characteristics of both the test and the patient being tested.[8-13]

The same type of reasoning—called *Bayesian analysis* after Thomas Bayes, the mathematician who developed it more than 200 years ago[14]—can also be used to clarify the meaning of the *P* value and other statistical terms. Although this application of Bayes' ideas has been discussed in epidemiologic and statistical literature,[15-18] it has received less attention in the journals read by clinicians. In this article, we begin with the basic aspects of the analogy between research studies and diagnostic tests, such as the similarity between the power of a study and the sensitivity of a test, and then examine more challenging issues, such as how a study with multiple hypotheses resembles a serum chemistry panel.

THE ANALOGY

An overview of the analogy between research studies and diagnostic tests is shown in Table 1. In this analogy, a

clinician obtains diagnostic data to test for the presence of a disease, such as breast cancer, and an investigator collects study data to determine the truth of a *research hypothesis*, such as that the efficacies of two drugs differ in the treatment of peptic ulcer disease. (The research hypothesis is often called the *alternative hypothesis* in standard terminology.) The absence of a *disease* (no breast cancer) is like the *null hypothesis* of no difference in the efficacy of the two drugs.

The term "positive" is used in its usual sense: to refer to diagnostic tests that are consistent with the presence of the disease and to studies that have statistically significant results. Similarly, "negative" refers to diagnostic tests consistent with the absence of disease and research results that fail to reach statistical significance. Thus there are four possible results whenever a patient undergoes a diagnostic test. Consider the use of fine-needle aspiration in the evaluation of a breast mass, for example (Table 2). If the patient has breast cancer, there are two possibilities: the test result can either be correctly positive or incorrectly negative. On the other hand, if the patient actually does not have cancer, then the result will either be correctly negative or incorrectly positive. Similarly, there are four possible results whenever an investigator studies a research hypothesis (Table 3). If the efficacies of the two drugs really do differ, there are two possibilities: the study can be correctly positive if it finds a difference or incorrectly negative if it

Table 1.—The Analogy Between Diagnostic Tests and Research Studies

Diagnostic Test	Research Study
Absence of disease	Truth of null hypothesis
Presence of disease	Truth of research (alternative) hypothesis
Positive result (outside normal limits)	Positive result (reject null hypothesis)
Negative result (within normal limits)	Negative result (fail to reject null hypothesis)
Sensitivity	Power
False-positive rate (1 − specificity)	*P* value
Prior probability of disease	Prior probability of research hypothesis
Predictive value of a positive (or negative) test result	Predictive value of a positive (or negative) study

Table 2.—The Four Possible Results of a Diagnostic Test

		If Breast Mass is Actually:	
		Malignant	**Benign**
And Result of Fine-Needle Aspirate is:	**Positive**	This is a true-positive test: result is correct	This is a false-positive test: result is incorrect
	Negative	This is a false-negative test: result is incorrect	This is a true-negative test: result is correct

Table 3.—The Four Possible Results of a Research Study

		If Research Hypothesis is Actually:	
		True (Efficacy of Drug A and Drug B Differ in Treatment of Ulcer Disease)	**False** (Drug A Has Same Efficacy as Drug B in Treatment of Ulcer Disease)
And Result of Study is:	**Positive**	This is a true-positive study: result is correct	This is a false-positive study: result is incorrect
	Negative	This is a false-negative study: result is incorrect	This is a true-negative study: result is correct

misses the difference. If the two drugs actually have the same efficacy, then the study can either be correctly negative if it finds no difference or incorrectly positive if it does find one.

The relationships between the four possible outcomes of a diagnostic test are usually expressed as the *sensitivity* and *specificity* of the test, which are determined by assuming that the presence or absence of the disease is known. Sensitivity is the likelihood that a test result will be positive in a patient with the disease. Specificity is the likelihood that a test result will be negative in a patient without the disease. If the result from a fine-needle aspiration is positive in 80 of 100 women with breast cancer, and negative in 95 of 100 women without cancer, the test would have a sensitivity of 80% and a specificity of 95%. There is another term that is useful in the analogy: the false-positive rate (1 − specificity), which is the likelihood that a test result will be (falsely) positive in someone without the disease. In this example, the false-positive rate is 5%: of 100 women without breast cancer, five will have falsely positive test results.

Similarly, the relationships between the four possible outcomes of a research study are usually expressed as the *power* and *P value* of the study, which are determined by assuming that the truth or falsity of the null hypothesis is known. Power is the likelihood of a study being positive if the research hypothesis is true (and the null hypothesis is false); it is analogous to the sensitivity of a diagnostic test. The *P* value is the likelihood of a study being positive when the null hypothesis is true; it is analogous to the false-positive rate (1 − specificity) of a diagnostic test. A study comparing two drugs in the treatment of ulcers that has an 80% chance of being correctly positive if

there really is a difference in their efficacies would have a power of 0.80. A study with a 5% chance of being incorrectly positive if there is no difference between the drugs would have a *P* value of .05. (Conventionally, when the *P* value is less than a certain predetermined "level of statistical significance," usually .01 or .05, the results are said to be "statistically significant.")

Knowing the sensitivity and specificity of a test is not sufficient, however, to interpret its results: that interpretation also depends on the characteristics of the patient being tested. If the patient is a 30-year-old woman with several soft breast masses, a positive result from a fine-needle aspiration (even with a false-positive rate of only 5%) would not suffice to make a diagnosis of cancer. Similarly, if the patient is a 60-year-old woman with a firm solitary breast mass, a negative aspirate result (with a sensitivity of 80%) would not rule out malignancy.[19] Clinicians use these sorts of patient characteristics to estimate the *prior probability* of the disease—the likelihood that the patient has the disease, made prior to knowing the test results. The prior probability of a disease is based on the history and physical findings, previous experience with similar patients, and knowledge of alternative diagnostic explanations. It can be very high (breast cancer in the 60-year-old woman with a single firm mass), very low (breast cancer in the younger woman), or somewhere in between. Although they may not realize it, clinicians express prior probabilities when using phrases such as "a low index of suspicion" or "a strong clinical impression."

In the same way, knowing the power and the *P* value of a study is not sufficient to determine the truth of the research hypothesis. That determination also depends on the characteristics of the hypothesis being studied. Suppose

one drug is diphenhydramine hydrochloride (Benadryl) and the other is chlorpheniramine maleate (Chlor-Trimeton): a positive study (at $P = .05$) would not ensure that one of the drugs is effective in the treatment of ulcers. Similarly, if one drug was ranitidine hydrochloride (Zantac) and the other a placebo, a negative study (even with power of 0.80) would not establish the ineffectiveness of ranitidine. The characteristics of a research hypothesis determine its prior probability—an estimate of the likelihood that the hypothesis is true, made prior to knowing the study results. The prior probability of a hypothesis is based on biologic plausibility, previous experience with similar hypotheses, and knowledge of alternative scientific explanations. Analogous to the situation with diagnostic tests, the prior probability of a research hypothesis can be very high (that an H_2-blocker, such as ranitidine, is more effective than placebo in the treatment of ulcers), very low (that the efficacies of two H_1-blockers, such as diphenhydramine and chlorpheniramine, differ in the treatment of ulcer disease), or somewhere in between. Authors of research reports indicate prior probabilities with terms like "unanticipated" or "expected" when they discuss their results.

The advantage of Bayesian analysis in interpreting diagnostic tests is that it can determine what the clinician really wants to know—the likelihood that the patient has the disease, given a certain test result. Bayesian analysis combines the characteristics of the patient (expressed as the prior probability of disease), the characteristics of the test (expressed as sensitivity and specificity), and the test result (positive or negative) to determine the predictive value of a test result. The *predictive value of a positive diagnostic test* is the probability that given a positive result, the patient actually has the disease. (The *predictive value of a negative test* is the probability that given a negative result, the patient does not have the disease.)

As an example, recall the 60-year-old woman with a firm breast mass. The prior probability that the mass is malignant is moderate, say 50%. A positive result from a fine-needle aspirate (with a specificity of 95% and a sensitivity of 80% for cancer) results in a very high predictive value for malignancy, about 94% (Figure). Next, consider the 30-year-old woman with multiple soft masses. The prior probability of cancer is low, say 1%. Even given a positive aspirate result, the likelihood that she has breast cancer is still small (about 14%).

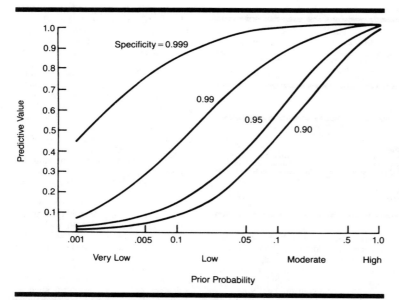

Relationship between prior probability and predictive value of positive result of diagnostic test with sensitivity of 0.80, at several specificities. Figure can also be used to estimate predictive value of positive research study with power of 0.80 by substituting (1 – P value) for specificity, and prior probability of hypothesis for prior probability of disease (see "Limitations" section).

A Bayesian approach can also be used to determine what the reader of a research study really wants to know—the likelihood that the research hypothesis is true, given the study results. It combines the characteristics of the hypothesis (expressed as prior probability), the characteristics of the study (expressed as power and the P value), and the study results (positive or negative) to determine the predictive value of a study. The *predictive value of a positive study* is the probability that a positive result, the research hypothesis is actually true. (The *predictive value of a negative study* is the probability that given a negative result, the research hypothesis is false.)

The predictive value of a research study, however, is usually harder to estimate than the predictive value of a diagnostic test (see "Limitations" section). Nonetheless, the basic analogy remains valid: the prior probability of the hypothesis must be combined with the power and the P value of the study to determine the likelihood that the research hypothesis is true. In the next section, we discuss how this analogy can be used to understand several statistical concepts.

IMPLICATIONS
Specificity and the P Value

How low must a P value be for it to be accepted as evidence of the truth of a

research hypothesis? This question is analogous to asking: how high must the specificity of a test be to accept a positive test result as evidence of a disease? Requiring that a P value be less than .05 before it is "significant" is as arbitrary as requiring that a diagnostic test have a specificity of at least 95%. A more important criterion, but one that is not as easy to quantitate, is whether the results of the study combined with the prior probability of the research hypothesis are sufficient to suggest that the hypothesis is true. Consider the hypothesis, tested in the Lipid Research Clinics Primary Prevention Trial,[20] that cholestyramine resin decreases the incidence of coronary heart disease in hypercholesterolemic men. This research hypothesis had at least a low to moderate prior probability, based on previous evidence. Even with a "nonsignificant" P value of .094 (the two-sided equivalent of the controversial one-sided P = .047 reported by the investigators), the hypothesis is likely to be true.

It is also a mistake to *believe* a research hypothesis just because a P value *is* statistically significant. Consider a study that found that drinking two or more cups of coffee a day was associated with pancreatic cancer (P < .05).[21] This hypothesis had a very low prior probability: the authors called the association "unexpected." Thus,

finding a significant P value did not establish the truth of the hypothesis; subsequent studies, including one by the same authors, failed to confirm the association.[22-27]

Of course, many diagnostic test results are not simply reported as "positive"; they also indicate how abnormal the result is. The more abnormal that result, the less likely that it is just a chance finding in a normal person. If the upper limit of normal for a serum thyroxine level at a specificity of 95% is 12.0 μg/dL (154 nmol/L), then a thyroxine level of 18.0 μg/L (232 nmol/L) is almost certainly abnormal. The question becomes whether it represents hyperthyroidism, another disease, or a laboratory error. By analogy, if the cutoff for calling a study positive is a P value less than .05, then a P value of .0001 means chance is an extremely unlikely explanation for the findings. The question becomes whether the results indicate the truth of the research hypothesis or are a result of confounding or bias (see "Laboratory Error and Bias" and "Alternative Diagnoses and Confounding Explanations" sections). Because the P value is analogous to the false-positive rate (1 – specificity), a study with a very low P value is like a test with very high specificity: both give few false-positive results due to chance, but may require careful consideration of other possible explanations.

Sensitivity and Power

When the result of a diagnostic test that has a high sensitivity is negative, such as a urinalysis in the diagnosis of pyelonephritis, it is especially useful for ruling out a disease. Similarly, when a powerful research study is negative, it strongly suggests that the research hypothesis is false. However, if the sensitivity of a test is low, such as a sputum smear in a patient with possible tuberculosis, then a negative result does not rule out the disease.[9] In the same way, a negative study with inadequate power cannot disprove a research hypothesis.[28,29]

Laboratory Error and Bias

When unexpected or incredible results on a diagnostic test are found, such as a serum potassium level of 9.0 mEq/L (mmol/L) in an apparently well person, the first possibility to consider is laboratory error: Was the test adequately performed? Did the sample hemolyze? Was the specimen mislabeled? Similarly, readers of a research study, such as a trial of biofeedback in the treatment of hypertension, must always consider the possibility of bias, especially if the study yields surprising results: Was the study adequately designed and executed? Did the investigators assign subjects randomly? Was blood pressure measured blindly?[30] Improperly performed tests and biased studies do not yield reliable information, no matter how specific or significant their results.

Alternative Diagnoses and Confounding Explanations

Even if a diagnostic test is adequately performed, there may be several explanations for the result. An elevated serum amylase level, for example, has a high specificity to distinguish patients who have pancreatitis from those with nonspecific abdominal pain. However, there are extrapancreatic diseases (such as bowel infarction) that elevate the amylase level and that must be considered in the differential diagnosis. In the same way, although a low P value may indicate an association between an exposure and a disease (like the association between carrying matches and lung cancer), a confounder (cigarette smoking) may actually be responsible. Readers of research studies should always keep in mind potential confounding explanations for significant P values.

Better Tests and Bigger Studies

Increasing the sample size in a research study is similar to using a better diagnostic test. Better diagnostic tests can have more sensitivity or specificity or both; large studies can have greater power or lower levels of statistical significance or both. Often the choice of a diagnostic test is a matter of practicality: biopsies are not feasible in every patient for every disease. Similarly, power or the significance level may be determined by practical considerations, since studies of 20 000 or more subjects cannot be done for every research question. Of course, bigger studies may find smaller differences, just like better tests may detect less advanced cases of a disease. A small but statistically significant difference in a research study is like a subtle but definite abnormality on a diagnostic test; its importance is a matter of judgment.

Intentionally Ordered Tests and Prospective Hypotheses

A positive result on a single intentionally ordered test is more likely to indicate disease than the same result that turns up on a set of routine admission laboratory tests. Similarly, the P value for a research hypothesis stated in advance of a study is usually more meaningful than the same P value for a hypothesis generated by the data. The reason is that clinicians usually order tests and investigators state hypotheses in advance when the prior probability is moderate or high. Thus the

predictive values of positive results are generally greater for intentionally ordered tests and prospectively stated hypotheses.

Not all unexpected results, however, have low prior probabilities. Occasionally, clinicians or investigators are just not smart or lucky enough to consider the diagnosis or hypothesis in advance. For example, a house officer caring for a patient with fatigue and vague abdominal symptoms might ignore a serum calcium level of 10.5 mg/dL (2.62 mmol/L) until the attending physician mentions the possibility of hyperparathyroidism in rounds the next morning. Similarly, researchers might disregard the association between smoking and cervical cancer until a plausible biologic explanation is suggested.[31-34] Estimating the prior probability of a hypothesis on the basis of whether it was considered prospectively is a useful, but not infallible, method. The truth, elusive though it sometimes may be, does not depend on when a hypothesis is first formulated.

Multiple Tests and Multiple Hypotheses

Most of us are intuitively skeptical when one of 50 substances on a checklist is associated with a disease at $P<.05$ because of the likelihood of finding such an association by chance alone. A standard technique for dealing with this problem of testing multiple hypotheses is to use a more stringent level of statistical significance, thus requiring a lower P value.[35,36] This approach is simple and practical, but it leads to some unsatisfying situations. It seems unfair, for example, to reduce the required significance level for a reasonable hypothesis just because other, perhaps ridiculous, hypotheses were also tested. What if the disease was mesothelioma and one of the exposures was asbestos: should a more stringent level of statistical significance be required because 49 other substances were also included? Should the level of significance be reduced when testing the main hypothesis of a study whenever additional hypotheses are considered? Need statistical adjustments for multiple hypothesis testing be made only when reporting all of the hypotheses in a single publication?

This vexing problem of multiple hypothesis testing resembles the interpretation of a serum chemistry panel. When a clinician evaluates a patient with a swollen knee, a serum uric acid level of 10.0 mg/dL (0.6 mmol/L) has the same meaning no matter how many other tests were also performed on the specimen by the autoanalyzer. However, an unanticipated abnormal value on another test in the panel is likely to

be a false-positive: that is because the diseases it might represent usually have low prior probabilities, *not* because several tests were performed on the same sample of serum. Similarly, testing multiple hypotheses in a single study causes problems because the prior probabilities of such hypotheses tend to be low: when investigators are not sure of what they are looking for, they test many possibilities. The solution is to recognize that it is not the number of hypotheses tested, but the prior probability of each of them, that determines whether a result is meaningful.[37]

Confirmatory Tests and Pooled Studies

When a single diagnostic test is insufficient to make a diagnosis, additional tests are often ordered, some results of which may be positive and some negative. The clinician revises the probability of the disease by combining these results, often weighting them by the tests' characteristics. In a patient with a swollen leg, for example, a normal result from a Doppler study would lower the probability of deep venous thrombosis, but an abnormal result of a fibrinogen scan might raise it sufficiently to make the diagnosis. In the same way, it may be necessary to combine the results of several research studies, weighting them by the characteristics of each study. This process, known as *pooling*, allows studies with both significant and nonsignificant P values to change incrementally the likelihood that a research hypothesis is true. However, just as only those tests that are relevant to the diagnosis in question should be combined, only those research studies that address the same research hypothesis should be pooled.

Confidence Intervals

There is no ready diagnostic test analogy for confidence intervals from research studies (the concept of test precision comes closest). But because confidence intervals are commonly misinterpreted as expressions of predictive value, they merit a short discussion. The term "confidence interval" is unfortunate, because it leads many people to believe that they can be confident that the interval contains the true value being estimated. Actually, confidence intervals are determined entirely by the study data: the prior probability that the true value lies within that interval is not at all considered in the calculations. A 95% confidence interval is simply the range of values that would *not* differ from the estimate provided by the study at a statistical significance level of .05.[38,39]

Confidence intervals are useful because they define the upper and lower limits consistent with a study's data. But they do not estimate the likelihood that the results of the research are correct. A confidence interval provides no more information about the likelihood of chance as an explanation for a finding than does a P value.[40] As an example, suppose a well-designed study finds that joggers are twice as likely as nonjoggers to develop coronary heart disease, with a 95% confidence interval for the relative risk of 1.01 to 3.96. (This is equivalent to rejecting the null hypothesis of no association between jogging and heart disease at $P = .05$.) Despite a 95% confidence interval that excludes 1.0, there is obviously not a 95% likelihood that joggers are at an increased risk of coronary heart disease. There are many other studies that have found that exercise is associated with a reduced risk of heart disease. Given the low prior probability of the hypothesis that jogging increases the risk of coronary heart disease, chance (or perhaps bias) would be a more likely explanation for the results.

LIMITATIONS

While it provides several useful insights, the analogy between diagnostic tests and clinical research is not perfect. It is easier to determine the prior probability of a disease, based on the prevalence of the disease in similar patients, than the prior probability of a hypothesis, based on the prevalence of the truth of similar hypotheses. Similarity in patients can be defined by characteristics known to be associated with a disease, such as age, sex, and symptoms.[11] But what defines similar hypotheses? Thus the prior probability of most research hypotheses tends to be a subjective estimate (although, in practice, estimates of the prior probability of a disease are generally subjective as well).

Second, as long as there is a gold standard for its diagnosis, a disease is either present or absent: there are only these two possibilities. If a group of patients known to have the disease is assembled, a single value for the sensitivity of a test can be determined empirically. But there is no single value for the power of a research study: it depends on the sample size, as well as the magnitude of the actual difference between the groups being compared. A study comparing IQ in internists and surgeons, for example, might have a power of only 50% to detect a difference between them if surgeons actually scored five points higher than internists, but a power of 98% if surgeons actually scored ten points higher. Since the actual difference is unknown, a

unique value for power cannot be calculated.

CONCLUSIONS

Clinicians do not simply decide that a patient has a disease when a diagnostic test result is positive or rule out the disease when the test result is negative. They also consider the sensitivity and specificity of the test and the characteristics of the patient being tested. In the same way, readers should not believe or disbelieve the research hypothesis of a study on the basis of whether the results were statistically significant. They should also take into account the study's power and P value and the characteristics of the hypothesis being tested.

Thus, all significant P values are not created equal. Just as the accuracy of a diagnosis depends on how well the clinician has estimated the prior probability and considered alternative diagnoses and laboratory errors, the interpretation of a research study depends on how well the reader has estimated the prior probability and considered confounders and biases. Knowing the power and P value (or the confidence interval) for a study's results, like knowing the sensitivity and specificity of a diagnostic test, is necessary but not sufficient. This Bayesian approach requires the active participation of the reader and emphasizes the importance of scientific context in the interpretation of research.

This project was supported by a grant from the Andrew W. Mellon Foundation.

References

1. Schade DS, Mitchell WJ, Griego G: Addition of sulfonylurea to insulin treatment in poorly controlled type II diabetes: A double-blind, randomized clinical trial. JAMA 1987;257:2441-2445.
2. Cramer DW, Goldman MB, Schiff I, et al: The relationship of tubal infertility to oral contraceptive use. JAMA 1987;257:2446-2450.
3. Bennett KJ, Sackett DL, Haynes RB, et al: A controlled trial of teaching critical appraisal of the clinical literature to medical students. JAMA 1987;257:2451-2454.
4. Chaiken BP, Williams NM, Preblud SR, et al: The effect of a school entry law on mumps activity in a school district. JAMA 1987;257:2455-2458.
5. Diamond GA, Forrester JS: Clinical trials and statistical verdicts: Probable grounds for appeal. Ann Intern Med 1983;98:385-394.
6. Nugent CA, Warner HR, Dunn JT, et al: Probability theory in the diagnosis of Cushing's syndrome. J Clin Endocrinol Metab 1964;24:621-627.
7. Crapo L: Cushing's syndrome: A review of diagnostic tests. Metabolism 1979;28:955-977.
8. Vecchio TJ: Predictive value of a single diagnostic test in unselected populations. N Engl J Med 1966;274:1171-1173.
9. Boyd JC, Marr JJ: Decreasing reliability of acid-fast smear techniques for detection of tuberculosis. Ann Intern Med 1975;82:489-492.
10. Jones RB: Bayes' theorem, the exercise ECG, and coronary artery disease. JAMA 1979;242:1067-1068.
11. Diamond GA, Forrester JS: Analysis of probability as an aid in the clinical diagnosis of coronary-artery disease. N Engl J Med 1979;300:1350-1358.

12. Griner PF, Mayewski RJ, Mushlin AI, et al: Selection and interpretation of diagnostic tests and procedures: Principles and applications. Ann Intern Med 1981;94:553-600.
13. Havey RJ, Krumlovsky F, delGreco F, et al: Screening for renovascular hypertension: Is renal digital-subtraction angiography the preferred noninvasive test? JAMA 1985;254:388-393.
14. Bayes T: An essay towards solving a problem in the doctrine of chances. Philos Trans R Soc Lond 1763;53:370-418.
15. Phillips LD: Bayesian Statistics for Social Scientists. New York, Crowell, 1974.
16. Donner A: A Bayesian approach to the interpretation of subgroup results in clinical trials. J Chronic Dis 1982;35:429-435.
17. Pater JL, Willan AR: Clinical trials as diagnostic tests. Controlled Clin Trials 1984;5:107-113.
18. Thomas DC, Siemiatycki J, Dewar R, et al: The problem of multiple inferences in studies designed to generate hypotheses. Am J Epidemiol 1985;122:1080-1095.
19. Mushlin AI: Diagnostic tests in breast cancer: Clinical strategies based on diagnostic probabilities. Ann Intern Med 1985;103:79-85.
20. Lipid Research Clinics Program: The Lipid Research Clinics Coronary Primary Prevention Trial results: I. Reduction in incidence of coronary heart disease. JAMA 1984;251:351-364.
21. MacMahon B, Yen S, Trichopolous D, et al: Coffee and cancer of the pancreas. N Engl J Med 1981;304:630-633.
22. Jick H, Dinan BJ: Coffee and pancreatic cancer. Lancet 1981;2:92.
23. Goldstein HR: No association found between coffee and cancer of the pancreas. N Engl J Med 1982;306:997.
24. Wynder EL, Hall NEL, Polansky M: Epidemiology of coffee and pancreatic cancer. Cancer Res 1983;43:3900-3906.
25. Kinlen LJ, McPherson K: Pancreas cancer and coffee and tea consumption: A case-control study. Br J Cancer 1984;49:93-96.
26. Gold EB, Gordis L, Diener MD, et al: Diet and other risk factors for cancer of the pancreas. Cancer 1985;55:460-467.
27. Hsieh C, MacMahon B, Yen S, et al: Coffee and pancreatic cancer (chapter 2). N Engl J Med 1986;315:587-589.
28. Frieman JA, Chalmers TC, Smith H Jr, et al: The importance of beta, type II errors and sample size in the randomized control trial: Survey of 71 'negative' trials. N Engl J Med 1978;299:690-694.
29. Young MJ, Bresnitz EA, Strom BL: Sample size nomograms for interpreting negative clinical studies. Ann Intern Med 1983;99:248-251.
30. Sackett DL: Bias in analytic research. J Chronic Dis 1979;32:51-63.
31. Winkelstein W Jr: Smoking and cancer of the uterine cervix: Hypothesis. Am J Epidemiol 1977;106:257-259.
32. Wright NH, Vessey MP, Kenward B, et al: Neoplasia and dysplasia of the cervix uteri and contraception: A possible protective effect of the diaphragm. Br J Cancer 1978;38:273-279.
33. Harris RWC, Brinton LA, Cowdell RH, et al: Characteristics of women with dysplasia or carcinoma in situ of the cervix uteri. Br J Cancer 1980;42:359-369.
34. Lyon JL, Gardner JW, West DW, et al: Smoking and carcinoma in situ of the uterine cervix. Am J Public Health 1983;73:558-562.
35. Godfrey K: Comparing the means of several groups. N Engl J Med 1985;313:1450-1456.
36. Cupples LA, Heeren T, Schatzkin A, et al: Multiple testing of hypotheses in comparing two groups. Ann Intern Med 1984;100:122-129.
37. Cole P: The evolving case-control study. J Chronic Dis 1979;32:15-27.
38. Fleiss JL: Statistical Methods for Rates' and Proportions, ed 2. New York, John Wiley & Sons Inc, 1981, p 14.
39. Rothman KJ: A show of confidence. N Engl J Med 1978;299:1362-1363.
40. Browner WS, Newman TB: Confidence intervals. Ann Intern Med 1986;105:973-974.

Index

Page numbers in *italics* denote figures; those followed by "t" denote tables.

Accuracy, 36–39. *See also* Measurement
Adjustment, 107
 advantages, 107
 disadvantages, 107
 example, 208–209
Alpha, 132–133, 139–143, 147–148

Beta, 132–133, 139–143, 147–148
Bias. *See also* Errors
 attribution, 38
 avoiding spurious associations due to, 99t,
   98–101, *100*
  analysis phase strategies, 101
  design phase strategies, 102, 103t
 differential, 37
  controlling in case-control studies, 83
 instrument, 34, 37
 measurement, 94–95
 observer, 36
 prevalence/incidence, 78
 reporting, 95
 sampling, 93
  controlling in case-control studies, 81–83
 subject, 34, 36
 survivor, 70
Blinding, 37–38
 attribution bias, 38
 in case-control studies, 83t, 83–84
  as to case-control status, 83
  as to risk factor being studied, 84
 in diagnostic test studies, 87
 differential bias, 37–38
 ethical considerations, 155–156. *See also* Ethics in
   research
 partial, 122
 quality control
  of drug interventions, 177
  of laboratory procedures, 177
 randomized blinded trial, 87, *111*, 111–122. *See
   also* Experimental studies
 single- vs. double-blind strategies, 37
 triple blind strategy, 118
BMDP statistical program, 166
 example of use, 224–225

Case-control studies, *78*, 78–84
 definition, 75
 designing, 79, 204–205
  odds ratio, 80, 142, 206
 ruling out effect-cause, 101

strengths, 80
 efficiency for rare outcomes, 80
 generating hypotheses, 80
structure, 78–79
summary, 84
use of multiple controls per case, 149
weaknesses, 80–84
 controlling differential measurement bias, 83
  by blinding, 83t, 83–84
   as to case-control status, 83–84
   as to risk factor being studied, 83–84
  by use of data recorded before the outcome
    occurred, 83
 controlling sampling bias, 80–82, *81*
  by selection of cases, 81
  by selection of controls, 81–82
   matching, 82
   sampling cases and controls in same way,
     81–82
   using a population-based sample, 82
   using two or more control groups, 82
 increased susceptibility to bias, 80
Categorical variables. *See* Variables
Causal inference. *See* Inference, causal
Cause-effect relationship. *See* Inference, causal
Chi square test, 119, 141
Coefficient of variation, 34
Cohort studies, 63–74
 analysis, 73–74
  choice of statistical tests and models, 73
  incidence of outcomes, 73
  relative risk statistics, 73, 142
 double-cohort studies and external controls, 69,
   71
  selecting subjects, 71
  strengths, 69
  structure, 68–69
  weaknesses, 69
 experiments. *See* Experimental studies
 following subjects, 71, 72t
 measuring outcomes, 73
 nested case-control designs, *67*, 67–68
  strengths, 68
  structure, 68–69
  weaknesses, 68
 planning, 69–74
  choosing among cohort designs, 70–71
  measuring predictor and confounding
    variables, 71
  selecting subjects, 71

239

Cohort studies, planning—*continued*
  when to use a cohort design, 69–70
    avoiding survivor bias, 70
    describing incidence and natural history of
      condition, 70
    establishing temporal sequence of variables,
      70
    studying numerous outcome variables,
      70
  prospective, 63, 63–65
    definition, 63
    strengths, 64–65
      measurement of confounding variables, 65
      studying antecedents of fatal diseases, 64, 65
    structure, 63, 64, *64*
      internal vs. external control groups, 64
    weaknesses, 65
  purposes, 63
    analytic, 63
    descriptive, 63
  retrospective, 63, 65–67, *66*
    strengths, 66
    structure, 65–66
    weaknesses, 65–67
  ruling out effect-cause, 102
  summary, 73–74
  variations, 63
Collaborative studies, 180
  governance of study, 180
  use of distributed data processing systems, 180
Computers. *See also* Data analysis; Data
    management
  data storage on floppy discs vs. hard disc,
    165–166
  mainframe vs. microcomputers, 160–161
  software
    for data analysis, 166
    for data entry, 161–164
Confidence intervals, 93, 144, 145, 169
Confidence levels, 144–145
Confidentiality, 154. *See also* Ethics in research
Confounding, 102, 207
Confounding variables. *See* Variables
Consent. *See also* Ethics in research
  constrained, 152–153
  informed, 153–154
    checklist, 223
    sample form, 221–222
Continuous variables. *See* Variables
Correlation coefficient, 34–35, 143
  sample size required per group, 218
Cox regression analysis, 119
Cross-sectional studies, 2, 3, 75–78
  definition, 75
  designing, 76–77
    prevalence, 76–77, 77t
    relative prevalence, 77
  ruling out effect-cause, 102
  strengths, 77
  structure, 75–76, *76*
    describing variables, 75
    examining associations, 75–76
  weaknesses, 77–78
    prevalence/incidence bias, 78
Cutoff point, determining, 89–90, *90*

Data analysis
  interpreting results, 166–170, 168t

analytic statistics, 168t, 168–169
  with other predictor and outcome variables,
    170, 226
  with two categorical variables, 168t, 168–170
    confidence interval, 169
    two-by-two table, 168
  with two continuous variables, 169
    scatterplot, 169, *169*
descriptive statistics, 166–168
  freezing data set, 167
  frequency distribution, 167, *167*
  parametric vs. nonparametric statistics, 168
secondary data sets, 53–62
  advantages and disadvantages, 53
  choice of approach, 57–60
    finding data sets to fit a research question,
      58–60, 59t
    finding research questions to fit the data,
      57–58, 58t
  definition, 53
  fixed sample size, 145–146
  summary, 61
  types of, 53–57, 55t–56t
    aggregate, 53–54
      ecological fallacy, 54
      use of hospital discharge records, 54
      use of published statistics, 54–55
    individual, 55–57
      data previously collected at same
        institution, 55
      death certificate registries, 56–57
      large regional and national data sets, 55
      National Death Index, 56–57
      tumor registries, 56
  types of study design, 60
statistical analysis system, 166–169
  software programs, 167 for mainframe, 166
    example of use of DMDP system, 224–
      225
    for microcomputers, 166
  summary, 170–171
tertiary data sets, 60–61
  definition, 60
  pros and cons of pooling data, 60–61
Data management, 159–166
  computers, 161
    mainframe vs. microcomputers, 161
  data entry, 161–164, 162t, 163t, 179
    data base programs, 163–165
      advantages, 164–165
      disadvantages, 165
    rules for, 160
      coding the variables, 160, 161t
      editing data, 162, 179
    spreadsheet programs, 161–162, 162t
      disadvantages, 163
      logic checks, 162
      range checks, 162
    statistical programs, 164
  designing system, 164–166, *165*
    pretesting, 173t, 178
  storage on floppy discs vs. hard disc, 165–166
  use of study log, 166
  quality control, 177–180, 179t. *See also* Quality
    control
Department of Health and Human Services
    guidelines for human research, 151–154,
    152t

exemptions from, 155, 155t
Design of study, 5–6
    case-control studies, 78–84. *See also* Case-control
        studies
    choice of subjects, 6, 18–30. *See also* Subjects
    choice of variables, 6–7
    choosing among designs, 84, 85
    classifying, 3–4
    cohort studies, 63–74. *See also* Cohort studies
    cross-sectional studies, 2, 3, 75–78. *See also* Cross-
        sectional studies
    diagnostic test studies, 87–97. *See also* Diagnostic
        test studies
    effect of design errors, 6, 7
    experimental studies, 2, 3, 110–126. *See also*
        Experimental studies
    longitudinal study, 2, 3
    observational study, 2, 3
    questionnaires, 42–52. *See also* Questionnaires
    from research question to study plan, 6, 6
    serial surveys, 78
    study sequence
        analysis, 3
        description, 3
        experiment, 3
Diagnostic test studies, 87–97
    analysis, 88–92, 89t
        choice of cutoff point, 89–90, 90
        determining sensitivity and specificity, 89, 89t
        likelihood ratios, 91–92, 92t
        posterior probability, 91
        predictive value of negative test, 91, 92t
        predictive value of positive test, 91, 92t
        prevalence, 90–91
        prior odds of disease, 92
        prior probability, 91, 92t
        use of receiver operator characteristic (ROC)
            curves, 90, 90
    concept of usual clinical practice, 88
    limitations and strategies, 92–95
        random error, 92–93
            increasing usefulness of summary measure,
                93
            use of confidence intervals, 93
        systematic error, 93–95
            measurement bias, 94
            reporting bias, 95
            sampling bias, 93
    planning and performing, 92t, 95–97
    structure, 88
        disease as outcome variable, 88
        use of gold standard, 88
        test result as predictor variable, 88
    summary, 96
    use of randomized blinded trial, 87
    vs. prognostic test studies, 87
Dose-response relationship, 108

Ecological fallacy, 54
Effect size, 132, 139, 143, 148
Errors, 8, 8–9
    design errors and preventive strategies, 27, 28,
        28t
    effect of design errors, 6, 7
    implementation errors and preventive strategies,
        27–28, 28t
    intended vs. actual measurements, 7, 7–8
    intended vs. actual sample, 7, 7

measurement, 9
random, 8, 8–9, 29, 29t, 169
    avoiding spurious associations due to, 98–99,
        99t
    effects on precision, 34
    enhancing precision, 9, 34t, 35
sampling, 9
systematic, 8, 8–9, 29, 29t, 169
    effects on accuracy, 36–37
    enhancing accuracy, 9, 35, 37, 38t
technical mistake, 29, 29t
Ethics in research, 15, 23, 151–154
    deception of subjects, 156
    elaborating in research proposal, 190
    federal guidelines for human research, 151–154,
        152t
        exemptions from, 155, 155t
        informed consent, 153–154
            legal considerations, 154
            process of consent, 153
            surrogate consent, 154
            what information must be disclosed, 153,
                223
            written consent forms, 153–154, 221–222
        privacy and confidentiality, 154
            strategies for protecting, 154
        risks and benefits, 152
        selection of subjects, 152–153
            constrained consent, 152–153
            vulnerable populations, 153
    institutional review boards, 154–155
    nonrandomized between-group studies, 122
    principles
        beneficence, 151
        justice, 151
        respect for persons, 151
    randomized blinded trials, 155–156
        analysis of preliminary data, 156
        enrolling adequate number of subjects, 156
        use of placebo controls, 155–156
    role of investigator, 156–157
    summary, 157
    withholding treatment of control groups, 116
Experimental studies, 2, 3, 110–124
    advantages and disadvantages, 124, 125t
    definition, 110
    randomized blinded trial, 87, 111, 111–119
        analyzing results, 119
            early stopping rules, 119, 214
            intention-to-treat analysis, 119, 212–213
            subgroup analyses, 119, 213–214
        applying intervention, 114–117
            choice of comparison group, 116–117
                assuring compliance, 117
                tests of equivalence, 117
                withholding treatment, 116
            choice of experimental treatment, 115–116
                importance of generalizability, 116
                problems with combination treatments, 116
            importance of blinding, 114–115, 115t
                difficulties in carrying out, 115
                specifying and standardizing intervention,
                    114–115
                unintended intervention, 114
        factorial design, 119–120, 121
        group (cluster) randomization, 121
        measuring baseline variables, 112–113
            avoid collecting too many data, 113

Experimental studies,
    randomized blinded trial—*continued*
     characterize study cohort, 112
     consider measuring outcome variable, 112
     measure predictors of outcome, 112–113
    measuring outcome, 117–119
     appropriateness to research question, 117
     complete follow-up, 118–119
     outcome variables, 118
      importance of blinding, 118
     statistical characteristics
      accuracy and precision, 117
      continuous vs. dichotomous variables,
       117–118
    randomizing before obtaining consent, 120
    randomizing matched pairs, 120
    randomizing study subjects, 113, *113*
     equal vs. disproportionate allocation, 114
     for small or moderate sample sizes, 114, 210–
      211
     tamperproof allocation procedure, 113–114
     true random allocation procedure, 113
    run-in design, 119, *120*
     measuring intermediary variable, 119
    selecting study subjects, 111–112. *See also*
     Subjects, choice of determine sample
     size, 112
     exclusion criteria, 112
     inclusion criteria, 111–112
     plan recruitment, 111–112
    steps in designing, 111, *111*
    summary, 124–126
    types of design, 110–111
     between-group, 110–111
     crossover design, 124
     natural experiments, 124
     nonblinded between-group designs, 122–123
     nonrandomized between-group designs, 122
     repeated measures strategy, 124
     time series designs, *123*, 123–124
     within-group, 110–111
Extrapolation, 174

Frequency distributions, 167–168, *167*, 179
Funding for research, *192–193*, 192–196
    corporate support, 195
    foundation grants, 194–195
    intramural support, 195
    NIH grants and contracts, *193–194*, 192–194
     application review process, 193–194
     institute-initiated proposals, 192–193
     institutes and DRG study sections, 230–231
     investigator-initiated applications, 192–193

Grants. *See* Funding for research
Guttman scales, 48. *See also* Measurement,
    questionnaires

Hypotheses, 128–131, *130*, 139–144, 147–148
    characteristics of good hypothesis, 129, *130*
     in advance vs. after-the-fact, 129
     simple vs. complex, 129
     specific vs. vague, 129
    generation
     in case-control studies, 80
     by the study, 137

    multiple, 136–137
     advantages of, 136
     Bonferoni approach, 136
     single primary, 136–137
    purpose, 129
    types of, 129–131
     alternative, 129–130
     null, 129
     one-tailed, 130–131, 134
     two-tailed, 130, 134
    when needed, 129

Implementation of study, 5, 7–8, 172–183, *173*
    errors and preventive strategies, 28t, 28–29, 29t
    pretesting, 49, 172–174
     of data management system, 174
     as dress rehearsal for actual study, 174
     as guide for development of measurement
      approaches, 173t, 173–174
     as guide for subject recruitment, 173, 173t
     purpose, 172–173
    quality control, 172, 174–180
     of clinical procedures, 175t, 175–177
      leadership and supervision of research team,
       176
      operations manual, 175, 201
       contents of, 175, 227
       necessity for, 175
      performance reviews of team members, 176
       peer observation, 176
      periodic data tabulations and reports, 177
      special procedures for drug interventions,
       177
      staff meetings, 176
      training and certification of researchers,
       175–176
      use of role-playing, 176
     of collaborative studies, 180, *180*
      governance of study, 180
      use of distributed data processing systems,
       180
     of data, 177–180, 179t
      collecting and entering data, 179, 228–229
      collecting too many data, 177–178
      designing forms, 178–179. *See also*
       Questionnaires quality control
       coordinator, 180
     of laboratory procedures, 177, 178t
      blinding the observer, 177
      labeling specimens, 177
      use blinded duplicates or standard pools of
       specimens, 177
     need for, 174–175
      inaccurate and imprecise data, 174–175
      missing data, 174
       use of interpolation and extrapolation, 174
    revising study protocol, 172, 181–182
     minor revisions, 182
     substantive revisions, 181–182
    summary, 182
Incidence, definition, 77
Inference, *5*
    causal, 8, 98–109
     analysis strategies for dealing with confounding
      variables, 106t, 106–107
      adjustment, 107

advantages, 107
disadvantages, 107
example, 208–209
stratification, 106–107
advantages, 106–107
disadvantages, 107
avoiding spurious associations, 98–101
due to bias, 99t, 99–101, *100*
analysis phase strategies, 101
design phase strategies, 99–101
due to chance (random error), 98–99, 99t
by increasing sample size, 99
by testing statistical significance, 99
choosing strategy to deal with confounding
variables, 107–108
design strategies for dealing with confounding
variables, 102–105, 103t
matching, 103–106, *105*, 107–108
advantages, 104
disadvantages, 104–105
specification, 102–103, 107
disadvantages, 103
positive evidence for causality, 108
biologic plausibility, 108
consistent, strong association, 108
dose-response relationship, 108
ruling out real associations other than cause-
effect, 101t, 101–102
effect-cause relationships, 102
effect-effect relationships (confounding), 102,
207
summary, 108–109
external validity (generalizability), 5, *5*
internal validity, 5, *5*
Institutional review boards, 154–155. *See also* Ethics
in research
Instrument. *See* Measurement
Interpolation, 174
Interviews
enhancing reliability of, 50–51
vs. questionnaires, 42–43, 43t
Iterative process, 15–16
in writing research proposal, 186

Legal considerations. *See* Ethics in research
Life table techniques, 119, 144
Likelihood ratios, 91–92, 92t
Likert scales, 48. *See also* Measurement,
questionnaires
Linear regression analysis, 169
Logistic regression tests, 143

Matching, 82, 103–106, 107–108, 144
advantages, 104
disadvantages, 104–105
overmatching, 105
Measurements, 31–42, *32*
accuracy, 36–39
assessment of, 37
distinction from precision, 36, *36*, 36t
external validity of abstract variables, 39
criterion-related validity, 39
existing vs. new instruments, 39
face validity, 39
predictive validity, 39
strategies for enhancing, 9, 37, 38t

automating instruments, 35
blinding, 37–39
attribution bias, 38
differential bias, 37–38
single- vs. double-blind strategies, 37–39
calibrating instrument, 37
making unobtrusive measures, 37
refining instruments, 35
standardizing measurement methods, 35
training and certifying observers, 35
systematic error, 36
instrument bias, 37
observer bias, 36–37
subject bias, 37
characteristics
efficiency, 40
of individual measurements, 39–40
adequate distribution of responses, 40
appropriate, 40
objective, 40, 40t
sensitive, 39–40
specific, 40
supplementation, 40–41
definition, 31
intended vs. actual, 7, 7–8
interviews
enhancing reliability of, 50
vs. questionnaires, 43–44, 44t, 49
paired, 148
precision, 34–36
assessment of, 35
coefficient of variation, 35
correlation coefficient, 3, 143
inter- and intraobserver consistency, 35
internal consistency, 35
standard deviation, 35
test-retest consistency, 35
random error effects, 34
sources, 34
instrument variability, 34
observer variability, 34
subject variability, 34
strategies for enhancing, 9, 34t, 35–36, 147–148
automating instruments, 35
refining instruments, 35
repetition, 35
standardizing measurement methods, 35
training and certifying observers, 35
pretesting, 173t, 173–174
questionnaires, 42–52. *See also* Questionnaires
scales, 31–33, 32t
categorical variables, 32–33
dichotomous, 32
nominal, 32
ordinal, 32
continuous variables, 31–32
discrete, 32
how to choose, 32–33
summary, 41

National Death Index, 56–57
National Institutes of Health
grants. *See* Funding for research
institutes and DRG study sections, 230–231
Nonparametric statistics, 168. *See also* Statistics
Nonparametric tests, 144

Objectivity, of individual measurements, 40, 40t
Odds ratio, 80, 142, 206
Operations manual, 10, 175
  content of, 175, 227
  example, 202
  necessity for, 175
Outcome variables. *See* Variables

P value, 133–134, 232–236
Parametric statistics, 167. *See also* Statistics
Population. *See also* Subjects
  accessible, 18
  target, 18
  vulnerable, 153
Posterior probability, 92
Power, 132–133, 133t, 139–150
Precision, 34–36. *See also* Measurement
Predictive value, 91–92, *92*
Predictor variables. *See* Variables
Pretesting, 49, 172–174, 190
  of data management system, 174
  as dress rehearsal for actual study, 174
  as guide for development of measurement
      approaches, 173t, 173–174
  as guide for subject recruitment, 173, 173t
  purpose, 172–173
  in writing research proposal, 186
Prevalence
  definition, 77
  in diagnostic test studies, 90–91
Prevalence studies. *See* Cross-sectional studies
Privacy, 154. *See also* Ethics in research
Probability. *See* Statistics, P value
Prognostic test studies, vs. diagnostic test studies,
      87
Protocol. *See* Study protocol

Quality control, 174–180
  of clinical procedures, 175t, 175–177
    leadership and supervision of research team,
        176
    operations manual, 10, 175
      contents of, 175, 227
      example, 201
      necessity for, 175
    performance reviews of team members, 176
      peer observation, 176
    periodic data tabulations and reports, 177
    special procedures for drug interventions, 177
    staff meetings, 176
    training and certification of researchers,
        175–176
      use of role-playing, 176
  of collaborative studies, 180, *180*
    governance of study, 180
    use of distributed data processing systems, 180
  of data, 177–180, 179t
    collecting and entering data, 179, 228–229
    collecting too many data, 177–178
    designing forms, 178–179. *See also*
        Questionnaires
    quality control coordinator, 180
  elaborating in research proposal, 189
  of laboratory procedures, 177, 178t
    blinding the observer, 177
    labeling specimens, 177

use of blinded duplicates or standard pools of
    specimens, 177
  need for, 174–175
    inaccurate and imprecise data, 174–175
    missing data, 174
    use of interpolation and extrapolation, 174
Questionnaires, 42–52
  administration of, 51–52
    methods, 44
    strategies for minimizing missing data and
        errors, 51–55
  design of, 44t, 44–49, 178–179
    branching questions, 44–45
    codes, scores, and scales, 46–47
      cumulative (Guttman) scales, 47
      summative (Likert) scales, 47–48
    instrument format, 44–45
    open- vs. closed-ended questions, 43–44
    revising, 181
    wording, 45–46, 179
      clarity, 45
      double-barreled questions, 45
      neutrality, 45
      of potentially sensitive questions, 45–46
      setting time frame, 45–46
      simplicity, 45
  example, 202–203
  steps in writing, 48–50
    administer pretests, 49, 179
    combine existing and new questions, 48–49
    decide between interviews and questionnaires,
        48
    list variables, 48
    precode responses, 50, 178
    revise draft, 49
    shorten and revise again, 49
    write draft, 48
  summary, 51–52
  vs. interviews, 42–43, 43t
Question(s)
  branching, 44–45
  double-barreled, 45
  open- vs. closed-ended, 43–44
  potentially sensitive, 45–46
  research. *See* Research question

Randomized blinded trial, 87, 111–124, *111*
Receiver operator characteristic (ROC) curves, *90*,
    90
Relative risk, 73, 142, 169, 206
Research. *See also* Design of study; Errors;
        Implementation of study; Measurement;
        Research question; Study protocol
  how it works, 5–9, *9*
    drawing causal inference, 8
    errors, 8–9, *8*
    implementing study, 5, 7–8
    inferences, 5
    study design, 6–7
      from research question to study plan, 6, *6*
    summary of elements, 11
Research proposal, 184–196
  characteristics of good proposals, 190–191, *190*
    scientific quality of research plan, 190
    technical quality of proposal, 190
  definition, 184

elements of, 186–190, 186t
  abstract, 186–187
  appendices, 190–191
  biosketches of investigators, 187–188
  budget, 187
  ethical considerations, 189. *See also* Ethics in
    research
  goals and rationale, 188
    preliminary studies and competence of
      investigators, 188
    pilot studies, 188
    significance, 188
    specific objectives, 188
  references, 190
  resources available, 187
  role of consultants, 189
  scientific methods, 188–189, *189*
    data management and quality control, 189.
      See also Data management
    measurements, 189. *See also* Measurements
    organizational chart, 189, *190*
    overview of design, 188, *190*
    pretests, 189. *See also* Pretesting
    statistical issues, 189. *See also* Statistics
    study subjects, 189. *See also* Subjects
    timetable, 189, 189t
  table of contents, 187
  title, 186
finding research funding, *193–194*, 192–196
  corporate support, 195
  foundation grants, 194–195
  intramural support, 195
  NIH grants and contracts, *193–194*, 192–195
    application review process, *193*, 193–194
    institute-initiated proposals, 192–193
    institutes and DRG study sections,
      230–231
    investigator-initiated applications, 192–193
steps in writing, 185–186
  develop outline, 185, 186t
  establish timetable and meet periodically, 185
  follow guidelines of funding agency, 185
    contact with scientific administrator, 185
  organize team and designate leader, 184–185
    principal investigator, 184–185
  review, pretest, and revise, 186
  review other successful and unsuccessful
    proposals, 185
summary, 195–197
Research question, 1–2, 12–17, *13*
  characteristics, 14t, 14–15
    ethical, 15
    feasible, 14–15
      number of subjects, 14
      scope, 14–15
      technical expertise, 14
      time and money costs, 14
    interesting, 15
    novel, 15
    relevant, 15
  definition, 12
  development of, 15–17
    hypothetical example, 198–199
    primary and secondary questions, 16–17
      advantages and disadvantages, 16
    problems and solutions, 15–16, 16t
      importance of good advice, 15

  use of iterative process, 15–16
origins of, 12–14
  experience, 12
    apprenticeship, 12
    scholarship, 12
  imagination, 13–14
  new ideas, 13
    patient observation, 13
    professional meetings, 13
    skeptical attitude, 13
    technologic changes, 13
  "so what" test, 2
  summary, 17
  vague vs. specific, 2
Review boards, 154–155. *See also* Ethics in research

Sample size. *See* Subjects, number of
Sampling, 21, *21*, 24–26. *See also* Subjects, choice of
SAS statistical program, 166
Scatterplot, 169
Sensitivity
  of diagnostic test studies, 89, 89t
  of individual measurements, 39–40
Serial surveys, 78
Software, 161–164, 162t. *See also* Data analysis; Data
    management
  data base programs, 163–165
  spreadsheet programs, 162–163, 163t
  statistical
    for data analysis, 166
    for data entry, 164
Specification, 4, 21–24, 102–103, 106–107. *See also*
    Subjects, choice of
Specificity
  of diagnostic test studies, 89, 89t
  of individual measurements, 40
SPSS statistical program, 166
Standard deviation, 35
Statistics
  alpha, beta, and power, 131t, 131–134, 232–236
  analytic, 168t, 168–169
    other predictor and outcome variables, 169
    two categorical variables, 168–169
    two continuous variables, 169, 170
  correlation coefficient, 35, 143
    sample size required per group, 218
  descriptive, 166–168
    frequency distribution, 166–167, 167
    parametric vs. nonparametric statistics, 167
  effect size, 132, 139–143, 148, 169
  elaborating in research proposal, 189
  in experimental studies, 117
  level of statistical significance, 99, 131–132,
    168–169
  P value, 133–134, 232–236
  t test, 140–141, 169
    sample size required per group, 215
  Type I (false-positive) error, 132
    causes of, 132
  Type II (false-negative) error, 132
    causes of, 132
  z statistic, 141–142
    distinction from chi square test, 141
    sample size required per group, 216–217
Statview statistical program, 166
Stratification, 106–107
  advantages, 107

Stratification—*continued*
  disadvantages, 107
Study protocol, 1–5, 2t
  AIDS example, 198
  design, 2–4, *3*, 21, *21*, 27–29. *See also* Design of
      study
  development of, 9–10, 15–17, 16t
    complete protocol, 10
    operations manual, 10, 175, 201
    revisions, 172, 181–182
      minor, 181
      substantive, 181–182
    study outline, 2t, 9–10
    study question, 10
  implementation. *See* Implementation of study
  inclusion in research proposal, 184. *See also*
      Research proposal
  research question, 1–2, 12–17, *13*. *See also*
      Research question
  significance, 2
  statistical issues, 4–5. *See also* Statistics
    developing hypothesis, 4
    sample size estimation, 4–5
  subjects, 4, 18–30. *See also* Subjects
  trade-offs, 10–11
  variables, 4. *See also* Variables
Subjects
  choice of, 6, 18–30
    accessible population, 18
    errors, 27–29
      design errors and preventive strategies, 28,
        28t
      implementation errors and preventive
        strategies, 28–29, 29t
      random error, 28–29
      systematic error, 29
      technical mistake, 29
    ethical guidelines, 151. *See also* Ethics in
      research
    generalizing study findings, 19–21, *20*
    for randomized blinded trial, *111*, 111–119. *See*
      also Experimental studies
    approaches, 27
      recruitment, 26–27
      pretesting, 172–173, 173t
      enhancing response rate, 27
      effects of nonresponse, 27
      repeated contact attempts, 27
    goals of, 26–27
      adequate sample size, 26
      unbiased sample, 26–27
    representative of population, 18, *19*
    sampling, 4, 21, *21*, 24–26
      advantages and disadvantages, 27
      choosing among sampling design options,
        25–26, *26*
      nonprobability sampling, 25
        consecutive, 25
        convenience, 25
        judgmental, 25
      probability sampling, 24–25
        cluster, 24–25
        random, 24
        stratified random, 24
        systematic, 24
      studying entire population, 24

    specification, 4, 21–24, 102–103, 108
      choosing accessible population, 23–24
        hospital/clinic-based samples, 23
        population-based samples, 23
      establishing exclusion criteria, 23
      establishing inclusion criteria, 21–23, 22t
        clinical characteristics, 21–22
        demographic characteristics, 22
        geographic and temporal characteristics, 23
      revising, 181
    steps in designing study protocol, 21, *21*, 29–30
    summary, 29–30
    table of random numbers, 200
    target population, 18
  number of
    estimating, 14, 139–150
      in analytic studies and experiments, 139–144
        with categorical variables, 143–144
        correlation coefficient, 35, 143, 218
        logistic regression tests, 143
        matched designs, 144
        nonparametric tests, 143
        statistical tests for, 140t
        steps in estimating, 139–140
        survival analysis techniques, 144
        t test, 140–141, 215
        z statistic, 141–142, 216–217
      in descriptive studies, 144–145
        confidence intervals, 144–145
        confidence levels, 144–145
        with continuous variables, 144–145, 220
        with dichotomous variables, 145, 219
      summary, 150
      when there is insufficient information,
        149–150
        dichotomize variable, 145
        make educated guess, 150
        search for previous findings, 149
    fixed sample size, 145–149
    planning, 128–138
      confounding variables, 136
      dropouts, 136
      hypotheses, 128–131, *130*, 136–138, 147–148.
        See also Hypotheses
        characteristics of good hypotheses, 130, *130*
        multiple, 136–137
        those generated by the study, 137
        types of, 129–130
      sampling units, 135–136
      statistical principles, 131t, 131–134. *See also*
        Statistics
      summary, 137
      variability, 134–135, *135*, 139
    strategies for minimizing, 146–148
      make technical adjustments, 146
      use a more common outcome, 149
      use continuous variables, 146–147
      use more precise variables, 147–148
      use paired measurements, 148
      use unequal group sizes, 148–149
Survival analysis, 144
SysStat statistical program, 166

t test, 120, 140–141
  sample size required per group, 215
  use with paired measurements, 148

Time series studies, 122–123, *123. See also*
    Experimental studies
Two-by-two table, 168, 168t

Validity
  external, 5, *5*
    of abstract variables, 39
      criterion-related validity, 39
      existing vs. new instruments, 39
      face validity, 39
      predictive validity, 39
  internal, 5, *5*
Variability, 134–135, *135*, 139–143
Variables, 4
  categorical, 32, 143–144
    analytic statistics, 168
    data analysis, 166–170
    dichotomous, 32, *33*
    nominal, 32, *33*
    ordinal, 32, *33*
  choice of, 6–7
  confounding, 4
    in cohort studies double-cohort studies, 70–71
      measurement of, 71
      prospective studies, 65
    effect-effect relationships and, 102, 207
    in planning sample size, 137
    strategies for dealing with analysis phase, 106t,
      106–107
      adjustment, 107–108, 208–209
      stratification, 106–107

    choice of, 107–108
    design phase, 102–105, 103t
      matching, 103–105, *105*
      specification, 102–103
    time dependent, 124
  continuous, 31–32, 144
    analytic statistics, 169
    data analysis, 167–169
    in descriptive studies, 144–145, 220
    discrete, 32
    in randomized blinded trial, 119
    use to minimize sample size, 146–147
  dichotomous, 144, 145, 168–169, 219
    in randomized blinded trial, 119
  increasing precision of, 34–36, 147–148
  individual, 4
  intermediary, 119
  outcome, 4, 71–72, 89, 143
    in randomized blinded trial, 119
    in studies of diagnostic tests, 87
  predictor, 4, 89, 144
    intervention, 4
    measurement in cohort studies, 71–72. *See also*
      Cohort studies
    in studies of diagnostic tests, 89
    vs. outcome, in cross-sectional studies, 77
  relationships among, 4

z statistic, 141–142
  distinction from chi square test, 141
  sample size required per group, 216–217